TREATING CHILDHOOD BEHAVIORAL AND EMOTIONAL PROBLEMS

Treating Childhood Behavioral and Emotional Problems

A Step-by-Step, Evidence-Based Approach

Edited by Andrew R. Eisen

THE GUILFORD PRESS
New York   London

© 2008 The Guilford Press
A Division of Guilford Publications, Inc.
72 Spring Street, New York, NY 10012
www.guilford.com

Printed in the United States of America

This book is printed on acid-free paper.

Last digit is print number: 9 8 7 6 5 4 3 2 1

The authors have checked with sources believed to be reliable in their efforts to provide information that is complete and generally in accord with the standards of practice that are accepted at the time of publication. However, in view of the possibility of human error or changes in medical sciences, neither the authors, nor the editor and publisher, nor any other party who has been involved in the preparation or publication of this work warrants that the information contained herein is in every respect accurate or complete, and they are not responsible for any errors or omissions or the results obtained from the use of such information. Readers are encouraged to confirm the information contained in this book with other sources.

Library of Congress Cataloging-in-Publication Data

Treating childhood behavioral and emotional problems : a step-by-step, evidence-based approach / edited by Andrew R. Eisen.
    p. ; cm.
Includes bibliographical references and index.
ISBN-13: 978-1-59385-564-2 (hardcover : alk. paper)
ISBN-10: 1-59385-564-8 (hardcover : alk. paper)
1. Adjustment disorders in children—Treatment. I. Eisen, Andrew R.
[DNLM: 1. Child Behavior Disorders—therapy. 2. Affective Symptoms—therapy. 3. Child. WS 350.6 T763v 2007]
    RJ506.A33T74 2007
    618.92'89—dc22
                                                                200702136

To Linda—loving partner, dedicated collaborator,
and unceasing supporter

—A. R. E.

About the Editor

Andrew R. Eisen, PhD, is Associate Professor in the School of Psychology and Director of the Child Anxiety Disorders Clinic at Fairleigh Dickinson University. His research and clinical interests include childhood anxiety and related problems, learning disorders, and sensory integration issues, with an emphasis on developing individualized treatments for these populations. Dr. Eisen has published numerous articles and chapters, and is on the editorial board of the *Journal of Clinical Child and Adolescent Psychology*. He has coauthored or coedited seven books, including *Separation Anxiety in Children and Adolescents: An Individualized Approach to Assessment and Treatment*, *Helping Your Child Overcome Separation Anxiety or School Refusal: A Step-by-Step Guide for Parents*, and *Helping Your Socially Vulnerable Child: What to Do When Your Child Is Shy, Socially Anxious, Withdrawn, or Bullied*. Dr. Eisen maintains a private practice with children and their families in Bergen County, New Jersey (*www.childanxieties.com*).

Contributors

Kimberly D. Becker, PhD, is currently enrolled in the Clinical Studies Respecialization Program at the University of Hawaii and is receiving internship training through the Kennedy Krieger Institute's Behavioral Psychology Department at The Johns Hopkins University School of Medicine. Dr. Becker's research interests include child and adolescent psychopathology, evidence-based treatments, and family violence. Dr. Becker was awarded a Harry Frank Guggenheim Foundation Dissertation Fellowship for her research on the emotional and physiological arousal of children exposed to family violence.

Steven J. Bottjer is a graduate student in child clinical psychology at The Pennsylvania State University. He is currently conducting research on the relationships between sleep problems and daytime behavior.

Daniel M. Cheron is a doctoral student in the clinical psychology program at Boston University and a clinician at the Center for Anxiety and Related Disorders. His research interests include examining the role of family factors in youth diagnosed with anxiety disorders, as well as providing empirically supported treatment to anxious youth and their families.

Bruce F. Chorpita, PhD, is Professor of Clinical Psychology, Clinical Adjunct Professor of Psychiatry, and Codirector of the Center for Cognitive Behavior Therapy at the University of Hawaii. Dr. Chorpita has also served as the Clinical Director of the Hawaii Department of Health's Child and Adolescent Mental Health Division. Dr. Chorpita has authored over 75 publications on anxiety disorders and children's mental health, including the book *Modular Cognitive-Behavioral Therapy for Childhood Anxiety Disorders*. Dr. Chorpita is the recipient of multiple honors and awards for his work and has held research and training grants with the National Institute of Mental Health, the Hawaii Departments of Education and Health, and the John D. and Catherine T. MacArthur Foundation.

Kristen Davidson, PhD, is a clinician in the Departments of Psychiatry and Pediatrics at the University of Rochester Medical Center. Dr. Davidson has published in the areas of assessment and treatment of childhood mood disorders and maintains a part-time private practice with children, adolescents, and their families.

Andrew R. Eisen, PhD (see "About the Editor").

Mary A. Fristad, PhD, ABPP, is Professor of Psychiatry and Psychology at The Ohio State University, and directs Research and Psychological Services in the Division of Child and Adolescent Psychiatry. Dr. Fristad has over 125 publications addressing the assessment and treatment of childhood-onset depression, suicidality, and bipolar disorder (manic–depression), including a book for families entitled *Raising a Moody Child: How to Cope with Depression and Bipolar Disorder.*

James B. Hale, PhD, is Associate Professor and Associate Director of Clinical Training in the School Psychology Program at Philadelphia College of Osteopathic Medicine. His interests include the neuropsychological characteristics of children with attention-deficit/hyperactivity disorder and learning disabilities, combining response to intervention with school neuropsychological assessment techniques, and making assessment results meaningful for individualized interventions. Dr. Hale has published numerous articles and chapters, and the book *School Neuropsychology: A Practitioner's Handbook.*

Rebecca Hashim is a doctoral fellow in clinical psychology at Fairleigh Dickinson University and clinical research coordinator of the Child Anxiety Disorders Clinic. Her research interests include anxiety and related disorders, with an emphasis on adolescent adjustment issues.

Jennifer L. Hudson, PhD, is Millennium Research Fellow in the Department of Psychology, Macquarie University, Sydney, Australia. Her research focuses on anxiety disorders in children and adolescents, specifically the role of parents in the etiology of anxiety disorders in youth and the treatment of internalizing disorders using cognitive-behavioral therapy. Dr. Hudson has received early career awards from the Australian Psychological Society, the Anxiety Disorders Association of America, the Australian Association for Cognitive and Behaviour Therapy, and the Australian Institute of Political Science. She has published her research in international journals and published two books, *Psychopathology and the Family* and *Treating Anxious Children and Adolescents: An Evidence-Based Approach.*

Sony Khemlani-Patel, PhD, is Executive Director of the Bio-Behavioral Institute in Great Neck, New York. Dr. Khemlani-Patel is a behavioral and cognitive therapist whose primary research interest is in the field of obsessive–compulsive spectrum disorders, including body dysmorphic disorder and trichotillomania. She has published numerous peer-reviewed articles and several book chapters with Fugen Neziroglu. She is a member of and has presented at various professional organizations. At the Bio-Behavioral Institute, Dr. Khemlani-Patel provides direct therapeutic services to children, adolescents, and adults, and supervises interns and postdoctoral students.

James Lock, MD, PhD, is Associate Professor of Child Psychiatry and Pediatrics in the Department of Psychiatry and Behavioral Sciences at Stanford University School of

Medicine, and Director of the Eating Disorders Program. His major research and clinical interests are in psychotherapy research, especially in children and adolescents, and specifically for those with eating disorders. Dr. Lock has published over 100 articles, abstracts, and book chapters. He is the author, along with Daniel le Grange, W. Stewart Agras, and Christopher Dare, of the only evidence-based treatment manual for anorexia nervosa, *Treatment Manual for Anorexia Nervosa: A Family-Based Approach*. He has also recently published a book for parents, *Help Your Teenager Beat an Eating Disorder*. Dr. Lock is the recipient of a National Institute of Mental Health (NIMH) Career Development Award, and an NIMH Mid-Career Award, both focused on enhancing psychosocial treatments of eating disorders in children and adolescents. He is the principal investigator (at Stanford) on a multisite trial funded by the National Institutes of Health comparing individual and family approaches to anorexia nervosa in adolescents.

Heidi J. Lyneham, PhD, is research fellow at Macquarie University, Sydney, Australia, where she focuses on improving accessibility of assessment and treatment for anxious children and adolescents, predictors of treatment success, and improving the fit between individual children's difficulties and the treatment they are offered. Dr. Lyneham has authored the treatment manual and client workbooks for the *Cool Kids* program, a cognitive-behavioral treatment for child and adolescent anxiety disorders.

Merry McVey-Noble, PhD, is an adjunct Professor in the Department of Psychology, Hofstra University, and a staff psychologist at the Bio-Behavioral Institute in Great Neck, New York, where she treats children, adolescents, and adults within the obsessive–compulsive spectrum; provides consultation to various school districts; and supervises interns and postdoctoral students. Dr. McVey-Noble lectures frequently at hospitals, schools, and local mental health organizations on topics including self-injury, eating disorders, and obsessive–compulsive spectrum disorders in children and adolescents. She recently coauthored her first book, *When Your Child Is Cutting: A Parent's Guide to Helping Children Overcome Self-Injury*.

Fugen Neziroglu, PhD, is Professor of Psychology, Hofstra University, and Clinical Professor of Psychiatry, New York University. Dr. Neziroglu is a board-certified behavior and cognitive psychologist who has been involved in the research and treatment of anxiety disorders and depression for many years. She is a scientist and clinician who has presented and published over 100 papers in scientific journals and has written numerous book chapters and 13 books. Dr. Neziroglu is Clinical Director of the Bio-Behavioral Institute in Great Neck, New York, where she provides direct therapeutic services, supervises assistant psychologists and psychology interns, sponsors doctoral dissertations, and conducts research. She is a member of many national and international societies, is on the Scientific Advisory Board of the Obsessive–Compulsive Foundation, and is a consultant to the Bio-Behavioral Institute in Buenos Aires, Argentina.

Donna B. Pincus, PhD, is Associate Professor at Boston University and Director of the Child and Adolescent Fear and Anxiety Treatment Program at the Center for Anxiety and Related Disorders. Dr. Pincus has focused her clinical research career on developing new, evidence-based treatments for children and adolescents with anxiety disorders. She has given numerous talks and workshops on child anxiety to parents, teachers, students, and health care professionals. Dr. Pincus created the Child Anxiety Network (*www.childanxiety.net*), which presents state-of-the-art information on child anxiety to the public and to health care professionals. Dr. Pincus has appeared on NBC's *Today Show*, National Geographic Channel, Women's Lifetime Television, *Nick News*, and the ABC News program *20-20 Downtown*.

Brian Rabian, PhD, is Associate Professor in the Department of Psychology at The Pennsylvania State University and Director of Child and Adolescent Services at the Pennsylvania State Psychological Clinic. Dr. Rabian has published numerous articles and chapters on the topic of child psychopathology, particularly child anxiety. He received funding from the National Science Foundation for work on pediatric sleep problems in infants and is currently engaged in research on both sleep and anxiety.

Ronald M. Rapee, PhD, is Professor in the Department of Psychology, Macquarie University, Sydney, Australia, and Director of the Centre for Emotional Health. Dr. Rapee has been involved in an advisory capacity with DSM-IV and DSM-V, and is a member of several international advisory boards. He is on the editorial board of several international journals and is associate editor for *Behaviour Research and Therapy*. Dr. Rapee received an Early Career Award from the Australian Psychological Society (APS) in 1990 and the Ian Mathew Campbell Prize from the Clinical College of the APS in 1996. He has published extensively in the areas of child and adult anxiety and anxiety disorders, and has written and edited books for professionals and for the general public.

Linda A. Reddy, PhD, is an Associate Professor and Director of the Child/Adolescent ADHD and ADHD-Related Disorders Clinic at Rutgers University, Piscataway, New Jersey. Her clinical and research interests include the assessment and treatment of children with emotional and behavioral disorders, attention-deficit/hyperactivity disorder, and learning disabilities; test validation; and parent and teacher consultation. Dr. Reddy has published numerous articles, chapters, and several books, including *Empirically Based Play Interventions for Children*.

Megan Roehrig, PhD, is a postdoctoral research associate at the Yale Obesity and Eating Disorders Research Program in the Yale University School of Medicine. Her clinical interests broadly include the treatment of eating disorders, obesity, and body image disturbance. Her research focuses on risk factors, treatment, and prevention of eating disorders and obesity as well as bariatric surgery outcome. She has coauthored several peer-reviewed journal articles and book chapters on these topics.

Lauren C. Santucci is a doctoral student in clinical psychology at Boston University. Her research interests include the development and dissemination of treatments for emotional disorders in early childhood and adolescence. Currently she is working on examining the efficacy of parent–child interaction therapy adapted for young children with separation anxiety disorder.

Steffanie Sperry is a doctoral student in clinical psychology at the University of South Florida. Her research focuses on sociocultural influences on body image and eating disorders. Her past research has focused on factors influencing the efficacy of body image intervention programs. She has an additional interest in cosmetic surgery as it relates to body image. Clinically, her interests include the treatment of body image and eating disturbances across the lifespan.

J. Kevin Thompson, PhD, is Professor of Psychology at the University of South Florida. His research interests over the past 25 years have focused on body image and eating disorders. He has authored, coauthored, or coedited six books on these topics and is on the editorial boards of the *International Journal of Eating Disorders* and *Eating Behaviors.*

Jose A. Yaryura-Tobias, MD, is Professor of Psychiatry at New York University and Medical Director of the Bio-Behavioral Institute in Great Neck, New York. He is a biological psychiatrist and an internist with over 40 years of experience, in addition to being a writer and a poet. He has pioneered research in the dopamine theory of schizophrenia and the serotonin theory of obsessive–compulsive disorder. Dr. Yaryura-Tobias has presented and/or published over 300 scientific papers and book chapters, and 15 books. He is a member of numerous national and international societies, and a founding member of the International College of Psychosomatic Medicine, the Argentine Society of Biological Psychiatry, the World Federation of Biological Psychiatry, and the Society of Obsessive–Compulsive Disorders. He is on the scientific advisory board of the Obsessive–Compulsive Foundation and a consultant to the Bio-Behavioral Institute in Buenos Aires, Argentina.

Preface

Practicing child clinicians receive frequent referrals from parents, teachers, school counselors, and mental health and medical professionals expressing concerns that children are "easily distracted," "moody," or "socially anxious," to name a few. Trying to make sense of these vague symptom complaints can be remarkably challenging given the frequent overlap of childhood disorders at both symptom and diagnostic levels. Thus, it is not surprising that misdiagnosis in the form of both under- and overidentification is a common phenomenon.

As a result, identifying common symptom dimensions across childhood disorders is becoming increasingly important. Instead of focusing solely on diagnostic criteria, targeting symptom dimensions allows for a broader examination of the cognitive, behavioral, physical, and social characteristics underlying emotional and behavioral problems in youth. Such an approach also permits qualified practitioners to develop individualized case formulations and treatment plans tailored to the unique needs of their child and adolescent clients.

For this reason, unlike other books that target common childhood disorders such as obsessive–compulsive disorder or attention-deficit/hyperactivity disorder, this volume emphasizes in each chapter core symptom dimensions such as "obsessive thoughts," "moodiness," or "inattentiveness." Doing so allows for a careful examination of both primary and comorbid behavior problems.

Each chapter in this volume begins with a discussion of relevant symptom dimensions as they relate to specific childhood disorders, and is followed by an intricate examination of the process of differential diagnosis. A conceptual model of assessment and treatment is then introduced in the context of a comprehensive, real-life case example. The authors provide careful guidance through the step-by-step process of assessment, keeping in mind the content and use of commonly employed assessment measures, as well as the role of assessment data in treatment decision making. Most chapters include both handouts and excerpts of therapeutic dialogue to guide implementation of evidence-based assessment.

The heart and soul of the book, however, is the comprehensive description of the step-by-step treatment process. Now, for the first time in a single volume, qualified practitioners have a source that demonstrates how to treat a broad range of symptoms, disorders, and comorbid conditions that emerge during the developmental span of childhood and adolescence.

To accomplish these objectives, the treatment section of each chapter begins with an overview of the outcome literature. For example, following a general discussion of goals and considerations, the context of treatment (e.g., child, family, and therapist variables), as well as a description of evidence-based interventions, is examined. Next, clinicians are provided a session-by-session account of how to treat effectively a challenging clinical case in which the child or adolescent experiences overlapping symptom dimensions and disorders. As in the assessment section, most chapters include excerpts of therapeutic dialogue as well as relevant handouts to help implement evidence-based treatment procedures. The nuances of the therapeutic process are carefully examined, as are strategies for overcoming resistance and addressing relapse. Regardless of their own theoretical orientation, clinicians will be able to integrate the strategies presented into their own treatment approaches.

The chapters in this volume reflect our most current knowledge, the latest developments in the field, and the expert clinical wisdom of the contributors. I thank my contributors, world-renowned leaders in their respective areas, for taking the time and effort to describe carefully their unique conceptual frameworks and treatment programs. It is my hope that clinicians will be equally grateful as their own approaches become inherently more powerful in producing positive treatment outcomes in children, adolescents, and their families.

I will always be indebted to my mentors David H. Barlow, Ronald S. Drabman, Charles E. Schaefer, and Wendy K. Silverman, as well as to countless colleagues and students, for their profound influence on my thinking and ideas that ultimately led to this book. Special thanks to Kitty Moore, Executive Editor of The Guilford Press, for giving me the opportunity to take on this ambitious project, and for her thoughtful guidance, support, and patience throughout every phase of this work. Finally, as always, my heartfelt thanks to the charter members of my fan club for making everything I do worthwhile.

ANDREW R. EISEN

Contents

CHAPTER 1 ✿ Seeking Safety   1
Andrew R. Eisen, Donna B. Pincus, Rebecca Hashim,
Daniel M. Cheron, and Lauren C. Santucci

CHAPTER 2 ✿ Social Anxiety   53
Jennifer L. Hudson, Heidi J. Lyneham,
and Ronald M. Rapee

CHAPTER 3 ✿ Obsessive Thoughts   102
Fugen Neziroglu, Merry McVey-Noble,
Sony Khemlani-Patel, and Jose A. Yaryura-Tobias

CHAPTER 4 ✿ Inattentiveness   156
Linda A. Reddy and James B. Hale

CHAPTER 5 ✿ Negative Affect   212
Kimberly D. Becker and Bruce F. Chorpita

CHAPTER 6 ✿ Moodiness   264
Kristen Davidson and Mary A. Fristad

CHAPTER 7 ✿ Eating Problems   309
Megan Roehrig, Steffanie Sperry, James Lock,
and J. Kevin Thompson

CHAPTER 8 ✿ Sleep Problems   365
Brian Rabian and Steven J. Bottjer

Index   411

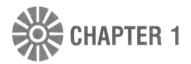 **CHAPTER 1**

Seeking Safety

*Andrew R. Eisen, Donna B. Pincus, Rebecca Hashim,
Daniel M. Cheron, and Lauren C. Santucci*

When it comes to anxiety disorders, comorbidity with other internalizing and externalizing disorders is the norm. In this chapter, we present a conceptual framework that unifies anxiety disorders based on core symptom dimensions and seeking safety behaviors. In doing so, we present an assessment tool that allows qualified practitioners to design and implement case formulations tailored to the individual needs of their child and adolescent clients. Until now, treatment protocols for anxious youth have emphasized anxiety reduction and elimination of phobic avoidance through gradual exposure and cognitive-behavioral coping strategies. But what happens when comorbid externalizing symptoms or disorders are present? Parent–child interaction therapy (PCIT) has long been considered the treatment of choice for youth with oppositional defiant disorder. Recently, PCIT has been adapted for youth with separation anxiety disorder (Pincus, Eyberg, Choate, & Barlow, 2005). Now, for the first time, we demonstrate the broad applicability of PCIT as we take you through the case of "Julie," a young child experiencing separation and generalized anxieties, obsessive–compulsive symptoms, and oppositional defiant behaviors. Practitioners will obtain much valuable knowledge here to guide their own approaches.—A. R. E.

INTRODUCTION

Worry and somatic complaints are characteristic of anxiety disorders in children and adolescents (Last, 1991; Weems, Silverman, & LaGreca, 2000) and present to varying degrees in normative samples (Egger, Costello, Erkanli, &

1

Angold, 1999; Silverman, LaGreca, & Wassertein, 1995). Because of developmental constraints, however, children are less likely to experience full-fledged disorders such as panic or obsessive–compulsive disorder (OCD; Nelles & Barlow, 1988). When diagnostic criteria are met for anxiety disorders, comorbidity with other internalizing and/or externalizing disorders occurs approximately 80% of the time (Kendall, Brady, & Verduin, 2001). Even within specific anxiety disorder categories, heterogeneity of symptoms is the norm. For instance, some children with separation anxiety disorder (SAD) are primarily afraid to be alone, whereas others are more concerned about being abandoned. Similarly, children with OCD may experience obsessions, compulsions, or both, and the form (e.g., washing, checking, repeating, or counting), developmental progression, and function of their rituals may vary widely (see March & Mulle, 1998).

Given these issues, the importance of identifying symptom dimensions for specific adult (Barlow, 2002; Brown, Chorpita, & Barlow, 1998; Chorpita, Albano, & Barlow, 1998) and childhood emotional disorders (Chorpita, 2006; Eisen & Schaefer, 2005; Eisen & Silverman, 1993, 1998; Kearney, 2001) is being recognized. In this chapter, the conceptual framework we present for assessing and treating anxious youth emphasizes core symptom dimensions and safety needs. First, we discuss the basis for these symptom dimensions and their relationship to specific anxiety disorders in which seeking safety is prominent.

Nature of Symptom Dimensions

A number of symptom dimensions are associated with anxiety disorders in children and adolescents (see Eisen & Schaefer, 2005). These include a fear of physical illness (FPI), worry about calamitous events (WCE), phobic avoidance (PA), and seeking safety behaviors.

Somatic complaints may occur in anticipation of anxiety-provoking situations, seemingly "out of the blue," and/or as a means of attracting the attention of significant others (Eisen & Kearney, 1995). Most youth can handle the periodic experience of uncomfortable physical feelings. What is more difficult to manage, however, is the fear of serious consequences stemming from these feelings, such as vomiting, choking, or illness. This FPI is common across DSM-IV anxiety disorders (Hajinlian et al., 2003).

Like somatic complaints, worry is ubiquitous in children and adolescents. Common spheres of worry include school performance, family, friends, health, and personal safety. Children with anxiety disorders, however, experience more frequent and intense worries, emphasize potential calamitous events that affect the self (e.g., being kidnapped or abandoned) and significant others (e.g., illness or death), and/or are preoccupied with worldly concerns (e.g., natural disasters, terrorism, war).

FPI and/or WCE may cause significant disruptions to child, family, school, and social functioning through varied forms of PA. At its most basic level, FPI may result in interoceptive avoidance, that is, avoiding activities such as exercise or sports that trigger dreaded physical sensations (Barlow, 2002). FPI may also result in avoidance of situations or places where physical illness could occur. Similarly, WCE may lead to avoidance of activities that trigger excessive apprehensive expectation and more importantly, to situations that generate uncontrollable worry that the personal safety and well-being of the child and/or significant others may be in jeopardy. Overall, the symptom dimensions of FPI and WCE singly or in combination may result in widespread PA of social, extracurricular, and/or school-related events, unless, of course, the child seeks safety.

Given the frightening nature of FPI and WCE, it is not surprising that anxious youth seek safety. Safety signals are persons, places, actions, and objects that help children feel more secure in anticipation of and/or during anxiety-provoking encounters (Barlow, 2002; Craske, 1999; Eisen & Schaefer, 2005). Common safety signals associated with anxiety are presented in Table 1.1.

Seeking safety typically occurs when avoidance of an anxiety-provoking situation or event is not possible. For example, a child who is fearful of sleeping alone in his or her room can do so if a "safe" parent is present. Similarly, an adolescent may venture far from home if he or she has access to safe objects, such as a water bottle (to prevent possible choking) or cell phone. These safety signals allay anxious apprehension and create an illusion that the child or adolescent is coping effectively. In actuality, however, without them, the child or adolescent would engage in avoidance behavior and/or endure intense anxiety.

It is important to keep in mind that safety signals may serve useful functions (e.g., transitional objects) and are often considered developmentally appropriate. The presence of safety signals may also help a child or adolescent confront anxiety-provoking situations that he or she ordinarily would have avoided. Only excessive reliance is problematic, because it may interfere with habituation during *in vivo* exposures (Barlow, 2002). Our conceptual framework calls for the identification and gradual elimination of seeking safety

TABLE 1.1. Common Safety Signals in Youngsters with Anxiety

Persons	Places	Objects	Actions
Primary caregiver	Home	Night light	Calling a parent
Parent/guardian	Relative's house	Blankie	Specific promises
Relative	Best friend's house	Special toy	Shadowing
Sibling/pet	Parent's room	Stuffed animal	Sleeping with others
Best friend	Sibling's room	Book	Staying with nurse
Teacher/nurse/ coach	Familiar place	Food/drink	Engaging in favorite activity

Note. From Eisen and Schaefer (2005). Copyright 2005 by The Guilford Press. Reprinted by permission.

behaviors. More important, however, is to replace unhealthy safety signals by learning effective coping strategies.

The Anxiety disorders in the *Diagnostic and Statistical Manual of Mental Disorders*, fourth edition, text revision (DSM-IV-TR; American Psychiatric Association [APA], 2000) that best exemplify our framework and involve a prominent seeking safety component include SAD, panic disorder (PD), generalized anxiety disorder (GAD), OCD, and posttraumatic stress disorder (PTSD).

Relationship to Specific Disorders

Separation Anxiety Disorder

The central feature of SAD is unrealistic and excessive anxiety upon separation, or anticipation of separation, from major attachment figures (APA, 2000). Separation is dreaded because of the possibility of potential harm to the child (e.g., being kidnapped) and/or to major attachment figures (e.g., a car accident). PA may be prompted by FPI and/or WCE, and is often manifested as a fear of being alone, sleeping alone, and/or being abandoned. Children may avoid situations such as attending or staying in school, being dropped off at a friend's house, extracurricular activities, or social events. When avoidance is not possible, it is not surprising that children with SAD seek safety.

For example, a child who refuses to be alone (when family members are somewhere else in the house) may do so if he or she has access to a "medical monitor" (Eisen & Engler, 2006)—someone who agrees to remain nearby, just in case physical illness occurs. Similarly, a child who fears being abandoned may stay in school or attend play dates and extracurricular activities as long as he or she has access to a "lifeguard"—a safe person such as a parent, nurse, teacher, or coach who can prevent a personal catastrophe (Eisen & Engler, 2006; Eisen & Schaefer, 2005).

Panic Disorder

PD comprises two key criteria. The first requires the experience of recurrent, unexpected panic attacks. DSM-IV-TR defines a "panic attack" as a sudden episode of intense fear or discomfort that includes at least 4 of 13 physical (e.g., palpitations, shortness of breath, nausea) and/or cognitive symptoms (e.g., fear of dying, losing control). Common symptoms in youth with PD include pounding heart, nausea, hot–cold flashes, shaking, and shortness of breath (Kearney, Albano, Eisen, Allen, & Barlow, 1997). The second criterion requires at least 1 month of apprehensive expectation about having additional attacks or worry concerning the implications of these attacks (e.g., losing control or going crazy; APA, 2000). Given the unexpected nature of panic attacks, agoraphobic avoidance is common and may include restaurants, crowds, elevators, small rooms, parks, malls, and stores (Kearney et al., 1997). Panic attacks are often sustained by FPI and/or WCE, and youth frequently seek safety in the form of safe persons, places, objects, and actions.

Generalized Anxiety Disorder

The central feature of GAD is excessive anxiety and worry that is difficult to control. The worry must occur for at least 6 months, across multiple spheres, and is associated with somatic complaints. In adults, three of six (i.e., restlessness, easily fatigued, difficulty concentrating, irritability, muscle tension, sleep disturbance) symptoms are required, but for children, one is sufficient (APA, 2000).

Unlike SAD or PD, worry experienced by children with GAD is diffuse and focuses on both catastrophic and daily life events. Children with GAD worry about everything and appear to have minimal ability to stop their worrying. A child's awareness of frightening events, such as a neighborhood robbery or natural disaster, may immediately lead to the assumption of personal relevancy and become the basis for catastrophic worry. More typically, however, minor events, such as receiving a mediocre test grade, become a crisis, and the child goes from one crisis to another with minimal relief (Chorpita, Tracey, Brown, Collica, & Barlow, 1997).

The worry associated with GAD is chronic and debilitating, and as such "wears the child down" with fatigue, muscle tension, irritability, and sleep problems. Given the more frequent but less intense physical sensations, a child with GAD may not fear physical illness to the same extent as children with SAD and PD, but he or she may dwell on feeling physically uncomfortable much of the time, and as a result may engage in "self-pampering" and attempt to avoid school, social, and/or extracurricular activities (Eisen & Schaefer, 2005; Kearney, 2001). PA may also be expressed through distraction (keeping preoccupied) and mental blocking (see Friedberg & McClure, 2002). Children with GAD often seek safe persons for constant reassurance that their catastrophic worries (e.g., "What if" worries) will not come true.

Obsessive–Compulsive Disorder

Children with OCD experience obsessions and/or compulsions, typically both. "Obsessions" are intrusive thoughts, impulses, or images that are persistent and cause remarkable distress and anxiety. The most common obsessions in children focus on themes of contamination (e.g., germs, disgust), fears of harm to self or others, symmetry (a feeling of incompleteness), and excessive religiosity (a need to confess; APA, 2000; March & Mulle, 1998). Given the intense discomfort associated with obsessions, children often perform compulsions that temporarily neutralize their anxiety.

"Compulsions" are repetitive behaviors (e.g., hand washing or checking) or mental acts (counting, repeating words) that develop in response to the obsessions. Most children recognize their obsessions as senseless but still cannot help but follow through with their rituals in a rigid or stereotyped manner. It is not uncommon for children to involve family members in their rituals. For example, a child or adolescent may insist that all family members adhere to a strict standard of cleanliness or demand that his or her food be prepared a specific way. When rituals cannot be completed, a child can easily become argumentative, and at times, explosive.

DSM-IV-TR requires that obsessions and/or compulsions cause marked distress in the child's social, academic, and family functioning, and consume more than 1 hour per day (APA, 2000). Children with OCD may fear physical illness, especially if they struggle with contamination-related obsessions. WCE to self or others is common, typically in the form of intruder fears at night, being kidnapped, or car accidents. Children with OCD regularly seek safety in the form of safe persons, but more typically, safe actions (rituals).

Posttraumatic Stress Disorder

Until now, we have been discussing anxiety that is largely irrational. For instance, minimal or no evidence supports fears or worries regarding catastrophic outcomes. Children with PTSD, however, have experienced directly or vicariously (observing or learning about) overwhelming trauma that transcends general life stressors (e.g., illness or divorce) and greatly exceeds their coping abilities.

By definition, one's response to the traumatic event must be intense fear, helplessness, or horror (APA, 2000). Core symptom clusters of PTSD include persistent reexperiencing (of the trauma), avoidance of trauma-related stimuli, emotional numbness, and increased physiological arousal. Trauma in children, however, is typically expressed in the form of disorganization, agitation, repetitive play, frightening nightmares, regressive behaviors (bedwetting), somatic complaints, generalized anxiety, clinginess, fears of being alone, abandoned, and/or school refusal (Terr et al., 1999; Webb, 1994; Yule, 2001). PTSD in children is typically associated with being the victim (or witness) of a major accident; burglary; physical, emotional, or sexual abuse, including chronic bullying; kidnapping; man-made or natural disaster; terrorist attack, and the unexpected death or serious injury of a family member or close relative.

Children with PTSD may not fear physical illness, although they may have strong levels of generalized physiological arousal and be hypervigilant to any associations of the traumatic event. PA is likely to be strong to avoid trauma-related situations, but generalized (school, social). WCE may be ongoing and strong if cued by associations. Seeking safety is common in the form of safe persons and safe places.

Differential Diagnosis

Comorbidity is the norm when it comes to anxiety disorders in youth. In this section, we make some notable distinctions among disorders when differential diagnosis is challenging.

SAD versus PD

SAD is considered the most common anxiety disorder of childhood, with typical onset around 7 to 12 years of age (Compton, Nelson, & March, 2000; Keller et al., 1992). PD, on the other hand, is more closely associated with adolescence, with panic attacks initially emerging around 15 to 19 years of age (Kearney & Allan, 1995). However, given that both separation anxiety symptoms and panic attacks have been observed in children, often overlap, and are prevalent across DSM-IV-TR anxiety disorders, differential diagnosis can be challenging.

Although panic attacks have been observed in children (e.g., Burke, Burke, Regier, & Rae, 1990; Garland & Smith, 1991; Vitiello, Behar, Wolfson, & McLeer, 1990), whether their experience resembles the PD observed in adolescents and adults remains controversial (Kearney & Silverman, 1992). For instance, a child with SAD may experience a panic attack that is maintained by FPI. The intensity of fear and/or physical discomfort may also approximate adult panic (see Eisen & Schaefer, 2005). However, panic attacks are likely to be limited to one or two somatic complaints. In addition, characteristic cognitive symptoms, such as "losing control" or "going crazy," may not yet be evident (Nelles & Barlow, 1988). Most importantly, panic is likely to be triggered by situational cues rather than being unexpected or "out of the blue."

It is important to remember that PD, even in adolescents (from less than 1%; e.g., Wittchen, Reed, & Kessler, 1998), and SAD in community samples (as low as 3%; e.g., Anderson, Williams, McGee, & Silva, 1987) are relatively rare. Panic attacks (as high as 65%; Ollendick, Mattis, & King, 1994) and separation-anxious concerns (as high as 75%; Costello & Angold, 1995; Hajinlian et al., 2003), however, are remarkably prevalent in the general population. Thus, for our purposes, it makes sense to look at not only the overlap between these disorders but also, more importantly, their symptom dimensions.

High rates of comorbidity between SAD and PD have been reported (e.g., Alessi & Magen, 1988; Biederman, 1987; Moreau, Weissman, & Warner, 1989). At the symptom level, comorbid separation anxiety has been reported to be as high as 73% in youth with panic attacks (Masi, Favilla, Mucci, & Millepiedi, 2000). Studies have also demonstrated that childhood separation anxiety is associated with a lifetime history of PD (Silove & Manicavasagar, 1993; Silove et al., 1995), suggesting that separation anxiety may be a precursor to PD. Alternatively, however, other studies have failed to find this relationship (Aschenbrand, Kendall, & Webb, 2003). Thus, it remains unclear whether separation anxiety represents a specific risk factor for the development of PD or poses a general risk for adult anxiety.

Clinically, a number of markers may suggest one disorder over the other. For example, we know that panic attacks as part of PD, by definition, must be unexpected or uncued. Separation-related panic attacks are triggered in anticipation of being alone and/or abandoned (Hahn, Hajinlian, Eisen, Winder, & Pincus, 2003). Chances are, children age 10 and younger are experiencing cued panic attacks even when they seem unaware of the source. A little probing, coupled with a functional analysis, invariably reveals situational and/or cognitive triggers.

Although both panic and separation anxiety may be maintained by FPI, PD is associated with heightened anxiety sensitivity (Kearney et al., 1997). Youth with elevated anxiety sensitivity are not only frightened by bodily sensations but, more importantly, are worried about the consequences of these physical sensations (Reiss, Silverman, & Weems, 2001). For this reason, the Child Anxiety Sensitivity Index (CASI; Silverman, Fleisig, Rabian, & Peterson, 1991) may be a useful tool (see the "Assessment" section) in differentiating between PD and more general somatic complaints stemming from other anxiety disorders.

Of special note, PD is less likely than SAD to be comorbid with other disorders (about 50% vs. as high as 90%). The most frequent additional disorders with PD tend to be depression and/or other anxiety disorders (Kearney et al., 1997; Last & Strauss, 1989). SAD, however, is frequently comorbid with other disorders (as high as 90%), including GAD (Kendall et al., 2001), OCD (Geller, Biederman, Griffin, Jones, & Lefkowitz, 1996), panic attacks (Masi et al., 2000), specific and social phobias (Verduin & Kendall, 2003), PTSD (Fischer, Himle, & Thyer, 1999), and school refusal behavior (Kearney, 2001).

Some more general distinctions to consider are that SAD appears to be equally common in boys and girls, whereas PD is more likely in (adolescent) girls. In addition, PD is more likely than SAD to be associated with stressful life events (King, Ollendick, & Mattis, 1994). Both PD and SAD may stem from insecure parent–child attachments and/or behaviorally inhibited temperaments (see Ollendick, 1998). Family factors such as overprotectiveness, enmeshment, and/or elevated parental control have been found to be associated with both disorders, as well as anxiety in general (Eisen, Brien, Bowers, & Strudler, 2001; Hudson & Rapee, 2001).

Finally, within our conceptual framework, both SAD and PD may be maintained by FPI and/or WCE. PA for SAD typically centers around fears of being alone and/or being abandoned. PD, however, more likely resembles abandonment fears (i.e., afraid to venture away from home) unless, of course, nocturnal panic attacks are present. Most importantly, SAD is largely about youth having access to safe persons, whereas youth with PD tend to have broader safety needs that encompass persons, places, objects, or actions (for a full explication, see Eisen & Schaefer, 2005).

SAD versus PTSD

Because of the similarity of symptoms, trauma may be mistaken for separation fears that are irrational or that stem from insecure parent–child attachments. For instance, children with both SAD and PTSD frequently experience anxiety in the form of excessive worry; somatic complaints; and/or panic attacks (Alter-Reid, Gibbs, Lachenmeyer, Sigal, & Massoth, 1986; Cooke-Cottone, 2004); developmental regression (Pullis, 1998; Yule, 2001); fears of being alone, especially sleeping alone (Cohen, Berliner, & Mannarino, 2000); social withdrawal; and school refusal behavior (Terr et al., 1999; Yule, 2001).

As a first step, therefore, it is important to determine whether a child or close family member actually has experienced or continues to experience trauma-related exposure. Sometimes the trauma may remain unknown, for instance, if a child is fearful of potential repercussions stemming from sexual abuse. Research suggests that adolescents in particular are at increased risk for trauma-related exposures. For example, in a large national survey, 23% of adolescents reported being both a victim of assault and a witness to violence (Kilpatrick, Saunders, Resnick, & Smith, 1995). Second, irrespective of the stressor, the child or adolescent must respond with intense fear, helplessness, or horror (APA, 2000). Even when these elements are evident, a differential diagnosis may still be challenging given that multiple forms of exposure are often intermixed with features of PTSD, SAD, and/or depression (Pelcovitz, Kaplan, DeRosa, Mandel, & Salzinger, 2000). For this reason, we emphasize signs and symptoms most characteristic of PTSD.

For example, unlike fear-based separation anxiety, trauma-related symptoms are more likely to be varied and/or severe, and frequently result in serious disruptions in a child or adolescent's daily functioning. In addition to core DSM-IV-TR symptom clusters, trauma is more likely to be associated with self-destructive behavior (Johnson, 1998; Kiser, Heston, Millsap, & Pruitt, 1991) sexual problems (Dubowitz, Black, Harrington, & Verschoore, 1993), explosive outbursts and conduct problems (Cohen et al., 2000), confusion, impaired sense of trust, disruptive relationships, substance abuse, and suicidal behavior (Tufts New England Medical Center, Division of Child Psychiatry, 1984).

It is important to keep in mind that PTSD symptoms may have a delayed onset and first appear as intrusive thoughts, repetitive play, and regressive and/or socially inappropriate behaviors (Yule, 2001). These behaviors may be addressed while monitoring a child's overall adjustment and carefully evaluating any potentially trauma-related experiences.

A clinician who suspects that a child may have experienced trauma should consider administering the Children's PTSD Inventory (Saigh, 1998). Within our framework, in comparison to SAD, children with PTSD are more likely to worry about calamitous events, may exhibit strong and generalized PA, especially to PTSD-related stimuli, and may seek both safe persons and places to feel protected.

GAD, OCD, and SAD

Worry associated with GAD is excessive and varied (multiple spheres), difficult to control, and accompanied by somatic complaints. These worries are not viewed as senseless and are not resisted. Obsessions, however, are not simply excessive worries about everyday problems. Rather, by nature, they tend to be intrusive and bizarre. For example, common obsessions include thoughts or images of having serious diseases such as AIDS or getting rabies from accidentally stepping in animal feces. Children will do everything in their power to avoid these disturbing images. For instance, in the feces example, they may repeatedly check the soles of their shoes, clean their sneakers excessively, and/ or refuse to play outside.

GAD is highly comorbid with other anxiety disorders, most notably depression and adjustment problems (Keller et al., 1992; see Davidson & Fristad, Chapter 6, and Roehrig, Sperry, Lock, & Thompson, Chapter 7, this volume, for a full discussion of mood-related symptoms, disorders, and comorbidity). OCD is comorbid with not only other anxiety disorders and depression, but it is also more likely to be comorbid with behavior, learning, tic, and substance abuse disorders (Piacentini & Graae, 1997).

Both worry and obsessive thoughts tend to follow a developmental progression. For instance, worrisome thoughts do not become prominent until children are at least 8 years of age (Muris, Merckelbach, Gadet, & Moulaert, 2000). As children get older, worry typically becomes more pervasive and severe, and is often accompanied by depression during adolescence. Typical age of onset for GAD is around 10–14 years (Albano, Chorpita, & Barlow, 1996). Obsessive thoughts are rare in young children, and when OCD develops early (age 5–8), rituals typically develop in response to uncomfortable feelings or overwhelming urges (Piacentini & Graae, 1997). Early onset of OCD is also more likely to be associated with family histories of OCD, tic disorders, and Tourette syndrome (Swedo, Rapoport, Leonard, Lenane, & Cheslow, 1989). Typical age of onset for OCD is around 9–12 years (Hanna, 1995).

Both GAD and OCD are frequently comorbid with SAD. GAD co-occurs with SAD approximately one-third of the time (Kendall et al., 2001). Both disorders are associated with frequent worry and somatic complaints. The focus of worry for GAD is not limited to calamitous events affecting the self or others, and its course is more chronic. In addition, children with GAD are more likely to feel fatigued and physically uncomfortable rather than to fear physical illness. Children with GAD seek safe persons for reassurance that their "What if" worries will not come true. Children with SAD, however, seek safe persons to ensure that their own safety, as well as that of significant others, is not compromised. In our experience, SAD may develop subsequent to GAD. For example, when a worried child becomes aware of potential threats to other people's personal safety, from any number of sources (e.g., family members, friends, television broadcasts or movies), his or her worry often becomes overgeneralized and may lead to PA and/or seeking safety.

OCD co-occurs with SAD as much as 24–34% of the time (Geller et al., 1996; Valleni-Basile et al., 1994). In OCD, children seek safe persons for reassurance but rely more heavily on safe actions (compulsions) to neutralize their anxiety (Mesnik, Hajinlian, & Eisen, 2005). Seeking safety is triggered by obsessive thoughts, images, or impulses. Children with SAD seek safe persons and objects in anticipation of being alone and/or abandoned. Thinking about and/or enduring these situations trigger WCE and FPI. The combination of OCD and SAD is associated with earlier onset of PD (Goodwin, Lipsitz, Chapman, Manuzza, & Fyer, 2001).

In the following section, we illustrate how our conceptual framework permits individualized case formulation and treatment planning with a young child experiencing separation and generalized anxieties, obsessive–compulsive symptoms, and oppositional defiant behaviors. We then demonstrate in a step-by-step fashion how to implement parent–child interaction therapy (PCIT) effectively to manage both anxiety and disruptive behavior problems.

CASE FORMULATION: CONCEPTUAL MODEL OF ASSESSMENT AND TREATMENT

Case Presentation

Julie, a 6-year-old Caucasian female, arrives at our clinic with her father, who indicates that Julie is having an increasingly difficult time separating from him and is "acting out" in the classroom. Julie frequently begs and pleads with her father to stay with her when he must leave. She has trouble falling asleep alone at night, going to school or on the bus, and is also hesitant to have play dates with her peers if her father will not stay with her. In addition, Julie reportedly bosses, tries to control, and occasionally shoves her classmates to have her way.

Psychosocial History

Julie currently lives with her father, Tom, and older brother, Peter (age 10), as well as a new stepmother, Catherine. Approximately 1½ years ago, Julie's mother and father separated after years of marital discord. Julie's mother moved out of the family home and was joined by Julie's other brother, Owen, age 13. At that time, Julie's parents shared joint custody of her, and she spent half of her time with each parent. However, after approximately 6 months of this arrangement, Julie's mother took an extended trip to another country for approximately 3 months, during which time Julie did not have contact with her. Although her mother returned to the United States after her 3-month trip, her contact with Julie has been sporadic. Julie's worries about separating from her father began around this time and have continued to the present.

Julie's symptoms of separation reportedly include getting upset and tearful in any situation in which she must be away from her father. Julie begs her father to stay with her and becomes irritable when he leaves. This behavior is especially pronounced when Julie's father must leave on a business trip. Whenever he is out of the home, Julie repeatedly calls her father on his cellular phone to verify his health and well-being. At nighttime, Julie frequently leaves her bedroom to check on her father, verifying that he is in the adjacent room. If Julie's father attempts to return to the ground floor of the home while Julie is trying to go to sleep, then she begs him to join her on the upstairs floor. She also refuses to attend sleepovers with other friends, citing similar difficulties being away from her father. Julie also refuses to engage in certain daytime activities, such as gymnastics class, because she must be away from her father. Julie worries that during these times something bad will happen to her father, so that she will be unable to see him again, or that he will go away and not return. Furthermore, Julie states that she fears that something will happen to her, such as getting lost or being taken, and never see her father again.

Julie's separation fears become especially pronounced in the school setting. In the classroom, Julie often complains of extreme nervousness, and stomachaches, and frequently requests to visit the nurse. Julie attempts to get the nurse to call her father. However, the school nurse has recently been trying to reduce the occurrence of this behavior by sending Julie back to her classroom promptly. While with her peers, Julie engages in several oppositional behaviors, including kicking, pushing, and shoving other children, and demanding that they obey her commands. She reportedly rips toys out of the hands of other children. Episodes such as these reportedly last several minutes, after which Julie becomes emotionally fragile and remorseful. When asked about possible triggers for Julie's behavior, her father notes that undergoing "transitions," being frustrated, and being asked to do something she does not like evoke these behaviors.

In addition to her fears about separation from her father, Julie reportedly exhibits a number of persistent worries. According to her father, Julie often refuses to eat without an adult present, indicating that she might choke or vomit, and no one would be there to help her. Despite reassurance from other adults, she consistently refuses to eat by herself and will not eat certain foods, if she thinks they might be tainted. On occasion, Julie engages in repetitive spitting when she feels she has eaten something that might make her sick. However, this spitting behavior does not occur every day. She often worries that she will catch an illness or disease, and reportedly complains to her father about every little pain in her body, asking whether she will be "all right." Julie also performs several behaviors that her father has reported as "superstitious." For example, when Julie tries to throw things into the wastebasket, she says that if she can "make the basket" on three tries, her father will be OK forever. She also refuses to write the number "6," because she thinks it is bad luck. For instance, she has stated that her mother left on the sixth day of the month; therefore, it is now a bad number. She also constantly asks her father "worry questions," such as what time he will be home, what they would do if they ran out of gas for their car, whether their family will always have enough money, and so on. Julie's worries extend beyond worries about separation and include worries about her own health, her father's health, her family's safety, her school, and her friendships. She often asks "worry questions" that span each of these "worry spheres." Overall, Julie's father characterizes her as a child who is always "seeking safety and assurance."

Assessment

Intake and Functional Behavioral Analysis

An initial behavioral analysis for a child such as Julie must be thorough enough to ascertain all problematic behaviors, the particular situations in which these behaviors take place, and possible triggers for them. Therefore, initial assessment may require a significant amount of time to complete, so that the clinician is assured that the appropriate information is obtained. Relevant assessment techniques should include a clinical interview, self-report measures, medical evaluation, behavioral observation, and self-monitoring tasks.

CLINICAL INTERVIEW

The clinical interview serves as the backbone for the initial assessment, providing important diagnostic information and allowing for a functional analysis of presenting problems. The Anxiety Disorders Interview Schedule for DSM-IV—Child and Parent Versions (ADIS-IV-C/P; Silverman & Albano, 1996) is a particularly useful tool that has proved useful in diagnosing children with a range of anxiety disorders, including SAD, social phobia, specific phobias, GAD, and OCD in addition to mood disorders.

The ADIS-IV-C/P is a semistructured clinical interview for the diagnosis of childhood anxiety and related mood disorders. Previous research has demonstrated good to excellent test–retest reliability for anxiety disorders with the ADIS-IV-C/P (Silverman, Saavedra, & Pina, 2001), as well as support for the concurrent validity of the interview (Wood, Piacentini, Bergman, McCracken, & Barrios, 2002). It has been used extensively in the assessment of children with anxiety disorders (Silverman et al., 2001; Westenberg, Siebelink, Warmenhoven, & Treffers, 1999). The child and parents are interviewed separately by a single interviewer, and the diagnosis is based on composite information from both interviews (Silverman & Eisen, 1992; Silverman & Nelles, 1988). The initial goal of this assessment procedure is to gain precise knowledge of the child's presenting symptoms, including the frequency, intensity, and duration of the current symptoms from the perspective of both the child and the parents. The purpose of using an interview such as the ADIS-IV-C/P is twofold: It provides a clear approach to assessing particular problem behaviors and can appropriately differentiate between a variety of anxiety and mood disorders, which is key to proper treatment. This is particularly useful given that literature has indicated a developmental trend in anxiety symptoms (Keller et al., 1992).

In the context of this case, after briefly meeting with the family to discuss the assessment process, the therapist interviewed Julie alone. This may present an immediate problem for some anxious children, because the separation involved in this assessment may be a challenge. Certain strategies have proved to be useful, such as showing the child exactly where his or her parents will be during the interview or having the parents sit immediately outside the interview room. In certain instances, it may be necessary to have the parents in an adjacent room, where the child can see them during the interview. This may be accomplished quite easily if the interview location is equipped with windows or translucent mirrors. However, if these facilities are not available, leaving the interview room door ajar may be a suitable compromise. Julie preferred to be in a room adjacent to that of her father, where there was a one-way mirror, so she could see him whenever she wanted.

Additional constraints associated with this clinical interview include the prolonged period of time needed to administer the ADIS-IV-C/P. With Julie, her father, and her stepmother, the entire interview process took approximately 3½ hours. In Julie's case, occasional breaks and some snacks helped to sustain her attention and energy during the interview. However, whenever possible, continuity during the interview process should be emphasized.

Throughout the administration of the ADIS-IV-C/P, Julie's particular difficulties became apparent. Her fear and anxiety around separation situations and the significant interference it causes in environments such as the school, the home, and with friends, warranted a diagnosis of SAD. Additionally, Julie's problems with persistent worry seemed to reach above and beyond the fear of separation. Although her fear of choking and catching an illness may have been related to a fear of separation, Julie's worries, frequent worry questions, and her subsequent behaviors indicated that a further diagnosis of GAD might be appropriate. Whereas some of Julie's behaviors may have suggested a diagnosis of OCD, such behavior did not seem to occur frequently enough to classify Julie in such a manner. Furthermore, the compulsive types of behaviors in which Julie engaged seemed more consistent with her fears of separation, because each of her "superstitious behaviors" was performed to keep her father "safe."

Self-Report Measures

In an effort to provide multiple modes of assessment, self-report measures should be collected from the parents and child, provided the child has the cognitive ability to respond to questionnaires in an appropriate manner. Additionally, in an ideal clinical situation, collateral reports from another parent, teacher, or any other person who has frequent contact with the child in situations where the child displays psychopathology, may provide a wealth of knowledge to aid diagnosis and treatment. However, more often than not, the nature of clinical practice inhibits collecting such information. At the very least, an effort should be made to collect both parent and child self-report measures. The following measures have proven to be very useful in the assessment and subsequent treatment of children presenting with separation anxiety and worries.

When addressing anxiety, precise assessment of avoidant behaviors is necessary to successful cognitive-behavioral treatment. Although clinicians may observe various events during the office visit for the assessment, a wealth of information may be tapped by exploring the particular avoidant behaviors of individual clients.

FEAR AND AVOIDANCE HIERARCHY

Common in many cognitive-behavioral approaches in the treatment of anxiety, the fear and avoidance hierarchy (FAH) is a useful self-report tool. The FAH, which we have called the "Bravery Ladder" for the purposes of working with young children, is an empty scale that is to be filled by approximately 10 real-life situations that the anxious child is avoiding. These situations are ranked in order of anxiety intensity. To assist in these rankings, a 0- to 8-point Likert-type scale is utilized, where zero is *No anxiety at all* and eight is *Extreme anxiety*. It is recommended that children and their parents complete the FAH with the help of the clinician, who can assist in drawing out the appropriate situations that may need to be addressed in treatment. In addition to the anxiety rating, clinicians may find it helpful to assess the relative avoidance of such situations with the same 0- to 8-point scale. The addition of this avoidance rating may help the clinician later in treatment, when designing particular exposures for the child to attempt.

To help Julie to feel more invested in working from her Bravery Ladder (FAH), we had Julie color and decorate the Bravery Ladder before we filled in the situations. Julie's Bravery Ladder was populated with several situations in which her father had to leave the home. At the top of this hierarchy was having her father leave for a weeklong business trip, while Julie stayed with a relative. Below that situation was having her father leave for a weeklong business trip, while Julie stayed with her stepmother. Other situations included leaving for school without a "fuss," being away from her father for the evening, staying home with a babysitter, and going on a play date to her friend Ali's house. Each situation was listed on her FAH and rated by Julie and her parents according to the approximate level of anxiety caused by each situation. By completing the FAH in the beginning of treatment, the family is able to notice clearly the goals of treatment. For example, when Julie's stepmother and father saw the completed FAH, they stated, "Wow, we have our work cut out for us, but if Julie can accomplish each of these goals through these sessions, we think she will be a much happier child." Thus, we continually referred to the FAH throughout treatment. The family was given the original, decorated FAH to take home, and a copy was retained in the patient's file.

Once diagnostic impressions are in hand and the FAH is developed, the heart of individualized case formulation and treatment planning begins with our Separation Anxiety Assessment Scales—Child and Parent Versions (SAAS-C/P; see Eisen & Schaefer, 2005, for a copy of the scales, clinical norms, and scoring instructions).

Child Self-Report Measures

SEPARATION ANXIETY ASSESSMENT SCALE—CHILD VERSION

The Separation Anxiety Assessment Scale—Child Version (SAAS-C) is a 34-item, empirically derived self-report measure designed to assess separation anxiety and related anxiety symptoms. Frequency of symptoms extends from 1 (*Never*) to 4 (*All the time*) to indicate the relative frequency of a child or adolescent's problem behaviors. The SAAS-C comprises four key symptom dimensions (five items each), including a Fear of Being Alone (FBA; e.g., "How often are you afraid to sleep alone at night?"), Fear of Abandonment (FAb; e.g., "How often are you afraid to go on a play date at a new friend's house?"), Fear of Physical Illness (FPI; e.g., "How often are you afraid to go to school if you feel sick?"), and Worry about Calamitous Events (WCE; e.g., "How often do you worry that bad things will happen to you?"). The SAAS-C also contains a Frequency of Calamitous Events (FCE) subscale (e.g., "How often has a parent, family member, friend, or relative been in a serious car accident?") and a nine-item Safety Signals Index (SSI) that assesses a child's reliance on safe persons, places, objects, and actions (e.g., "How often do you need your mom or dad to stay with you so you can go on a play date, birthday party, or after school activity?"). FBA and FAb reflect PA for SAD and related anxiety disorders (PD, GAD, OCD, and PTSD) whereas FPI and WCE, singly or in combination, maintain them.

The SAAS-C goes beyond measuring the content of anxiety and related problems, and affords a framework for individualized assessment and treatment. Preliminary data support the psychometric properties of the scale, most notably its factor structure, reliability, validity, and clinical utility (Hashim, Alex, & Eisen, 2006; Hajinlian et al., 2003; Hajinlian, Mesnik, & Eisen, 2005; Hahn et al., 2003).

The SAAS-C was read aloud to Julie, and she was given additional explanations of the questions whenever needed. Although Julie was fearful of sleeping alone, her PA largely stemmed from her FAb. She received a raw score of 14 (out of 20), which is consistent with a diagnosis of SAD. Julie was avoiding a broad range of situations, including play dates, extracurricular activities, sleepovers, taking the school bus, and school. Her PA was maintained by both FPI (12/20) and WCE (11/20), consistent with diagnoses of SAD or GAD. She was terrified of vomiting or choking and worried about bad things happening to herself, father, and friends. Her SSI was elevated (24/36), which is consistent with SAD, PD, or OCD. Julie's safe persons included her father, a school nurse, and her best friend. Her safe places included her father's bedroom, her house, and the nurse's office. Her safe actions included visiting her father at night and the nurse at school, repeated phone calls to her father, parental promises to stay home or stay at an activity for the entire time, and refusal to eat (in anticipation of becoming ill). Julie's SAAS-C data set the stage for individualized treatment planning.

MULTIDIMENSIONAL ANXIETY SCALE FOR CHILDREN

The Multidimensional Anxiety Scale for Children (MASC; March, Parker, Sullivan, Stallings, & Connors, 1997) is a 39-item, empirically derived, multidomain self-report measure designed to assess a broad range of anxiety symptoms. Subscales on the MASC include Tense/Restless, Somatic/Autonomic, Total Physical Symptoms, Perfectionism, Anxious Coping, Total Harm Avoidance, Humiliation/Rejection, Performance Fears, Total Social Anxiety, Separation/Panic, and Total MASC Score. A shorter, 10-item form (MASC-10) may also be used when appropriate. The MASC is a useful assessment tool because of the broad range of anxiety difficulties it addresses (see Curry, March, & Hervey, 2004). The MASC has significant empirical support demonstrating its validity and reliability, as well as its factor structure (March et al., 1997, 1999). Three-month test–retest reliability was found to be satisfactory to excellent, with all intraclass correlations above .60. Internal consistency was also found to be acceptable.

In Julie's case, the MASC was also read aloud to her. Her responses on the MASC help pinpoint specific anxiety difficulties. Only Julie's raw scores are reported, because her age precludes the use of *T*-scores. Julie's MASC Total Scale raw score was 72, indicating that she experiences a significant amount of overall anxiety. Additionally, Julie's Separation/Panic subscale raw score of 17 was also elevated, demonstrating her persistent anxiety around separation situations and reported feelings of panic. On the Anxious Coping subscale, Julie had a raw score of 13. This seems to be consistent with her reports of persistent worry in uncertain situations. Finally, Julie's Somatic/ Autonomic subscale score of 10 might suggest a particular difficulty with anxiety about bodily sensations, such as the physical feelings associated with vomiting. In addition to the SAAS-C, the MASC offers an additional perspective on Julie's particular anxiety concerns that can help facilitate treatment planning.

CHILD ANXIETY SENSITIVITY INDEX

The Child Anxiety Sensitivity Index (CASI; Silverman et al., 1991) is an 18-item, empirically derived self-report measure that assesses how aversive children view their physical sensations. Sample items include "It scares me when I feel like I'm going to throw up" or "It scares me when my heart beats fast." The CASI has excellent empirical support (e.g., Rabian, Peterson, Richters, & Jensen, 1993). Elevated scores are predictive of PD (Kearney et al., 1997). Julie's total CASI score of 32 (out of 54) was within normal limits, suggesting that her panic-like symptoms were not consistent with a full-fledged PD.

Other widely used rating scales to round out the assessment of anxiety and related problems in children and adolescents include the Fear Survey Schedule for Children—Revised (FSSC-R; Ollendick, 1983), Revised Child Manifest Anxiety Scale (RCMAS; Reynolds & Richmond, 1978), State–Trait Anxiety Inventory for Children (STAIC; Spielberger, Gorsuch, & Luchene, 1970), Children's Yale–Brown Obsessive–Compulsive Scale (CY-BOCS; Scahill et al., 1997), and the School Refusal Assessment Scale (SRAS; Kearney, 2001).

Parent Self-Report Measures

SEPARATION ANXIETY ASSESSMENT SCALE—PARENT VERSION

The Separation Anxiety Assessment Scale—Parent Version (SAAS-P) is similar to the child version in content, number, and structure of the questions. The SAAS-P contains the four key symptom dimensions, as well as the FCE and SSI. Preliminary data also support the psychometric properties of the scale (see Eisen & Schaefer, 2005).

Julie's father Tom and stepmom Catherine jointly completed the SAAS-P. Their report largely mirrored Julie's in the sense that FAb (13/20) was primary. However, both parents agreed that Julie's FBA, most notably her fear of sleeping alone, was more disruptive to their household than Julie reported (12/20 compared to 8/20). In addition, Julie's parents reported that FPI was largely maintaining her anxiety (12/20). Other than Julie's constant reassurance seeking, Tom and Catherine were not fully aware of the scope of their daughter's worries. As with Julie, Tom and Catherine reported a long list of seeking safety behaviors.

CHILD BEHAVIOR CHECKLIST

The Child Behavior Checklist (CBCL; Achenbach, 1991a) is a 120-item parent report questionnaire designed to assess children's behavioral and emotional functioning. Parents are asked to rate the how true these specific behaviors are in regard to their child on a 3-point scale from 0 (*Not true*) to 2 (*Very true*). A global index of psychopathology may be computed from the Total Behavior score, while the "Internalizing" and "Externalizing" scales reflect different patterns of maladjustment. The Internalizing scale comprises problems such as anxiety, depression, obsessions, and somatic complaints. The Externalizing scale comprises behavior and conduct problems such as oppositional behavior, aggression, hyperactivity, and delinquency. The CBCL provides further behavioral description through the utilization of eight subscales: Anxious/Depressed, Withdrawn/Depressed, Somatic Complaints, Social Problems, Thought Problems, Attention Problems, Rule-Breaking Behavior, and Aggressive Behavior.

The CBCL also provides useful information on the social and recreational activities and skills of the child, and probes the child's school functioning. Questions such as these operationalize the specific behaviors and environments where children suffering from anxiety seek safety, and identify subsequent areas to be addressed by treatment. Additional teacher report versions are available to provide collateral information relevant to the child's behavior in the school setting. The goal of such an assessment tool is to gain a broad perspective that allows the clinician to tailor treatment to the specific problem behaviors identified by the CBCL.

The internal consistency of the CBCL measure ranges from .78 to .97. The test–retest reliability ranges from .95 to 1.00. Additionally, criterion validity was assessed and found to be acceptable (Achenbach, 1991b). In clinical studies, the CBCL was found to be a reliable and valid measure of behavioral problems (Daughtery & Shapiro, 1994; Lowe, 1998). Considerable recent research supports the CBCL's capability to distinguish between children with anxiety disorders and normal nonclinical controls, as well as children with anxiety disorders and those with externalizing disorders. However, this same research found less evidence to support the CBCL's ability to distinguish between children with anxiety disorders and those with affective disorders, and cautions against use of the CBCL alone for diagnostic decisions, instead stressing the use of the CBCL as a supplement to careful diagnostic interviewing (Seligman, Ollendick, Langley, & Baldacci, 2004).

Julie's Total Problems scale T-score of 72 (98th percentile) was in the clinical range for girls her age, indicating a significant level of overall behavioral problems. Her total Internalizing scale T-score of 72 (98th percentile) on her father's report was also in the clinical range for girls her age, suggesting that she experiences elevated levels of anxiety and sadness. Julie's Externalizing scale T-score of 72 (98th percentile) was in the clinical range for girls her age also, suggesting that Julie often engages in "acting out" or aggressive behavior. Particularly elevated subscales included the Anxiety/Depression subscale ($T = 78$, > 97th percentile), the Social Problems subscale ($T = 72$, 97th percentile), and the Aggressive Behavior subscale ($T = 82$, > 97th percentile).

EYBERG CHILD BEHAVIOR INVENTORY

The Eyberg Child Behavior Inventory (ECBI; Eyberg & Pincus, 1999) is a 36-item parent self-report questionnaire that attempts to assess behavioral problems in children ages 2–16. The ECBI provides a quick, reliable measure of conduct problems, indicating both the frequency of a variety of behaviors and whether these behaviors interfere with the family unit. The ECBI offers significantly more information than the responses collected by the CBCL for many reasons. First, the ECBI Frequency of Behavior scale extends from 1 (*Never*) to 7 (*Always*) to indicate the relative frequency of a child's problem behaviors (e.g., "How often does your child refuse to do chores when asked?"). This extended response range provides more specificity for parents, as well as a broader range of data points for later analysis. The ECBI may prove particularly useful in measuring treatment changes because of this larger range.

Furthermore, the ECBI also collects information on the relative interference caused by these behaviors in the child's family unit. The ECBI inquires whether the specified behavior is "a real problem" for the respondent. This information greatly aids the clinician during the assessment by providing parent-reported indicators of particular behavior problems that cause interference, effectively separating them from behaviors that are not as problematic. This allows the clinician to focus his or her treatment by targeting the specific behaviors that interfere most in the family's life.

Past literature on the ECBI demonstrated good psychometric properties (McMahon & Estes, 1997; Funderburk, Eyberg, Rich, & Behar, 2003; Rich & Eyberg, 2001). Additional literature provides further evidence that the ECBI is a reliable and valid measure of child disruptive behavior problems (Burns & Patterson, 2001).

The ECBI comprises two subscales, the Intensity subscale and the Problem subscale. The Intensity subscale assesses the frequency with which the child displays the problem behaviors. The Problem subscale assesses whether the parent considers the behavior to be a problem (Eyberg & Pincus, 1999). Julie's Intensity subscale *T*-score of 67 indicates a significant number of problem behaviors that occur relatively frequently. Julie's Problem subscale *T*-score of 62 is above the cutoff for children her age, indicating that these behaviors cause significant interference and distress according to her parents.

PARENTING STRESS INDEX

The Parenting Stress Index (PSI; Abidin, 1995) is a 101-item self-report measure that seeks to recognize dysfunctional parent–child systems. In addition to the 101 items, a 19-item Life Events Stress scale attempts to assess the relative stress of the underlying environment of the respondent. The ultimate goal of the PSI is to provide a reliable measure of parent characteristics, child characteristics, and situational factors that may lead to dysfunctional parent–child interactions, children with emotional or behavioral problems, and dysfunctional parenting (Abidin, 1995). Subscales in the parent domain include Depression, Attachment, Role Restriction, Sense of Competence, Social Isolation, Relationship with Spouse, and Parental Health. Subscales in the child domain include Adaptability, Acceptability, Demandingness, Mood, Distractibility/Hyperactivity, and Reinforces Parent.

The PSI may be useful to clinicians assessing and treating an anxious young child by identifying the parenting problems and child adjustment difficulties that occur in the family system. Knowledge of these factors is vital in tailoring the treatment to the individual family. Each family has unique parent–child interactions. Some families may have a high proportion of negative interactions, whereas others may exhibit a general lack of interactions as a whole. By administering the PSI, clinicians can ascertain what behaviors may need to be improved to increase the frequency of healthy interactions.

Psychometric support for the use of the PSI is very extensive (see Abidin, 1997). Recent reviews have ascertained the feasibility of the PSI Short Form (PSI-SF) that comprises 36 questions spread across three factors (see Reitman, Currier, & Stickle, 2002). Data indicate very good to excellent internal consistency. Some researchers support the use of the PSI-SF, citing the prolonged period of time required to complete the full PSI (Reitman et al., 2002). However, the extra expenditure of time can yield a significant amount of data that are especially useful in tracking treatment progress and gains (Abidin, 1997).

On her father's report, Julie's PSI Total Scale score was elevated (in the 90th percentile). This indicates that, overall, this parent–child system is under a significant amount of stress and is subject to dysfunctional interactions. Julie's PSI scores on the child domain subscales were in the 99th percentile, indicating that she displays qualities that make it difficult for her parents to fulfill their parenting roles. In particular, Julie demonstrated an inability to adjust to changes in her physical and social environment, and to respond with appropriate affect. The scores also suggest that Julie places many demands on her parents and does not match the expectations that they have of her. These scores were consistent with information obtained during the interview.

Medical Evaluation

In addition to self-report data, a full and complete picture of the child's physical health, including any types of medical conditions or complications, should be undertaken (King, Leonard, & March, 1998). For example, episodes of extended sickness, severe injury, or chronic health problems may serve as instigating events for separation anxiety, resulting in prolonged absences from caregivers. Although the likelihood of extreme outcomes from many common childhood illnesses is low, it is critical to consider that children who have anxious tendencies may believe that the probability of a catastrophe such as death due to illness is high. Moreover, medical complications may be a continuous point of anxiety for children as they cope with the symptoms of their anxiety disorder. Children who require continuing medical care, often managed by their parents, have some grounded fears of separation and may feel they have "more to lose" in separation situations. Thus, proper recording of the child's medical history is of prime importance.

Collection of medical information need not be in any particular format. Often, for logistical reasons, a written parent report measure will suffice. In the process of a psychological assessment for anxiety, clinicians rarely have the time to engage in more than a brief investigation of complicating medical problems. When a medical problem does have a direct relationship with a child's anxiety difficulties (e.g., anxiety in situations where peers are eating peanut products and the child is severely allergic to peanuts), interview time should be spent conducting a precise survey of the presenting medical difficulties to make sure that treatment is both tailored to the child's needs and physically safe.

Such a medical history should assess serious illnesses, accidents, and other upsetting incidents, including a description of the incident's duration and the level of care the child requires. Significant allergies, fractures, and medication histories may also be collected through this parent questionnaire. Additionally, an inquiry into serious injuries and ongoing medical problems is necessary for assessment and treatment. It is also recommended that the medical history include an early life history assessing prenatal development, perinatal health, and any delivery complications. Supplementary information that may be useful includes reports of early developmental progress, behavioral contingencies in childhood, and a description of the child's family environment. A final addition to such a questionnaire should include a detailed history of any medical or psychosocial treatment for behavior problems. When inquiring into past treatment, it is helpful to collect information on the frequency and duration of the professional contact, as well as the primary focus of treatment, method or model of treatment provided, and the results obtained from the contact.

Julie had a relatively uncomplicated medical history. Her father did not report any significant illnesses or injuries during childhood except for the removal of her tonsils 1½ years ago. However, her father noted Julie's moderate chronic allergies for which she had an inhaler to be used as necessary. On one occasion while Julie was playing in a park, she reportedly developed an allergic reaction to pollen in the air and had significant trouble breathing. Although she did not need to be taken to the hospital, her father sat with her while she regained normal breathing. Following that incident, Julie was prescribed her inhaler and sometimes worries when she is left without it. No complications were reported during Julie's prenatal development or birth. Julie reportedly met all developmental milestones within normal limits. She responded only moderately to behavioral contingencies and could sometimes become uncontrollable, according to her father.

Behavioral Observations

Within a comprehensive psychological assessment, direct behavioral observation is extremely important and beneficial (Ciminero, 1986), especially with children (McMahon & Forehand, 1988). Such observations are necessary, because use of only self-report measures often produces incomplete results, especially when assessing inappropriate behavior (Hartmann & Wood, 1990), such as the avoidant behavior characteristic of children with SAD. Although direct observation is extremely beneficial to both assessment and treatment planning for children with clinical difficulties, several practical concerns often limit behavioral observations to a minimum in standard clinical assessments (see Bessmer, 1998). However, the development of the Dyadic Parent–Child Interaction Coding System (DPICS; Eyberg & Robinson, 1983) and the subsequent DPICS-II (Eyberg, Bessmer, Newcomb, Edwards, & Robinson, 1994) has provided the clinical community with a direct observational-based method to assess parent–child interactions. It is especially important to address these interactions in children with separation anxiety because, when maladaptive, these interactions form the core construct of the disorder. Psychometric data for the DPICS-II have prove to be good to excellent (see Deskin, 2005).

The DPICS-II contains 27 parent behavior and 25 child behavior categories. Parent categories include the occurrence of behavioral descriptions, informational descriptions, question asking, giving commands, offering labeled and unlabeled praise, criticism, warnings, and so on. The child behaviors include identical categories (see Bessmer, 1998). The DPICS-II is administered in a specific protocol in three phases that take place during a brief play interaction between the child and parent. The first phase (Child-Directed Interaction; CDI) is a parent–child interaction in which the child is encouraged to lead the play and the parent is encouraged to create a positive, nondirective environment. In the second phase of the interaction (Parent-Directed Interaction; PDI), the parent is to direct the play. In the final phase of the interaction (Cleanup; CU), the child is instructed to clean up the playroom (Eyberg et al., 1994).

The DPICS-II and its coding system have been recently modified, so that it particularly useful to clinicians working with young children with separation anxiety and their families (Pincus, Cheron, Santucci, & Eyberg, 2006). By adding a fourth observational phase (Separation; SEP), in which the parent is asked to leave the room for just a few minutes and the child must play with a confederate, the clinician can gain some firsthand knowledge of the types of behaviors that occur during periods of acute separation. This may be difficult to arrange in settings where a confederate is not readily available. In these situations, the clinician may serve as the confederate, observing the child's behavior directly. Such information is particularly useful to treatment planning, because it identifies particular child behaviors that must be addressed to reduce separation anxiety. The DPICS-II, as modified for children with separation anxiety, may be useful not only for assessment but also for monitoring treatment progress and outcome. It can be administered between different treatment phases, as well as at posttreatment and 3-, 6-, and 12-month follow-up points. Although such repeated administrations may be cumbersome, measuring observational change over time in this way can promote a better understating of specific treatment gains, as well as how these gains are maintained over time.

During Julie's initial assessment, she presented as particularly anxious when her father Tom had to leave the room during her portion of the assessment. When he returned to participate in the collaborative play task during which the DPICS-II was conducted, Julie became visibly calmer. During Phase 1 of the DPICS-II (CDI), it was evident that Julie's father displayed a significant amount of control over the direction of play, allowing Julie very few opportunities to direct the situation. Tom asked Julie a stream of questions and made continual suggestions regarding what she should play with or do. Although the interaction was enthusiastic and genuine at times, it became apparent that Julie had little control over the play time and received very little positive feedback from her father. In Phase 2 (PDI) Tom expressed several commands and became particularly agitated when Julie delayed in following these commands. Julie withdrew from the play situation quite notably when her father was directing the play. During Phase 3 (SEP), Julie began to cry when she was informed that her father had to leave the room. Tom reassured her for several minutes, pinpointing exactly where he was going to sit in the waiting room and offered to sit immediately outside the door of the playroom. Julie was inconsolable for several minutes and hardly engaged in play with the confederate. She carried out a considerable number of safety-seeking behaviors, repeatedly asking when her father would return. When Tom did return in Phase 4 (CU), Julie was elated and cleaned up readily.

Self-Monitoring

During the assessment phase, it can be extremely useful to monitor specific behaviors daily to aid in the functional behavioral analysis of children with SAD. Because the clinician spends only limited time with the child and parents during the assessment, further self-monitoring tasks may provide valuable data. One such monitoring task designed for children with SAD is the Weekly Record of Anxiety at Separation (WRAS; Choate & Pincus, 2001; see Eisen & Schaefer, 2005, for a copy), a daily measure of child anxiety symptoms that is completed by a parent or guardian. It assesses 22 behaviors common in children with SAD, measuring both their frequency and severity. The WRAS is designed to incorporate DSM-IV diagnostic criteria for SAD and requests that parents record such information. Such a monitoring form may help to strengthen a questionable diagnosis or provide further information for treatment planning.

Julie's father, Tom, noted several problem behaviors when he completed the WRAS during the assessment phase. He reported that Julie called him on his cellular phone nearly every 30 minutes while he was out on errands. Additionally, Julie would protest every day before going to school, claiming that she was scared to attend. According to the WRAS, Julie wanted her father to accompany her to the classroom and stay for nearly half an hour before she became calm enough to stay on her own. At nighttime, Julie needed her father to sit with her until she fell asleep for three of the seven nights in the week prior to the assessment. The other nights of the week, she needed her father to be on the same floor in her house as her bedroom. Julie also did not attend any afterschool activities unless her father was present.

Link between Assessment and Treatment

It is important that the assessment process be viewed as an integral part of each child's treatment. For example, in Julie's case, the pretreatment assessment provided some important information about which behaviors needed to be targeted during treatment. First, Julie's constant need for safety and reassurance was clearly the most disruptive aspect in her own life and that of family members. Julie's separation and generalized anxieties had persisted for years and her father, Tom, was desperate for some parenting skills to know better how to help her. Additionally, Julie displayed some oppositional behavior that we conceptualized as being somewhat related to separation anxiety from her father, and also possibly related to her anger regarding her mother leaving her so abruptly. Although we intended first to target Julie's anxiety-related struggles, we also planned to incorporate into treatment some time for Julie to express some of her sadness and feelings about her parents' breakup and her mother's departure. Information we received from the assessment indicated that her mother was indeed involved with drugs and alcohol, and was not likely to have a consistent role in Julie's life, because she had decided to move to a foreign country. Thus, we planned to focus our treatment on helping Julie to attach more securely to her father and stepmother, both of whom expressed a sincere desire to develop a close and warm bond with her.

It is important to keep in mind that the assessment process did not stop at pretreatment. Rather, is continued throughout the course of Julie's treatment program. For example, Julie's progress in treatment was assessed at multiple times throughout treatment. For example, specifically after each component of the treatment was introduced, we utilized various assessment measures (MASC, DPICS-II with separation situation) to determine the specific effects of that treatment component on Julie's progress. We also had one continuous monitoring measure (WRAS) that was completed every day by the parents to assess the frequency and intensity of separation incidents as they occurred. Finally, we also assessed Julie after her treatment was completed—at posttreatment, and at three follow-up points (3-, 6-, and 12-months posttreatment) with the SAAS-C/P. By doing this, we were able to track the maintenance of Julie's gains over the course of an entire year.

Treatment

Preview

We decided that the treatment of choice to utilize with Julie and her father and stepmother was to be parent–child interaction therapy (PCIT), which has recently been adapted specifically for children with SAD (Pincus et al., 2005). Because PCIT is also the treatment of choice for oppositional defiant disorder, and because it incorporates essential parenting skills for modifying maladaptive parent–child interactions, we determined that it would likely be effective in targeting both the separation and the oppositional concerns.

Julie's parents, Tom and Catherine, stated that they wanted to help Julie begin to enter new situations that she was enduring with distress, and also to learn to manage Julie's misbehavior when it occurred. Tom pointed out that it was at times difficult to tell the difference between separation anxiety and oppositional behavior, because he was not always sure whether Julie was simply avoiding doing new things due to anxiety or simply being oppositional. In addition, Julie's constant safety seeking demands were depleting both parents' patience and emotional resources. For these reasons, we hypothesized that PCIT would provide an excellent foundation of skills tailored to Julie's specific needs. Thus, PCIT was our chosen framework for beginning our treatment process.

Context of Treatment

Treatment sessions took place in a room with toys; a small, child-size table; and a one-way mirror that led to an observation room. We also utilized walkie-talkies with an earpiece microphone, so that we could coach Julie's father and stepmother as they began to implement the skills they were learning. A treasure box filled with stickers and other small, child-friendly items were used as rewards when Julie was successful at trying some new things. Sessions occurred weekly for approximately 1 hour each.

Description of Treatment Components

PCIT OVERVIEW

Numerous studies have demonstrated the effectiveness of PCIT in reducing child behavior problems (Eyberg & Robinson, 1982; Foote, Eyberg, & Schuhmann, 1998). These studies have documented change in the interaction style of parents in play situations with the child, as evidenced in increases in the proportion of praise and decreases in the proportion of criticism during play sessions with their child. These changes, which are reflected in significant improvements in child compliance and fewer disruptive behaviors, have been shown to generalize to the child's behavior at home and school (Boggs, Eyberg, & Reynolds, 1990). Additionally, parents' level of distress has been found to improve as the child's behavior improves. Maintenance of treatment gains has been demonstrated at 1-year follow-up for both children and parents.

Experimental evidence highlights the potential clinical utility of incorporating parents more centrally into the treatment of childhood anxiety disorders (Barrett, Dadds, & Rapee, 1996; Knox, Albano, & Barlow, 1996), yet few controlled studies have examined the effects of using parent-training procedures with young children with SAD. PCIT is one of the best-established, empirically supported parent training interventions for use with young children and their parents, yet it has never been applied to the treatment of young children with SAD. Although originally designed for use with oppositional children, PCIT incorporates each of the skills child anxiety researchers have identified as essential parent training components for reducing childhood anxiety, including enhancing parent attention, command training, differential reinforcement, and shaping. Thus, a revised PCIT protocol was expected to be effective in reducing children's separation anxiety behaviors and in promoting improved interactions between anxious children and their parents.

TREATMENT PHASES

PCIT, as developed for the treatment of SAD in young children, has three phases: Child-Directed Interaction (CDI), Bravery-Directed Interaction (BDI), and Parent-Directed Interaction (PDI). The CDI portion focuses on changing the quality of the parent–child relationship. Parents are taught nondirective interaction skills to provide a safe and therapeutic context that allows the child to experiment with change. Interpersonal factors such as parental warmth, attention, and praise serve as incentives that facilitate the child's development of internal attributions of self-control. Differential reinforcement of child behavior through praising the child's appropriate play and ignoring undesirable actions provides a positive form of behavior management.

The BDI phase provides psychoeducation to parents about anxiety and incorporates graduated exposure to feared separation situations. Fear of separation situations may be decreased by a properly managed and structured exposure program. The therapist works with the family to develop a hierarchy, as well as a reward list to reinforce the child's brave behavior. The child is instructed to create a "Bravery Ladder" that lists each situation he or she would like to enter but is currently avoiding.

In PDI, methods of incorporating clearly communicated and age-appropriate instructions to the child are taught to parents. Using techniques based directly on operant principles of behavior change, the therapist teaches parents to provide consistent positive and negative consequences following the child's obedience and disobedience. In addition, the therapist assists the parents in understanding how a child's behavior is shaped and maintained by the social environment.

MONITORING TREATMENT PROGRESS

Within the course of treatment, specific monitoring forms may be useful in tracking the child's progress through treatment. Within PCIT, weekly practice records for the CDI and PDI sections provide the clinician further information for treatment planning. Throughout treatment, parents are asked to practice 5-minutes of CDI during a play situation. These daily sessions, as well as toys used and problems encountered, are listed on the record form. The PDI practice record is used to monitor the use of PDI skills during the PDI phase, as well as any problems encountered during the implementation of the technique. Both forms increase accountability, thus enhancing implementation of the skills and, therefore, treatment effectiveness. Furthermore, recording problems that arise enables the discussion of more suitable methods of skills implementation during the subsequent session.

In addition to these monitoring forms, repeated administration of measures used during the assessment may also serve the clinician in tailoring PCIT to the individual client. Administration of the DPICS-II between treatment phases is recommended to ascertain the family's understanding and implementation of treatment concepts and techniques. By using the DPICS-II in this manner, clinicians may identify families needing additional skills training in particular treatment phases, and provide extra practice and assistance. Furthermore, the use of the WRAS and FAH, as described earlier, is beneficial in identifying particular separation worries that need to be targeted in treatment. Oftentimes in the course of treating children with difficulties like Julie's, avoidant behaviors may change as children learn to seek safety in new, more healthy, self-reliant ways. By administering these measures regularly during treatment, new separation situations that elicit anxiety may be identified and addressed, while those situations that are longer anxiety-provoking may serve as reinforcing examples of progress.

THE PROCESS OF TREATMENT: STEP-BY-STEP GUIDELINES

CDI Phase

Session 1: CDI Teaching Session

The goals of this first session, which is held with parents only whenever possible, are to establish rapport with the family, to teach parents the CDI skills, and to provide parents with the rationale underlying this component of treatment in such a way that each skill and the CDI phase as a whole, are seen as relevant to their child's functioning.

Founded on the skills that play therapists use to foster a safe environment and a warm relationship with a child, CDI aims to teach parents to communicate with their young children in a developmentally appropriate way that takes into account children's limited attention span. CDI skills are intended to alleviate frustration while improving the child's self-esteem and social skills. The result is a secure, warm relationship between parent and child, thus improving a connection that is often strained due to anxiety-driven oppositional behavior and the frustration parents' experience when disciplining such a child becomes ineffective.

After welcoming Julie's parents and providing a brief introduction to the session, we discussed any anticipated barriers to treatment. Even the most motivated family can encounter practical limitations in attending weekly treatment sessions, and one of the therapist's many roles includes identifying and preventing factors that may lead a family to discontinue therapy prematurely. Once a barrier is identified, a problem-solving approach should be used to generate acceptable solutions before any such problems arise. Like many families, both of Julie's caregivers were concerned about leaving their daytime commitments early to attend therapy. Tom worked full-time, while Catherine attended school as a full-time student. In addition to Julie, they had another child at home (Peter, age 10) who could not be left alone for an extended period. They were also concerned about pulling Julie out of school early given that she had become increasingly disengaged throughout the year. We agreed on a meeting time that accommodated the family's busy schedules and generated possible solutions if a scheduling conflict emerged. We also offered to have a research assistant watch the sibling in the waiting room while Julie was in session, if needed.

During the first session, it is important to provide the family with an overview of treatment and answer family members' pressing questions. In the PCIT protocol, it is particularly important to explain the phases of treatment. Doing so helps the family to integrate the various skills offered across phases; failure to describe the process often results in confusion as to why particular techniques are being taught, and how to integrate them with other skills. Julie and her family were given information about the nature of anxiety, as well as brief descriptions of CDI, BDI, and PDI. However, at the beginning of treatment, it is important to stress to families that these descriptions are brief, and that any questions they have will be addressed in the appropriate phase of treatment.

As a first step, we explained that CDI is introduced first as a way to lay the groundwork for the coming treatment phases that focus on anxiety concerns and behavior problems that are often more resistant to change. Once the warmth of the parent–child relationship is increased and the child begins to enjoy the special CDI time with the caregiver, it is easier for him or her to accept limits and discipline.

Following this explanation, the rules of CDI are introduced. These rules include what language and behavior to avoid, as well as what skills to use during this special playtime with the child. First, the parents are instructed to avoid using commands, which can reduce the child's sense of control over the play, and also to avoid asking questions of their child during this time. Questions can be interpreted as hidden commands and may suggest disapproval ("Are you sure you want to use the blue crayon?") or that the parent is not listening to the child. The parents are also instructed to avoid criticism during this special playtime to foster a supportive and positive environment for parent and child interaction. Last, the parents are asked to ignore completely all inappropriate behaviors. By doing so, undesirable behaviors are less likely to occur in the future. However, when children engage in dangerous behaviors (jumping off high furniture, placing toys in or near their eyes, etc.), it is important for parents to suspend CDI practice, address the dangerous behavior as they normally would, then reinitiate CDI practice.

Next, the "Do's" of this special playtime are described. The first skill PCIT attempts to foster is praise for appropriate behavior. Such praise usually results in an increase in the appropriate behavior. Parents who are able to praise their child successfully often have an easier time in the BDI phase, during which their child's attempts at brave behavior needs to be reinforced with praise. Another "Do" skill is reflecting appropriate talk. Parents who reflect their child's appropriate talk allow the child to lead the play and demonstrate that the parents both understand and accept their child's words. Furthermore, parents are asked to imitate and to describe appropriate behavior. Oftentimes, we have found that children may be confused about which behaviors are appropriate in certain situations. When we have parents imitate and describe these behaviors, children become more sure of their actions, subsequently building their confidence for other activities. Finally, these skills should be applied with enthusiasm to convey the degree to which the parent is enjoying the time spent with the child.

Like most parents in this treatment program, Tom felt that it would be challenging to avoid questions and commands while interacting with Julie. Oftentimes, conversing in this way does not come naturally to a parent. For this reason, PCIT treatment integrates both modeling by the therapist and coaching sessions with the family to facilitate the implementation of these skills. These CDI skills were role-played with both Tom and Catherine, who reported that the skills "felt awkward," that they "didn't have very much to say without using questions or commands," and that the resulting silence felt "uncomfortable." The parents were reassured that most families in their situation share these concerns, and that the CDI skills become more natural with time.

For homework, the parents were assigned 5 minutes of CDI playtime each day with Julie. They were also asked to monitor the frequency and intensity of Julie's separation-anxious behaviors throughout the week using the WRAS form.

Session 2: CDI Coaching Session 1

The goals of the first CDI coaching session, during which the child is present, are to strengthen the therapeutic relationship with the family, to reinforce the parents in their use of CDI skills over the previous week, and to enhance those skills through additional coaching.

We were fortunate that both Julie's father and stepmother were able to attend most treatment sessions. Their joint attendance allowed us to monitor each parents' use of the skills, while building an alliance between the parents in coping with Julie's anxiety, which in turn enables consistent implementation of the skills at home.

First, Tom was given a two-way walkie-talkie radio with an earpiece, which enabled us to communicate conveniently and discretely with him while he interacted with Julie. This piece of equipment, known as the "bug-in-the-ear" is very helpful for coaching parents from behind a one-way mirror. We asked Catherine to observe this interaction. Tom was instructed to play with Julie, using all the CDI skills he had been practicing, while we coached his response to her play. Because of the many different skills introduced in the previous week, it is most effective to emphasize only a few skills at a time during each coaching session. Once these are mastered, additional skills become the focus of coaching. During this session, coaching dealt primarily with Tom's use of behavioral descriptions, though he was praised when he implemented any additional CDI skills. While the two were drawing, Tom effortlessly praised Julie: "I love how you shared your crayons with me," and "You chose such pretty colors!" He also provided many descriptions of Julie's behavior, such as "You're drawing a princess with a hat on her head" and "You made me a birthday cake out of Play-Doh!" Tom displayed great enthusiasm in his play but had difficulty in refraining from asking questions (e.g., "What do you want to draw next?") and giving commands (e.g., "Please pass me the blue paper"). Although innocuous on the surface, these statements have the potential to remove Julie's control of the play and should be avoided during the special time. When Tom was told over the bug-in-the-ear to ask Julie to begin cleaning up, she exhibited distress and resistance. Tom was coached to ignore her negative behavior until she calmed down. Within 3 minutes, Julie's cheerful demeanor had returned, and she and her father were able to clean up the toys without incident.

Next, we coached Catherine over the bug-in-the-ear as she played with Julie. Catherine was new to the family, and whereas it was obvious that Julie cared a great deal for her, Catherine's relationship with Julie was not yet as cultivated as that between Julie and her father. This strain was evident during the playtime when Catherine did not often praise Julie's actions and evidenced difficulty generating conversation that did not contain questions or commands. Catherine also displayed difficulty relinquishing control of the play. We pointed out to Catherine over the bug-in-the-ear each question she posed to Julie, and praised her when she rephrased her question ("Is that a picture of your dad?") as an appropriate statement ("That's a picture of your dad"). Later, Catherine explained that she felt uncomfortable knowing that she was being watched. Therapists should make their best attempts to approximate a typical interaction between parent and child during the PCIT coaching sessions. However, it is important to acknowledge that the treatment setting may not enable a true replication of the interaction that typically occurs at home. For this reason, it is crucial that parents apply these skills at home throughout the week and bring to the session any "real-world" difficulties they encounter.

For homework, Tom and Catherine were asked to continue practicing CDI daily with Julie, and were encouraged to focus specifically on decreasing questions and increasing reflections during the playtime. The WRAS was also assigned to continue monitoring Julie's separation anxiety incidents over the week.

Session 3: CDI Coaching Session 2

The goals of the second CDI coaching session, during which the child is present, are to address the importance of homework and to continue shaping the parents' use of skills, with an emphasis on avoiding questions during CDI. This session should also be used to discuss modeling of appropriate behavior.

During homework review, Tom indicated that the frequency and intensity of Julie's separation-anxious incidents had greatly increased. Earlier that week, Julie said good-bye to her biological mother, who was moving out of the state indefinitely, and she had exhibited a range of distressing emotions since that time. In the session Julie appeared clingy and withdrawn, and was unwilling to discuss her mother's departure.

Given the circumstances, it is important to recognize the developmental appropriateness of Julie's spike in symptoms. Not surprisingly, her mother's departure exacerbated Julie's need to be close to her father and Catherine, as well as her heightened distress when this need could not be satisfied. This display of separation anxiety may not be inappropriate given the situation; thus, it should not necessarily be the focus of treatment. However, by continuing to foster the warmth and security of Julie's attachment to her father and to Catherine through the implementation of CDI skills, we hoped that these more acute symptoms would attenuate naturally.

After homework review, behavioral modeling was discussed as a way to teach Julie more appropriate behavior. Catherine and Tom were also informed of ways that anxious behaviors can inadvertently be modeled by parents. At this point, Catherine, new to the family and still learning how to discipline children effectively that were not her own, recognized that she had been modeling not only her own frustration but also her anxieties about being in charge of this often chaotic household. This discussion helped Catherine to gain insight into the way she reacted to stress, and well as implications of these reactions within the family. Moving forward, she expressed a commitment to be more sensitive to the behaviors she was modeling for Julie and her brother.

During the coaching portion of the session, Julie's father introduced fewer questions and commands relative to the previous session, and provided many behavioral descriptions, reflective statements, and labeled praises. Tom asked only one question, which he immediately changed into a statement. Similarly, Catherine evidenced great improvements, offering praise, reflections, and descriptions with much more ease than previously. The growing warmth in her relationship with Julie was becoming evident; Julie was increasingly receptive to Catherine's praise and frequently sought her contribution to drawings and the imaginary tales she enacted during the special playtime.

During a 5-minute coded interaction, both Tom and Catherine provided at least 10 behavioral descriptions, 10 reflections, 10 labeled praises, and less than 3 questions, commands, or criticisms. Thus, each parent had met the CDI phase mastery criteria and were therefore ready to move on to the BDI component of treatment. In the event that a family is unable to meet these mastery criteria, it is important to continue work on CDI until the family members become comfortable and competent at implementing CDI skills.

For homework, Tom and Catherine were asked to continue practicing CDI daily despite the fact that mastery criteria had been met. Continuing to utilize CDI skills not only strengthens the parent–child attachment but also facilitates Julie's ability to approach new situations during the next treatment phase.

Post-CDI Assessment

After the CDI portion of treatment, the family completed an assessment to determine the extent of change during the first treatment phase. The assessment included the self-report measures mentioned earlier and the administration of the DPICS-II, a behavioral coding system.

BDI

Session 4: BDI Teaching Session

The goals of the BDI teaching session include educating parents about the cycle of anxiety, specifically, the three components of cognitions, affect, and behaviors that maintain anxiety in children (see Barlow, 2002). Additionally, the clinician should explain the importance of using CDI skills in separation situations both to instill confidence and control in the child and to elicit appropriate behaviors. Furthermore, this session should be used to discuss the role that avoidance plays in anxiety. Parents are encouraged to prevent their child from avoiding situations that involve separation, despite the child's distress.

During the session, which is held with parents only whenever possible, Tom and Catherine were provided with information about anxiety. The task of breaking the cycle of anxiety was presented as a way to help reduce Julie's distress at separation. Framing anxiety as a natural, necessary, and harmless emotion proved particularly helpful. To demonstrate, Tom was asked to generate situations where the experience of anxiety had actually proven to be beneficial. They were told that the goal of treatment is not to rid Julie of her anxiety entirely, but to help her understand that feeling a little anxious will not hurt her, and that with repeated exposure to the situations she fears, Julie would experience a reduction in her anxiety.

Tom and Catherine were informed that separation anxiety can arise from many factors. It is likely that a combination of environmental factors, such as the inadvertent reinforcement of her fears when extra attention is given to Julie's symptoms, and biological vulnerabilities may underlie Julie's experience of anxiety. A self-described anxious person himself, Tom was relieved to hear that his "anxious genes" had not necessarily caused Julie's behavior.

After listening to this psychoeducation about anxiety, he expressed an understanding of Julie's symptoms as a product of many factors. Tom was now able to perceive how changes in Julie's environment, such as her mother's departure and entrance into school, may have contributed to the development of Julie's anxiety.

The three-component model of anxiety is then presented to teach parents how to break anxiety down into three elements: thoughts, feelings, and behaviors (see Barlow, 2002). Viewing anxiety as a global entity is not usually helpful, just as saying to a child, "Just relax" or "Stop worrying," never seems to bring about reductions in the anxiety. Instead, breaking anxiety down into its components can help parents become effective coaches for their children when feared situations arise. First, Tom and Catherine were asked to speculate what Julie was thinking during separation situations. These thoughts, including "I'll get lost," "I can't do this by myself," "My dad won't come back," and "Someone will take me," were written in the thoughts circle of a three-component model handout. Although some young children may not yet have the developmental capacity to reflect on their own thoughts, the previous examples are common to children experiencing separation anxiety. Whereas Julie may believe these thoughts to be fact, thus contributing to her feelings of fear, it is important for her parents to be aware that these thoughts may not be based in reality.

Feelings, or the physical sensations a child experiences during separation situations, make up the second component of the model. These sensations include racing heart, sweaty palms, dizziness, stomachaches, and headaches, among others. Such feelings are a natural part of the body's experience of anxiety and will not hurt the child. In fact, these sensations will attenuate when the child is able to remain in the feared situation, choosing to endure these feelings of anxiety rather than to avoid them. When having to separate from her parents, Julie often reported stomachaches, which she described as "bubbles in her stomach." In these situations, her parents were asked to explain to Julie that these feelings are a natural reaction to trying something new, and that they would eventually go away. Julie's "bubbles" may be her body's natural reaction to fear or danger. However, this feeling may also be triggered when no real danger is present. Luckily, in the natural process of preparing itself, the body will reduce these feelings of anxiety.

The last part of the model presented to parents, the behavior component, comprises the behaviors a child exhibits during anxiety-provoking situations. Common behaviors include clinging to parents, crying, yelling, complaining of physical ailments, or tantrums. Tom identified Julie's frequent outbursts as the most common behavioral manifestation of her anxiety. In this new context, the family was able to understand Julie's angry fits as a reaction to fear rather than deliberate misbehavior. Further psychoeducation focuses on avoidance as the most common behavior exhibited by anxious children. Avoidant behaviors commonly seen in youth with separation anxiety can take many forms, including visits to the school nurse, asking to be sent home, or refusing to attend a play date or birthday party without the company of one's mom or dad. According to her parents, Julie had become quite adept at avoiding her anxiety over the years. She visited the school nurse many times a week and her parents often allowed her to stay home from school due to the "bubbles in her stomach." Each time she received attention from the school nurse, Julie's avoidant behavior was inadvertently reinforced.

Armed with an understanding of the three components of anxiety, the parents were able to understand the interactions between these components in the PCIT protocol. In Julie's case, when faced with separation from her parents (e.g., school attendance), she reported thinking to herself, "I can't do this by myself. . . . What if Dad doesn't come back to get me?" As a result of these thoughts, she noted physical feelings of anxiety, including "bubbles in her stomach." Julie then engaged in tantrums to avoid going to school. When she was able to avoid attending school or a play date by staying home in the company of her parents, it became harder for her to go the next time, because her anxious thoughts had been reinforced. Julie no longer believed that she could attend school or play dates by herself, because she had previously been unsuccessful. Thus, her cycle of anxiety was maintained.

Oftentimes, parents recognize that intervening to reduce their child's anxiety in the short-term only makes the problem worse in the long term. However, it is often very for difficult for parents to refrain from helping their child avoid emotionally arousing experiences. The same was true for Tom and Catherine, who earnestly wanted Julie to be able to separate from them without fear but did not know whether they would have the strength to watch her increasing distress without intervening. Because PCIT requires Julie's parents to limit the attention that she usually gains when she stays home from school, it is important that they reallocated this attention to the times when Julie performs brave behaviors. Here, the relevance of CDI becomes apparent, because the special practice time during CDI provides reinforcement of these brave behaviors. Parents are instructed to use the CDI skills both when promoting and reinforcing brave behaviors, including labeled praise, reflection of emotion, and description of the situation.

At the end of session, Tom and Catherine were asked to apply the information they learned about the cycle of anxiety to Julie's symptoms by using other commonly occurring separation situations. In addition to what Julie might be thinking, feeling, and doing, they were asked to consider how anxiety was being reinforced in Julie's environment.

For homework, the parents were asked to continue implementing the CDI special playtime and to use the WRAS to record incidents of Julie's separation anxiety. In addition, they were encouraged to complete a cycle of anxiety worksheet for each separation incident that occurred. In doing this, Tom and Catherine would gain a better understating of Julie's symptoms and, therefore, know better how to break the cycle.

Session 5: BDI Coaching Session 1

An important goal of this session, which involves both the parents and the child, is to explain the purpose of the FAH, or "Bravery Ladder," to the child and encourage him or her to choose the first situation to practice over the next week. The next goal is to promote parents' use of CDI skills as they encourage their child to approach new situations and praise the child's efforts in taking a step on the Bravery Ladder. Additionally, this session is used to explain bravery points to both parents and the child. Each family is asked to come up with at least five rewards that have to do with the child earning time with the parents by practicing situations on the Bravery Ladder.

While Julie was given crayons and stickers to decorate her Bravery Ladder, we discussed with the parents which situations they would most like to see Julie achieve, as well as the rationale behind starting with easier items to build a sense of efficacy, before attempting more challenging items. Both the Bravery Ladder and the Reward Store were explained to Julie, whose eyes lit up at the thought of earning prizes. Together, Julie and her parents made a list of appropriate rewards for brave behavior, some of which included a picnic with her dad and stepmom, a pillow fight, a night that Julie would pick what they would eat for dinner and which movie they would watch, and a trip to her dad's office. It is important to note that these rewards need not have any monetary value. When constructing a reward list, children should be encouraged to think of prizes that will be highly motivating. However, it is important to keep rewards within reason, especially for families with limited means. In most instances, children who experience separation anxiety prefer the attention of their parents over any store-bought prize.

Once Julie was excited about her reward list, she more readily engaged in a discussion about items for her Bravery Ladder. Although it is often necessary to complete most of the Bravery Ladder with a parent due to a child's age or reluctance to discuss feared situations, it is beneficial to elicit the child's opinion in choosing the first item to attempt, even if the parents have generated the list. In doing so, the child feels a sense of control over the situation and is more likely to follow though with treatment. Despite her age and reluctance to discuss anything anxiety provoking at the start of treatment, Julie was able to generate many feared situations for her Bravery Ladder. At Julie's request, her father helped her make these situations into rhymes, causing her to howl with laughter. Such individual tailoring of the PCIT protocol to Julie and her family further evidenced the warm and responsive relationship between Julie and her father. At the bottom of her Bravery Ladder, she was to "Go to school while staying cool," meaning that Julie would not seek excessive reassurance or demonstrate clinging behaviors when it was time to separate for school. At the top, Julie was to have "A week away and I'll be OK," which referred to staying with Catherine while her father attended a weeklong business conference. At this point in treatment, Julie was unable to stay with a babysitter for any portion of the day, let alone be away from her father for an entire week. Julie first chose to attempt getting on the bus without seeking excessive reassurance, for which she would be rewarded an afternoon of baking and decorating cookies with Catherine.

For homework, Tom and Catherine were asked to continue daily CDI playtime and to use the WRAS to record instances of Julie's anxiety at separation. They were also asked to provide Julie with encouragement as she attempted her first situation on the Bravery Ladder, praising even small approaches toward the goal. Importantly, they were asked to discourage avoidance and to follow through with labeled praise after each successful attempt. As promised, Julie was to be rewarded for her brave behaviors. Julie's homework was to practice the brave activity she chose from the ladder. We empathized with her about the challenging nature of this task, yet expressed certainty about Julie's ability to accomplish it. Such reinforcement is often necessary in this section of PCIT as both the child and parent begin to challenge avoidance behavior.

Session 6: BDI Coaching Session 2

The first goal of this session is to review the previous week's homework and discuss whether the child was successful in entering the first situation on the Bravery Ladder. Next, the parents' reaction to the child's anxiety in this situation is explored, as well as their reaction to separation incidents that may have occurred since the last session. The therapist also praises the child's brave behaviors and applies stickers to the Bravery Ladder for any task accomplished. The last goal is to agree upon a new step to attempt on the Bravery Ladder in the upcoming week.

During homework review, Julie was asked what she felt most proud of during the previous week. She stated that she had boarded the bus without crying every day since the previous session. In addition, she had even started getting ready by herself in the morning—a task she chose to undertake, without being asked to do so by her parents. Her success in accomplishing the first task seemed to provide her with a sense of efficacy that she was eager to apply to new situations. Her parents identified being most proud of Julie's willingness to try more than what was asked of her in the previous week. In addition, they reported that Julie had not asked whether she would "be OK" as frequently as in weeks past. This reduction in reassurance-seeking behaviors seemed to be related to Julie's increased sense of security and strengthened attachment with her parents due to the family's implementation of CDI skills. At this point in the session, we discussed Tom's and Catherine's reactions to Julie's anxiety. As they encouraged Julie to get on the bus, both parents were surprised by the range of emotions they experienced in witnessing her newfound independence. Like many parents, they were eager to help reduce their daughter's anxiety but did not anticipate the feelings of loss that accompanied this change. For instance, they had become accustomed to Julie using them as safe persons, and she now needed this to a lesser degree.

Building on her successes, Julie was asked to choose new goals on her Bravery Ladder for the upcoming week. Julie decided that she was ready to attend a play date at a friend's without Catherine or Tom being present. In addition, she was willing to try going to bed without repeatedly getting up to be comforted. If successful, Julie would be rewarded with a picnic in the backyard with her dad and stepmom.

This session marked the end of the BDI phase for the family, although we explained to the parents that we would continue to set weekly goals from the Bravery Ladder. For homework, the family was asked to continue CDI playtime with Julie, to record her separation anxiety incidents on the WRAS, and to choose two more steps on Julie's Bravery Ladder to attempt over the next 2 weeks, because the following treatment session would be held with the parents alone.

Post-BDI Assessment

After the BDI portion of treatment, the family completed an assessment to determine the extent of change during the second treatment phase. The assessment included self-report measures and administration of the DPICS-II, a behavioral coding system.

PDI Phase

Session 7: PDI Teaching Session

The goals of the first session in the PDI phase, which is conducted without the child, are to teach the parents the PDI steps, a discipline method that emphasizes consistency, predictability, and follow through, as well as to provide parents with the rationale underlying each step. Although many children experiencing separation anxiety are not typically considered "problem kids" who evidence oppositional behavior, their reactions to a separation situation, whether it be leaving for school or staying with a babysitter, may be similarly disruptive. Furthermore, some parents find that disruptive behavior is amplified as children are asked to attempt increasingly difficult tasks on their Bravery Ladder. Although the technique is described in detail during this session, parents are asked to refrain from using the skills at home until the next session, during which the new rules are explained to the child and the family is coached to ensure correct execution.

At the start of the session, Julie's progress on her Bravery Ladder was discussed. Julie had continued working her way up the hierarchy, and in the past 2 weeks had attended a play date and on many nights was able to stay in her bed without seeking reassurance. Additionally, she stayed with a babysitter for 2 hours while Catherine and Tom went out. That night, Julie was also able to eat dinner without her father being present, a behavior she previously had avoided due to fear of choking or becoming ill. Her cycle of success was beginning to triumph over her cycle of anxiety as it related to both her separation fears and her GAD-related worries.

An overview of PDI was presented to Julie's parents. Tom and Catherine were informed that PDI should be used in situations when the parent needs the child to complete some task. As a result, PDI must first start with a command. However, within the PDI framework, commands should be direct rather than indirect. They should leave no question in the child's mind that he or she is being told to do something. Commands should not be stated like a question, which falsely suggests that a child has a choice ("Sit down" rather than "Would you like to sit down?"). Commands should always be positively stated, telling the child what to do rather than what not to do. Telling the child what not to do may be construed as a criticism of his or her behavior, and it is often possible to stop a negative behavior by telling the child to do a positive opposite task ("Please sit beside me" instead of "Stop running around"). Commands should be given one at a time, breaking down the task into more manageable pieces, and the child should be praised for each command he or she obeys. Commands should also be specific, with the parent telling the child exactly what he or she should do. Vague commands such as "Be careful" are nonspecific, and the child may not know what to do in order to comply. Commands should also be age-appropriate. To be fair in disciplining, the parent must be sure that the child can understand what is being asked. Parental commands should also be given politely and respectfully, as reflected in the parent's tone of voice. Parents whose commands are respectful avoid teaching a child to obey only when they yell at him or her. Furthermore, remaining calm even when frustrated demonstrates appropriate behavior to the child. Commands should be explained before they are given or after they are obeyed. The timing of the command is critical. For instance, an explanation that is given after the command but before it is obeyed interferes with compliance and calls attention to the problem behavior. Giving an explanation before the child complies often incites a debate between parent and child, with the child giving a counterexplanation as to why he or she should not obey. However, when the parent provides a reason after the command is obeyed, the child receives parental attention for compliance that can be combined with labeled praise, creating a positive atmosphere in which the child is likely to hear and understand the reason. Finally, commands should only be used when necessary. If a command is not important enough to require the parent to follow through with PDI consequences, it should not be given.

Tom and Catherine were asked to think of all the possible ways Julie might respond to a command. Commonly, Julie would comply with a command, but in a disrespectful or belligerent way. For example, when asked to turn off her TV before bed, she would scream, run away, slam the door in her father's face, then eventually comply. Situations like this are tricky, because the child is, in fact, complying, but the manner of doing so is inappropriate and certainly not worthy of praise. Tom and Catherine were told that they could phrase the command so that good behavior was embedded in its request, for instance, "Quietly turn off the TV," or "Nicely put your toys in the chest." Still specific, these commands have an added qualification necessary to improve upon Julie's typical behavior.

TIME-OUT PROCEDURES

Once parents understand the appropriate ways to give commands, they are informed of the "5-second rule" for dawdling, which occurs when the child does not immediately obey or disobey. After 5 seconds, the parent must decide whether the child has obeyed or refused to comply with the command. If the child obeys within this time frame, the parent offers an enthusiastic labeled praise (e.g., "Good job minding so quickly!") to reinforce the good behavior. If it seems that the child is continually disobeying after the 5-second rule expires, parents are to give a "chair warning" ("If you don't put your shirts into the hamper, you're going to have to sit in the chair"). It is important to use these exact words and not to repeat the command. Repeating the command tells the child that the parent was not serious the first time, thus reinforcing initial defiance. If the child obeys the warning, he or she is to be given a labeled praise. If the child does not obey after the command is given, parents are to guide the child to the chair, saying "You didn't do what I told you to do, so you have to sit in the chair." This precise phrase is important, because it clearly explains why the child is on the chair. After the child is placed on the time-out chair, the parent says, "Stay on the chair until I tell you to get off." At this point, the parent should persist with the time-out despite any willingness the child now expresses to obey the command. If these steps are not consistently implemented, parents may find that they need to follow up all commands with the threat of the time-out chair instead of gaining the child's immediate compliance. For the purpose of PCIT, a child is deemed to be "on the chair" if 50% of his or her weight is on it. Anything less is deemed noncompliance. The child must stay on the time-out chair for 3 minutes, plus 5 seconds of quiet. The 5 seconds of quiet prior to being released from the chair is vital. If the child engages in any behavior (yelling, whining, etc.) before being released, he or she may think that this behavior allowed for his or her release. Such learning is known as "superstitious learning."

A child who superstitiously learns that a behavior will release him or her from the chair will likely repeat this behavior during the next visit to the chair. Therefore, requiring 5 seconds of silence reinforces the child's good behavior while on the chair. After the silence, the parent approaches the chair and ask the child in a neutral voice, "Are you ready to put your shirts in the hamper?" If the answer is no, the child is to remain on the chair for an additional 3 minutes. If the answer is yes, expressed either verbally or physically by the child, the parent points to the task and says nothing until the child has complied. When the child obeys after being in the chair, the parent simply acknowledge the act and gives another, simple command ("Thank you for putting your shirt in the hamper. Now, put your socks in the hamper, too."). The child's compliance to this second command be followed by the parent's enthusiastic labeled praise ("Great job putting your socks in the hamper!") Thus, immediate compliance is reinforced, instead of compliance that occurred only after implementation of the time-out chair.

In the rare cases when a child gets off the chair before being allowed to do so, a "time-out room" is used as a behavioral strategy for encouraging compliance to the rules of the time-out chair. Parents are to say to the child, "If you don't stay on the chair, you will have to go to the time-out room." This statement is provided only once—with no exceptions. The child *will* remember that failure to comply with the time-out chair rules results in the time-out room, which ideally should be a completely stimulus-free area, separate from family activity. Although the time-out room may be unpleasant, it should not be aversive. The time-out room is not intended as a punishment. Rather, it is a place where the child can be removed from an overstimulating environment long enough to reevaluate his or her own behavior and comply with commands based on learned experience of consistent, predictable parenting behavior. The same 3 minutes of time-out plus 5 seconds of quiet are used for the time-out room. When compliant, the child is taken back to the time-out chair, because the time-out room is only used as a disciplinary method for the time-out chair. After the child returns to the time-out chair, the parent should then ask, again in a neutral voice, "Are you ready to put your shirts in the hamper?" If the answer is no, the child is to remain on the chair for an additional 3 minutes. If the answer is yes, the parents should acknowledge the compliance, provide an additional simple command, then provide enthusiastic praise when the task is completed.

When implementing PDI, it is crucial that parents use the technique consistently and to completion. To facilitate, parents are provided with a PDI command rules handout diagramming both the language and the steps to be taken based on the child's response. The lead therapist then coaches each parent, while the cotherapist plays the role of the child.

Tom was given the bug-in-the-ear and coached through the one-way mirror, while the cotherapist created situations in which the "child" obeys right away, requires a warning, disobeys the warning, complies after 3 minutes on the chair, refuses to comply after being on the chair, and finally, when the "child" gets off the chair before given permission to do so by the parent. Tom found it difficult to state the command only once—a struggle for many parents. So often, parents have grown accustomed to asking their child time and time again to do something, making multiple requests, and the child learns that he or she will have multiple chances to obey. Prior to initiating treatment, Tom and Catherine had begun using the "three strikes" rule with Julie, in that she would be given two warnings after initial disobedience to the request, after which she would be sent to time-out. By the third and final request, Julie usually obeyed. However, Julie's defiant behavior between the first and third request, including screaming, running away, and hitting, was exhausting both to her parents and to Julie herself. This new method alleviates the often-distressing steps in between and sends a clear message to the child that noncompliance will not be tolerated, and that it has immediate repercussions.

After coaching Catherine in the same way, we asked that she and Tom not practice PDI at home until we were able to coach them, with Julie present, in the next week's session. For homework, they were asked to study the PDI diagram, to continue daily CDI playtime with Julie, and to record her separation anxiety incidents on the WRAS. They were also reminded to encourage Julie to attempt the second task on her Bravery Ladder, which had been chosen during the previous week's session.

Session 8: PDI Coaching Session 1

The goal of this session is to coach the parents in the PDI technique, so that they implement it perfectly the first time it is experienced by the child. Parents should leave this session with the knowledge and confidence to apply the procedure, exactly as written, at home.

Both during her initial assessment and in the subsequent treatment sessions, it was evident that Julie often reacted to anxiety-provoking situations, as well as to other nonpreferred situations, with aggressive, oppositional behaviors. Initially not as impairing as her separation concerns, Julie's oppositional behavior became even less problematic as she had learned to better manage her anxiety. However, Julie's tantrums still occurred in an attenuated form. Thus, this phase of treatment was particularly appropriate for Julie's symptoms.

Prior to coaching, Julie's progress on her Bravery Ladder was discussed. She had nearly reached the top of her hierarchy; spending the week without her father was all that remained. Because Tom did not have plans to leave town in the immediate future, this task would have to be attempted after treatment ended. Many families encounter the same predicament, such that their schedules cannot easily accommodate each item on the Bravery Ladder while in treatment. In the meantime, Julie was encouraged to continue her bravery practices, even those that although successfully accomplished nevertheless remained challenging to her. Thus, when the time came for Tom to leave on business, Julie would feel prepared to take that next step.

This session also provides the opportunity to explain PDI to the child. Using role play, the therapist presents several instances of PDI using a child-friendly stuffed animal, doll, or action figure, such as Julie's friend "Mr. Bear." In session, Mr. Bear obeys and then disobeys a series of commands, and the consequences of each are demonstrated by praising Mr. Bear, giving him a warning, or sending him to the chair. This process is made fun and memorable for the child though the use of a stuffed animal and silly commands ("Mr. Bear, please sit on top of my head!"). While the therapist teaches the child about PDI, the role play with Mr. Bear also reinforces each step for the parents.

During the remainder of the session, each parent has the opportunity to be coached using PDI with Julie. First, CDI is coached for 5 minutes, both to reinforce CDI skills and to engage Julie in an activity she enjoys. Next, the parent is told to tell Julie, "Now I'm going to switch to my game," and to ignore Julie's fussing if any occurs, and give a simple command ("Hand me the Legos"). Each parent should try to give five commands during the session. Parents are also encouraged to use CDI skills in between each command–obey–praise sequence.

Both Tom and Catherine were able to implement both steps and the language of PDI quite well. However, Tom evidenced some frustration when attempting to make Julie stay on the chair. Through the bug-in-the-ear, he was coached to calmly and silently led Julie back to the seat the first time she left. It is important to avoid interacting with the child during this time, for any attention bestowed can reinforce the negative behavior. After being reseated, Julie was given the time-out room warning. Finally, Julie remained in the chair for the full 3 minutes and never again got off it on subsequent occasions during the session.

Following the coaching, parents are given feedback and homework instructions. For homework, Tom and Catherine were encouraged to continue practicing CDI for 5 minutes each day. In addition, they were assigned 10 minutes of daily PDI practice and were reminded to continue using CDI skills in between the command–obey–praise sequences. Last, Julie was asked to choose a task from her Bravery Ladder to attempt before the next session. Because she had previously attempted all but her most difficult task, we decided that she should work even harder the next week to stay in her bed at night, without seeking safety or reassurance.

Session 9: PDI Coaching Session 2

The goals of the second coaching PDI session, which involves parents and child, are to perfect each parent's use of the PDI procedure and to foster the use of these skills outside of the playroom. If the therapist believes that the family has appropriately adopted the skills, the parent–child interaction is coded to determine whether mastery criteria have been met.

Homework was first reviewed with the family, including Julie's approach of feared situations on her Bravery Ladder. Next, the implementation of PDI over the week was discussed. According to Tom, Julie only needed to go to the chair once. She had obeyed all other commands. However, both parents asked whether they could give any commands that did not require follow through using PDI consequences. In certain situations, Tom and Catherine felt that immediate compliance with their request was neither crucial nor warranted. Because consistency and follow through are crucial ingredients of PDI, we needed to make sure that these requests of lesser importance do not interfere with the effectiveness of PDI commands when given. Tom and Catherine were told to use only direct commands in situations where consequences for disobedience would be appropriate.

Consistent with the previous session, each parent was coached in using PDI with Julie. The interaction started with 5 minutes of coached CDI, after which the parent was to take control of the play and give an undesirable command. Both Tom and Catherine evidenced considerable improvements in both their implementation of the language and in following the PDI steps. After 10 minutes' coaching each, their interactions were coded for effective commands given (direct, positively stated, single commands) as well as correct follow through. It was evident that both Tom and Catherine had mastered the PDI technique and were ready for treatment termination.

At the end of session, the family members were praised for their perseverance and success. They were told that the termination session would take place the following week but were encouraged to continue using CDI skills when engaging in play, and to use BDI when separation situations arise. Additionally, they should use PDI when necessary to maintain Julie's appropriate behavior.

Termination Session

During the last session, we congratulated family members for their successful completion of the program, and presented Julie with a Bravery Certificate in recognition of her brave behaviors. Julie's progress was detailed, especially her accomplishment of completing nearly every step on her Bravery Ladder. Her improvement was striking. During the first session, Julie was unable to leave her father's lap without having a tantrum. Now, she was attending play dates, separating for school without incident, and remaining in her bed throughout the night, to name a few achievements. At the start of treatment, Julie averaged 15 separation-anxious incidents a week, all involving a great deal of distress.

During the last week of treatment, no anxiety at separation was reported. With the management of her anxiety, Julie's demeanor also greatly improved. The little girl who was reluctant to speak during the first session, withdrawing entirely from any conversation about her anxiety, was now able to engage in appropriate talk about her fears, as well as her progress. She was distinctly proud of what she had accomplished, which was reinforced by her parents' own enthusiasm and pride. Beyond her reduction in anxiety surrounding separation, Julie was no longer seeking safety in the form of safe persons (Tom, Catherine, school nurse, best friend), places (parent's bedroom, staying home), and actions (constant reassurance, parental promises, repeated phone calls). Her FPI and WCE from the SAAS-C/P had diminished considerably, as well as concerns that her foods were "tainted" and subsequent spitting. In addition, Julie was no longer exhibiting oppositional behavior at home or at school, and the reports from her teachers reflected this dramatic change. These changes were evident in her posttreatment ECBI scores. Finally, Tom and Catherine were pleased with Julie's progress, but more importantly, they were relieved of the intense stress that was depleting the parent–child system. Both the PSI Total score and the Child Domain subscale were now within normal limits.

CONCLUSION

Comorbidity, developmental constraints, and heterogeneity of symptoms create challenges in diagnosing youth with anxiety and related disorders. For these reasons, investigators are beginning to recognize the importance of targeting symptom dimensions in the treatment of emotional disorders in youth (Chorpita, 2006; Eisen & Schaefer, 2005; Kearney, 2001). In this chapter, we have presented a conceptual framework that unifies anxiety disorders on the basis of core symptom dimensions and seeking safety behaviors. We presented an assessment tool that permits individualized case formulation and treatment planning. By utilizing an adapted and modified form of parent–child interaction therapy, we were able to successfully treat a young child who was exhibiting significant symptoms of separation and generalized anxieties, obsessive–compulsive symptoms, and oppositional behaviors.

REFERENCES

Abidin, R. R. (1995). *Parenting Stress Index: Professional manual*. Odessa, FL: Psychological Assessment Resources.

Abidin, R. R. (1997). PSI: A measure of the parent–child system. In C. P. Zalaquett & R. J. Wood (Eds.), *Evaluating stress* (pp. 277–291). London: Scarecrow Press.

Achenbach, T. M. (1991a). *Integrative Guide to the 1991 CBCL/4–18, YSR, and TRF profiles*. Burlington: University of Vermont, Department of Psychology.

Achenbach, T. M. (1991b). *Manual for the Child Behavior Checklist/4–18 and 1991 profile*. Burlington: University of Vermont, Department of Psychiatry.

Albano, A. M., Chorpita, B. F., & Barlow, D. H. (1996). Childhood anxiety disorders. In E. J. Mash & R. A. Barkley (Eds.), *Child psychopathology* (pp. 196–241). New York: Guilford Press.

Alessi, N. E., & Magen, J. (1988). Panic disorder in psychiatrically hospitalized children. *American Journal of Psychiatry, 145*, 1450–1452.

Alter-Reid, K., Gibbs, M. S., Lachenmeyer, J. R., Sigal, G., & Massoth, N. A. (1986). Sexual abuse of children: A review of the empirical findings. *Clinical Psychology Review, 6*, 249–266.

American Psychiatric Association (APA). (2000). *Diagnostic and statistical manual of mental disorders* (4th ed., text rev.). Washington, DC: Author.

Anderson, J. C., Williams, S., McGee, R., & Silva, P. A. (1987). DSM-III disorders in preadolescent children. *Archives of General Psychiatry, 44*, 69–76.

Aschenbrand, S. G., Kendall, P. C., Webb, A., Safford, S. M., & Flannery-Schroeder, E. (2003). Is childhood separation anxiety disorder a predictor of adult panic disorder and agoraphobia?: A seven-year longitudinal study. *Journal of the American Academy of Child and Adolescent Psychiatry, 42*(12), 1478–1485.

Barlow, D. H. (2002). *Anxiety and its disorders: The nature and treatment of anxiety and panic* (2nd ed.). New York: Guilford Press.

Barrett, P. M., Dadds, M. R., & Rapee, R. M. (1996). Family treatment of childhood anxiety: A controlled trial. *Journal of Consulting and Clinical Psychology, 64*(2), 333–342.

Bessmer, J. (1998). The Dyadic Parent–Child Coding System II (DPICS II): Reliability and validity. *Dissertation Abstracts International, 58*(7B), 3961. (UMI No. AAM9800066)

Biederman, J. (1987). Clonazepam in the treatment of prepubertal children with panic-like symptoms. *Journal of Clinical Psychiatry, 48,* 38–41.

Boggs, S. R., Eyberg, S. M., & Reynolds, L. A. (1990). Concurrent validity of the Eyberg Child Behavior Inventory. *Journal of Clinical Child Psychology, 19,* 75–78.

Brown, T. A., Chorpita, B. F., & Barlow, D. H. (1998). Structural relationships among dimensions of the DSM-IV anxiety and mood disorders, and dimensions of negative affect, positive affect, and autonomic arousal. *Journal of Abnormal Psychology, 107,* 179–192.

Burke, K. C., Burke, J. D., Regier, D. A., & Rae, D. S. (1990). Age at onset of selected mental disorders in five community populations. *Archives of General Psychiatry, 47,* 511–518.

Burns, G. L., & Patterson, D. R. (2001). Normative data on the Eyberg Child Behavior Inventory and Sutter–Eyberg Student behavior inventory: Parent and teacher rating scales of disruptive behavior problems in children and adolescents. *Child and Family Behavior Therapy, 23*(1), 15–28.

Choate, M. L., & Pincus, D. B. (2001). *The weekly record of anxiety at separation: A home monitoring measure for parents.* Unpublished assessment measure, Boston University Center for Anxiety and Related Disorders.

Chorpita, B. F. (2006). *Modular cognitive-behavior therapy for childhood anxiety disorders.* New York: Guilford Press.

Chorpita, B. F., Albano, A. M., & Barlow, D. H. (1998). Cognitive processing in children: Relation to anxiety and family influences. *Journal of Clinical Child Psychology, 25*(2), 170–176.

Chorpita, B. F., Tracey, S. A., Brown, T. A., Collica, T. J., & Barlow, D. H. (1997). Assessment of worry in children and adolescents: An adaptation of the Penn State Worry Questionnaire. *Behaviour Research and Therapy, 35,* 569–581.

Ciminero, A. R. (1986). Behavioral assessment: An overview. In A. R. Ciminero, K. S. Calhoun, & H. E. Adams (Eds.), *Handbook of behavioral assessment* (2nd ed., pp. 3–11). New York: Wiley.

Cohen, J. A., Berliner, L., & Mannarino, A. P. (2000). Treating traumatizing children: A research review and synthesis. *Trauma, Violence, and Abuse, 1,* 29–47.

Compton, S. N., Nelson, A. H., & March, J. S. (2000). Social phobia and separation anxiety symptoms in community and clinical samples of children and adolescents. *Journal of the American Academy of Child and Adolescent Psychiatry, 39,* 1040–1046.

Cooke-Cottone, C. (2004). Childhood posttraumatic stress disorder: Diagnosis, treatment, and school reintegration. *School Psychology Review, 33,* 127–139.

Costello, E. J., & Angold, A. (1995). Epidemiology. In J. S. March (Ed.), *Anxiety in children and adolescents* (pp. 109–124). New York: Guilford Press.

Craske, M. G. (1999). *Anxiety disorders: Psychological approaches to theory and treatment.* Boulder, CO: Westview Press.

Curry, J. F., March, J. S., & Hervey, A. S. (2004). Comorbidity of childhood and adolescent anxiety disorders. In T. H. Ollendick & J. S. March (Eds.), *Phobic and anxiety disorders in children and adolescents: A clinician's guide to effective psychosocial and pharmacological interventions* (pp. 116–140). New York: Oxford University Press.

Daughtery, T. K., & Shapiro, S. E. (1994). Behavior checklists and rating forms. In T. H. Ollendick, H. Thomas, N. J. King, & W. Yule (Eds.), *International handbook of phobic and anxiety disorders in children and adolescents: Issues in clinical child psychology*. New York: Plenum Press.

Deskin, M. M. (2005). The Dyadic Parent–Child Interaction Coding System (DPICS II): Reliability and validity with school aged children. *Dissertation Abstracts International: Section B, Sciences and Engineering, 66*(4-B), 2302.

Dubowitz, H., Black, M., Harrington, D., & Verschoore, A. (1993). A follow-up study of behavior problems associated with child sexual abuse. *Child Abuse and Neglect, 17*, 743–754.

Egger, H. L., Costello, E. J., Erkanli, A., & Angold, A. (1999). Somatic complaints and psychopathology in children and adolescents. *Journal of the American Academy of Child and Adolescent Psychiatry, 38*, 852–860.

Eisen, A. R., Brien, L. K., Bowers, J., & Studler, A. (2001). Separation anxiety disorder. In C. A. Essau & F. Petermann (Eds.), *Anxiety disorders in children and adolescents* (pp. 111–165). East Sussex, UK: Brunner-Routledge.

Eisen, A. R., & Engler, L. B. (2006). *Helping your child overcome separation anxiety or school refusal: A step-by-step guide for parents*. Oakland, CA: New Harbinger.

Eisen, A. R., & Kearney, C. A. (1995). *Practitioner's guide to treating fear and anxiety in children and adolescents: A cognitive-behavioral approach*. Northvale, NJ: Aronson.

Eisen, A. R., & Schaefer, C. E. (2005). *Separation anxiety in children and adolescents: An individualized approach to assessment and treatment*. New York: Guilford Press.

Eisen, A. R., & Silverman, W. K. (1993). Should I relax or change my thoughts?: A preliminary examination of cognitive therapy, relaxation training, and their combination with overanxious children. *Journal of Cognitive Psychotherapy: An International Quarterly, 7*, 265–279.

Eisen, A. R., & Silverman, W. K. (1998). Prescriptive treatment for generalized anxiety disorder in children. *Behavior Therapy, 29*, 105–121.

Eyberg, S. M., Bessmer, J., Newcomb, K., Edwards, D., & Robinson, E. A. (1994). Dyadic Parent–Child Interaction Coding System–II: A manual. *Social and Behavioral Sciences Documents* (ms. no. 2897).

Eyberg, S. M., & Pincus, D. B. (1999). *Eyberg Child Behavior Inventory and Sutter–Eyberg Student Behavior Inventory: Professional manual*. Odessa, FL: Psychological Assessment Resources.

Eyberg, S. M., & Robinson, E. A. (1982). Parent–child interaction training: Effects on family functioning. *Journal of Clinical Child Psychology, 11*, 130–137.

Eyberg, S. M., & Robinson, E. A. (1983). Conduct problem behavior: Standardization of a behavioral rating scale with adolescents. *Journal of Clinical Child Psychology, 12*(3), 347–354.

Fischer, D. J., Himle, J. A., & Thyer, B. A. (1999). Separation anxiety disorder. In R. T. Ammerman, M. Hersen, & C. G. Last (Eds.), *Handbook of prescriptive treatments for children and adolescents* (pp. 141–154). Boston: Allyn & Bacon.

Foote, R., Eyberg, S. M., & Schuhmann, E. (1998). Parent–child interaction approaches to the treatment of child behavior disorders. In T. H. Ollendick & R. J. Prinz (Eds.), *Advances in clinical child psychology* (pp. 125–151). New York: Plenum Press.

Friedberg, R. D., & McClure, J. M. (2002). *Clinical practice of cognitive therapy in children and adolescents: The nuts and bolts*. New York: Guilford Press.

Funderburk, B. W., Eyberg, S. M., Rich, B. A., & Behar, L. (2003). Further psychometric evaluation of the Eyberg and Behar rating scales for parents and teachers of preschoolers. *Early Education and Development, 14*(1), 67–81.

Garland, E. J., & Smith, D. H. (1991). Simultaneous prepubertal onset of panic disorder, night terrors, and somnambulism. *Journal of the American Academy of Child and Adolescent Psychiatry, 30,* 553–555.

Geller, D., Biederman, J., Griffin, S., Jones, J., & Lefkowitz, T. (1996). Comorbidity of juvenile obsessive–compulsive disorder in children and adolescents: Phenomenology and family history. *Journal of the American Academy of Child and Adolescent Psychiatry, 35,* 1637–1646.

Goodwin, R., Lipsitz, J. D., Chapman, T. F., Manuzza, S., & Fyer, A. J. (2001). Obsessive–compulsive disorder and separation anxiety comorbidity in early onset panic disorder. *Psychological Medicine, 31,* 1307–1310.

Hahn, L., Hajinlian, J., Eisen, A. R., Winder, B., & Pincus, D. B. (2003, November). Measuring the dimensions of separation anxiety and early panic in children and adolescents: The Separation Anxiety Assessment Scale. In A. R. Eisen (Chair), *Recent Advances in the Treatment of Separation Anxiety and Panic in Children and Adolescents.* Paper Presented at the 37th annual convention of the Association for the Advancement of Behavior Therapy, Boston, MA.

Hajinlian, J., Hahn, L. G., Eisen, A. R., Zilli-Richardson, L., Reddy, L. A., Winder, B., et al. (2003, November). *The phenomenon of separation anxiety across DSM-IV internalizing and externalizing disorders.* Poster session presented at the 37th annual convention of the Association for the Advancement of Behavior Therapy, Boston, MA.

Hajinlian, J., Mesnik, J., & Eisen, A. R. (2005, November). *Separation anxiety symptom dimensions and DSM-IV anxiety disorders: Correlates, comorbidity, and clinical utility.* Poster presented at the 39th annual convention of the Association for Behavioral and Cognitive Therapies, Washington, DC.

Hanna, G. (1995). Demographic and clinical features of obsessive–compulsive disorder in children and adolescents. *Journal of the American Academy of Child and Adolescent Psychiatry, 34,* 19–27.

Hartmann, D. P., & Wood, D. D. (1990). Observational methods. In A. S. Bellack, M. Hersen, & A. E. Kazdin (Eds.), *International handbook of behavior modification and therapy* (2nd ed., pp. 107–139). New York: Pergamon Press.

Hashim, R., Alex, B., & Eisen, A. R. (2006, November). *Separation anxiety symptom dimensions as predictors of poor peer relations in older children and adolescents.* Poster presented at the 40th annual convention of the Association for the Advancement of Behavioral and Cognitive Therapies, Chicago, IL.

Hudson, J. L., & Rapee, R. M. (2001). Parent–child interactions with anxiety disorders: An observational study. *Behaviour Research and Therapy, 39,* 1411–1427.

Johnson, K. (1998). *Trauma in the lives of children: Crisis and stress management for counselors, teachers, and other professionals.* Alameda, CA: Hunter House.

Kearney, C. A. (2001). *School refusal in youth: A functional approach to assessment and treatment.* Washington, DC: American Psychological Association.

Kearney, C. A., Albano, A. M., Eisen, A. R., Allen, W. D., & Barlow, D. H. (1997). The phenomenology of panic disorder in youngsters: An empirical study of a clinical sample. *Journal of Anxiety Disorders, 11,* 49–62.

Kearney, C. A., & Allan, W. D. (1995). Panic disorder with or without agoraphobia. In A. R. Eisen, C. A. Kearney, & C. E. Schaefer (Eds.), *Clinical handbook of anxiety disorders in children and adolescents* (pp. 251–281). Northvale, NJ: Aronson.

Kearney, C. A., & Silverman, W. K. (1992). Let's not push the panic button: A critical analysis of panic and panic disorder in adolescents. *Clinical Psychology Review*, 12, 293–305.

Keller, M. B., Lavori, P. W., Wunder, J., Beardslee, W. R., Schwartz, C. E., & Roth, J. (1992). Chronic course of anxiety disorders in children and adolescents. *Journal of the American Academy of Child and Adolescent Psychiatry*, 31(4), 595–599.

Kendall, P. C., Brady, E. U., & Verduin, T. L. (2001). Comorbidity in childhood anxiety disorders and treatment outcome. *Journal of the American Academy of Child and Adolescent Psychiatry*, 40, 787–794.

Kilpatrick, D. G., Saunders, B. E., Resnick, H. S., & Smith, D. W. (1995). *The National Survey of Adolescents: Preliminary findings on lifetime prevalence of traumatic events and mental health correlates*. Charleston: Medical University of South Carolina, National Crime Victims Research and Treatment Center.

King, N. J., Ollendick, T. H., & Mattis, S. G. (1994). Panic in children and adolescents: Normative and clinical studies. *Australian Psychologist*, 29, 89–93.

King, R. A., Leonard, H., & March, J. S. (1998). Practice parameters for the assessment and treatment of children and adolescents with obsessive–compulsive disorder [Special Issue: Practice parameters]. *Journal of the American Academy of Child and Adolescent Psychiatry*, 37(Suppl. 10), 27S–45S.

Kiser, L. J., Heston, J., Millsap, P. A., & Pruitt, D. B. (1991). Physical and sexual abuse in childhood: Relationship with post-traumatic stress disorder. *Journal of the American Academy of Child and Adolescent Psychiatry*, 30, 776–783.

Knox, L. S., Albano, A. M., & Barlow, D. H. (1996). Parental involvement in the treatment of childhood obsessive–compulsive disorder: A multiple-baseline examination incorporating parents. *Behavior Therapy*, 27, 93–115.

Last, C. G. (1991). Somatic complaints in anxiety disordered children. *Journal of Anxiety Disorders*, 5, 125–138.

Last, C. G., & Strauss, C. C. (1989). Panic disorder in children and adolescents. *Journal of Anxiety Disorders*, 3, 87–95.

Lowe, L. A. (1998). Using the Child Behavior Checklist in assessing conduct disorder: Issues of reliability and validity [Special Issue: Assessment and treatment of youth and families]. *Research on Social Work Practice*, 8(3), 286–301.

March, J. S., Conners, C., Arnold, G., Epstein, J., Parker, J., Hinshaw, S., et al. (1999). The Multidimensional Anxiety Scale for Children (MASC): Confirmatory factor analysis in a pediatric ADHD sample. *Journal of Attention Disorders*, 3(2), 85–89.

March, J. S., & Mulle, K. (1998). *OCD in children and adolescents: A cognitive-behavioral treatment manual*. New York: Guilford Press.

March, J. S., Parker, J., Sullivan, K., Stallings, P., & Conners, C. K. (1997). The Multidimensional Anxiety Scale for Children (MASC): Factor structure, reliability, and validity. *Journal of the American Academy of Child and Adolescent Psychiatry*, 36(4), 554–565.

Masi, G., Favilla, L., Mucci, M., & Millepiedi, S. (2000). Panic disorder in clinically referred children and adolescents. *Child Psychiatry and Human Development*, 31, 139–151.

McMahon, R. J., & Estes, A. M. (1997). Conduct problems. In E. J. Mash & L. G. Terdal (Eds.), *Assessment of childhood disorders* (3rd ed., pp. 130–195). New York: Guilford Press.

McMahon, R. J., & Forehand, R. (1988). Conduct disorders. In E. J. Mash & L. G.

Terdal (Eds.), *Behavioral assessment of childhood disorders* (2nd ed., pp. 105–153). New York: Guilford Press.

Mesnik, J., Hajinlian, J., & Eisen, A. R. (2005, November). *Cautious partners: Safety signals and parental overprotection in children with separation anxiety and OCD.* Paper presented at the 39th annual convention of the Association for Behavioral and Cognitive Therapies, Washington, DC.

Moreau, D. L., Weissman, M., & Warner, V. (1989). Panic disorder in children at high risk for depression. *American Journal of Psychiatry, 146,* 1059–1060.

Muris, P., Merkelbach, H., Gadet, B., & Moulaert, V. (2000). Fears, worries, and scary dreams in 4 to 12 year-old children: Their content, developmental pattern, and origins. *Journal of Clinical Child Psychology, 29,* 43–52.

Nelles, W. B., & Barlow, D. H. (1988). Do children panic? *Clinical Psychology Review, 8,* 359–372.

Ollendick, T. H. (1983). Reliability and validity of the Revised Fear Survey Schedule for Children (FSSC-R). *Behaviour Research and Therapy, 21*(6), 685–692.

Ollendick, T. H. (1998). Panic disorder in children and adolescents: New developments, new directions. *Journal of Clinical Child Psychology, 27,* 234–245.

Ollendick, T. H., Mattis, S. G., & King, N. J. (1994). Panic in children and adolescents: A review. *Journal of Child Psychology and Psychiatry, and Allied Disciplines, 35,* 113–134.

Pelcovitz, D., Kaplan, S. J., DeRosa, R. R., Mandel, F. S., & Salzinger, S. (2000). Psychiatric disorders in adolescents exposed to violence and physical abuse. *American Journal of Orthopsychiatry, 70,* 360–369.

Piacentini, J., & Graae, F. (1997). Childhood OCD. In E. Hollander & D. Stein (Eds.), *Obsessive–compulsive disorder: Diagnosis, etiology, and treatment* (pp. 23–46). New York: Marcel Dekker.

Pincus, D. B., Cheron, D. M., Santucci, L. S., & Eyberg, S. M. (2006). *Dyadic Parent–Child Interaction Coding System–II: Modifications for use with separation-anxious children.* Unpublished manuscript, Boston University Center for Anxiety and Related Disorders.

Pincus, D. B., Eyberg, S. M., Choate, M. L., & Barlow, D. H. (2005). Adapting parent–child interaction therapy for young children with separation anxiety disorder. *Education and Treatment of Children, 28*(2), 163–181.

Pullis, M. (1998). Exposure to traumatic violence: Some lessons from Bosnia. *Education and Treatment of Children, 21,* 396–412.

Rabian, B., Peterson, R. A., Richters, J., & Jensen, P. S. (1993). Anxiety sensitivity among anxious children. *Journal of Clinical Child Psychology, 22,* 441–446.

Reiss, S., Silverman, W. K., & Weems, C. F. (2001). Anxiety sensitivity. In M. W. Vasey & M. R. Dadds (Eds.), *The developmental psychopathology of anxiety* (pp. 92–111). New York: Oxford University Press.

Reitman, D., Currier, R. O., & Stickle, T. (2002). A critical evaluation of the Parenting Stress Index—Short Form (PSI/SF) in a Head Start population. *Journal of Clinical Child and Adolescent Psychology, 31,* 384–392.

Reynolds, C. R., & Richmond, B. O. (1978). What I Think and Feel: A revised measure of children's manifest anxiety. *Journal of Abnormal Child Psychology, 6*(2), 271–280.

Rich, B. A., & Eyberg, S. M. (2001). Accuracy of assessment: The discriminative and predictive power of the Eyberg Child Behavior Inventory. *Ambulatory Child Health, 7,* 249–257.

Saigh, P. (1998). *Children's PTSD Inventory (DSM-IV version)*. New York: Department of Psychology, City University of New York.

Scahill, L., Riddle, M. A., McSwiggin-Hardin, M., Ort, S. I., King, R. A., Goodman, W. K., et al. (1997). Children's Yale–Brown Obsessive–Compulsive Scale: Reliability and validity. *Journal of the American Academy of Child and Adolescent Psychiatry, 36*, 844–852.

Seligman, L. D., Ollendick, T. H., Langley, A. K., & Baldacci, H. B. (2004). The utility of measures of child and adolescent anxiety: A meta-analytic review of the Revised Children's Anxiety Scale, the State–Trait Anxiety Inventory for Children, and the Child Behavior Checklist. *Journal of Clinical Child and Adolescent Psychology, 33*(3), 557–565.

Silove, D., Harris, M., Morgan, A., Boyce, P., Manicavasagar, V., Hadzi-Pavlovic, D., et al. (1995). Is early separation anxiety a specific precursor of panic disorder-agoraphobia?: A community study. *Psychological Medicine, 25*, 405–411.

Silove, D., & Manicavasagar, V. (1993). Adults who feared school: Is early separation anxiety specific to the pathogenesis of panic disorder? *Acta Psychiatrica Scandinavica, 88*, 385–390.

Silverman, W. K., & Albano, A. M. (1996). *The Anxiety Disorders Interview Schedule for DSM-IV—Child and Parent Versions*. San Antonio, TX: Psychological Corporation.

Silverman, W. K., & Eisen, A. R. (1992). Age differences in the reliability of parent and child reports of child anxious symptomatology using a structured interview. *Journal of the American Academy of Child and Adolescent Psychiatry, 31*, 117–124.

Silverman, W. K., Fleisig, W., Rabian, B., & Peterson, R. A. (1991). Childhood Anxiety Sensitivity Index. *Journal of Clinical Child Psychology, 20*, 162–168.

Silverman, W. K., La Greca, A. M., & Wasserstein, S. (1995). What do children worry about?: Worries and their relation to anxiety. *Child Development, 66*(3), 671–686.

Silverman, W. K., & Nelles, W. B. (1988). The Anxiety Disorders Interview Schedule for Children. *Journal of the American Academy of Child and Adolescent Psychiatry, 27*(6), 772–778.

Silverman, W. K., Saavedra, L. M., & Pina, A. A. (2001). Test–retest reliability of anxiety symptoms and diagnoses with the Anxiety Disorders Interview Schedule for DSM–IV: Child and Parent Versions. *Journal of the American Academy of Child and Adolescent Psychiatry, 40*, 937–944.

Spielberger, C. D., Gorsuch, R. L., & Luchene, R. E. (1970). *State–Trait Anxiety Inventory*. Palo Alto, CA: Consulting Psychology Press.

Swedo, S. E., Rapoport, J. L., Leonard, H., Lenane, M., & Cheslow, D. (1989). Obsessive–compulsive disorder in children and adolescents: Clinical phenomenology of 70 consecutive cases. *Archives of General Psychiatry, 46*, 335–341.

Terr, L. C., Bloch, D. A., Michel, B. A., Hong, S., Reinhardt, J. A., & Metayer, S. (1999). Children's symptoms in the wake of Challenger: A field study of distant-traumatic effects and an outline of related conditions. *American Journal of Psychiatry, 156*, 1536–1544.

Tufts New England Medical Center, Division of Child and Adolescent Psychiatry. (1984). *Sexually exploited children: Service and research project* [Final report for the Office of Juvenile Justice and Delinquency Prevention]. Washington, DC: U.S. Department of Justice.

Valleni-Basile, L., Garrison, C., Jackson, K., Waller, J., McKeown, R., Addy, C., et al. (1994). Frequency of obsessive–compulsive disorder in a community sample of young adolescents. *Journal of the American Academy of Child and Adolescent Psychiatry, 33*, 782–791.

Verduin, T. L., & Kendall, P. C. (2003). Differential occurrence of comorbidity within childhood anxiety disorders. *Journal of Clinical Child and Adolescent Psychology, 32*, 290–295.

Vitiello, B., Behar, D., Wolfson, S., & McLeer, S. U. (1990). Diagnosis of panic disorder in prepubertal children. *Journal of the American Academy of Child and Adolescent Psychiatry, 29*, 782–784.

Webb, N. B. (1994). School-based assessment and crisis intervention with kindergarten children following the New York World Trade Center bombing. *Crisis Interventions, 1*, 47–59.

Weems, C. F., Silverman, W. K., & LaGreca, A. M. (2000). What do youth referred for anxiety problems worry about?: Worry and its relation to anxiety and anxiety disorders in children and adolescents. *Journal of Abnormal Child Psychology, 28*(1), 63–72.

Westenberg, P. M., Siebelink, B. M., Warmenhoven, N. J. C., & Treffers, P. D. A. (1999). Separation anxiety and overanxious disorders: Relations to age and level of psychosocial maturity. *Journal of the American Academy of Child and Adolescent Psychiatry, 38*(8), 1000–1007.

Wittchen, H. U., Reed, V., & Kessler, R. C. (1998). The relationship of agoraphobia and panic in a community sample of adolescents and young adults. *Archives of General Psychiatry, 55*(11), 1017–1024.

Wood, J. J., Piacentini, J. C., Bergman, R. L., McCracken, J., & Barrios, V. (2002). Concurrent validity of the anxiety disorders section of the Anxiety Disorders Interview Schedule for DSM–IV: Child and Parent Versions. *Journal of Clinical Child and Adolescent Psychology, 31*(3), 335–342.

Yule, W. (2001). Posttraumatic stress disorder in the general population and in children. *Journal of Clinical Psychiatry, 62*, 23–28.

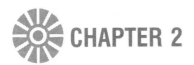 CHAPTER 2

Social Anxiety

Jennifer L. Hudson, Heidi J. Lyneham,
and Ronald M. Rapee

Shyness is a common phenomenon and may be present in as much as 40 to 50% of the population (Henderson & Zimbardo, 2001). In children, being shy per se is not viewed as problematic. In fact, in the eyes of some parents and teachers, shyness in the form of kindness, compliance, or respect, is most desirable. Social anxiety is often equated with shyness. As such, the necessity for intervention can easily be overlooked. It doesn't help that the dimensions of social anxiety are largely cognitive. We take for granted routine tasks such as starting a conversation or asking for help. But for the socially anxious child, the mental anguish associated with these acts can be overwhelming. Social anxiety (and social phobia) can lead to serious disruptions in a child's or adolescent's social, emotional, and/or academic functioning, and have lifelong implications. In this chapter, the authors of the "Cool Kids" program, one of the most powerful cognitive-behavioral treatments available, show us through the case of "Hailey" how to manage effectively the many dimensions of social anxiety and related problems.—A. R. E.

INTRODUCTION

Issues concerning clinical presentations of social anxiety in children are the focus of this chapter. First, we provide a description and theoretical discussion of the nature of social anxiety, identifying diagnostic presentations and frequent comorbid conditions. A comprehensive description of the assessment and treatment of social anxiety is provided, outlining current tools and techniques. Descriptions are accompanied by case material from a typical yet complex presentation. Finally, we provide step-by-step guidelines for the assessment, case formulation, and treatment of the aforementioned case.

Nature of Symptom Dimensions

The dimension of social anxiety is often also referred to under a variety of related labels, including shyness, embarrassability, heterosocial anxiety, performance anxiety, or dating fear. Some terms, such as "dating fear" or "performance anxiety" refer to a more limited dimension, highlighting a specific aspect of social anxiety, whereas other terms, most notably "shyness," are often used interchangeably with social anxiety. Despite the breadth of labels, social anxiety is probably one of the most easily identified and defined dimensions of human personality, as exemplified by the large number of measures of it and related constructs, all of which cover essentially similar descriptors.

Theoretically, most researchers in the field would agree that social anxiety lies along a dimension or continuum (Briggs, 1988; Chavira, Stein, & Malcarne, 2002; Rapee & Spence, 2004). The dimension is expected to be relatively normally distributed throughout the population, with few individuals lying at the very highest and lowest extremes. In terms of life interference and subsequent help seeking, generally the higher ends of the continuum are associated with the concept of disorder, largely due to the personal distress associated with these behaviors.

Descriptively, social anxiety refers to social fear and distress in response to social cues, especially characterized by self-consciousness and expectations of negative evaluation. As with all forms of anxiety, it is characterized by symptoms in four areas. Emotionally, people with high levels of social anxiety are easily embarrassed and experience intense discomfort and distress when placed in situations where they may be the focus of attention or evaluation. Physiologically, high levels of social anxiety are associated with many symptoms of autonomic arousal. Of greatest relevance are the highly visible symptoms, including blushing, shaking, sweating, or muscular "freezing" (Beidel, Turner, & Dancu, 1985). Probably of greatest salience are the behavioral features, which include social withdrawal and avoidance of situations involving other people, and the potential for observation and evaluation. People with high levels of social anxiety tend to avoid meeting and interacting with others, are reticent to perform in front of other people (e.g., public speaking, sports, working, or eating in front of others), and frequently appear awkward or diffident with others due to what has been referred to as "subtle avoidance behaviors" (Rapee & Heimberg, 1997) such as withholding opinions, averting their gaze, or minimizing interactions.

Finally, some authors have argued that the defining features of social anxiety are cognitive. People with high social anxiety levels report frequent beliefs that others are evaluating them negatively and will judge them to be less than competent, unfriendly, unattractive, or unintelligent. They also tend to judge themselves as poor in socially important features, including social performance, attractiveness, and personal traits (Rapee & Abbott, 2006; Wallace & Alden, 1991; Wilson & Rapee, 2006). In fact, most of this research has shown that the self-perceptions of adults with high levels of social anxiety are considerably more negative than the perceptions of others. However, as yet, these findings have not generally been extended to child-hood. High levels of social anxiety are also characterized by a strong sense of self-consciousness. Socially anxious individuals commonly describe an obser-vational self-focus and a shift in their attentional resources toward themselves, often to the detriment of task-focused performance (Bogels & Lamers, 2002; Buss, 1980; Hackmann, Surawy, & Clark, 1998).

Developmental Course

Social anxiety is one of the few dimensions that has been shown to occur rela-tively consistently across the lifespan. Levels of the core social concern appear to be experienced consistently from at least 6 years of age into late adoles-cence (Campbell & Rapee, 1994). In later years, social threat concerns remain consistent across most of the adult years, declining only to some extent in later adulthood (Lovibond & Rapee, 1993). In the earliest stages of development, social fears have been identified as one of the core dimensions of tempera-ment.

In the influential classification by Thomas and Chess (1977), a tempera-ment labeled "approach" was one of their nine core dimensions and referred to the extent to which a child would approach or withdraw from novel situa-tions, most of which were social in nature. A similar dimension of sociability has been empirically demonstrated by other researchers (Buss & Plomin, 1984; Prior, 1992). For example, Sanson, Pedlow, Cann, Prior, and Oberklaid (1996) identified a temperament dimension that they labeled "approach" or "shyness" in children as young as 4 months of age, and demonstrated that the construct could be reliably identified and remained moderately stable from at least 1 year of age. A wealth of research has also focused on a closely related construct of social withdrawal (Rubin & Asendorpf, 1993). Withdrawal is generally described behaviorally and refers purely to a tendency for children to fail to engage with other children.

Subsequent research has shown that socially withdrawn behavior may be motivated by several characteristics, with perhaps the most common being shyness and social fearfulness (Asendorpf, 1990; Harrist, Zaia, Bates, Dodge, & Pettit, 1997; Kim, Rapee, Oh, & Moon, 2007). One of the most influential descriptors of temperament of relevance to clinical issues has been the con-struct of behavioral inhibition (Kagan, Reznick, Clarke, Snidman, & Garcia-Coll, 1984). Whereas behavioral inhibition most likely refers to a somewhat broader dimension than pure social anxiety, its assessment is generally heavily loaded with social withdrawal and shyness-related measures. Hence, its operationalization is closely akin to social anxiety.

Kagan and colleagues have generally measured behavioral inhibition in children as young as 21 months through observation of withdrawn and anx-ious behaviors when confronted by strange adults and same-age peers (Kagan,

Reznick, & Snidman, 1987). In our own research with preschool children, we have also assessed the dimension of behavioral inhibition during interactions with peers and strange adults (Rapee, Kennedy, Ingram, Edwards, & Sweeney, 2005). The behaviors that most strongly differentiate between children rated high and low on the dimension include approaches to peers, approaches to strangers, and amount of talking (Rapee, 2002). The close relationship with social anxiety is obvious.

Thus, from a developmental perspective, one can see social anxiety emerging from a very early age. Clearly, assessment of the construct at these early stages is based heavily on observation of behaviors. As children develop, the construct itself is unlikely to be very different; however, assessment (hence, definition) begins to include more subjective and cognitive elements. From middle childhood, measures of social anxiety begin to include subjective descriptions of distress, as well as descriptors of negative thoughts. The constructs of fear of negative evaluation, self-denigration, and self-consciousness become more heavily emphasized (Beidel, Turner, & Morris, 1995; La Greca, Dandes, Wick, Shaw, & Stone, 1988; Spence, 1997). Negative social beliefs, especially fears of negative evaluation, have been shown to form a strong and clear factor that is independent of other dimensions of children's negative beliefs, even in very young children (Schniering & Rapee, 2002; Spence, Rapee, McDonald, & Ingram, 2001).

As described earlier, the fundamental dimension of social anxiety does not change greatly with age. Hence, social threat concerns have been shown to remain at a relatively steady level across middle childhood and adolescence (Bruch & Cheek, 1995; Campbell & Rapee, 1994). Similarly, social threat beliefs have also been shown to change little across middle childhood to adolescence (Schniering & Rapee, 2002). Interestingly, however, associated diagnostic entities do appear to change across this period of development. Diagnosis of the related disorder of social phobia increases in adolescence, based on retrospective reports, with the mean age of onset of social phobia in early to midadolescence (Otto et al., 2001). Prevalence data for social phobia also indicate that this disorder is more common in adolescence than in childhood (Cohen, Cohen, & Brook, 1993; Strauss & Last, 1993).

Similarly, the prevalence of major depression increases dramatically following puberty, especially in girls (Hankin, Abramson, Silva, McGee, & Moffitt, 1998). How does one reconcile these apparently discrepant findings? The answer very likely lies in the life interference and personal distress afforded by social anxiety (Rapee & Spence, 2004). For instance, Rapee and Spence have argued that definition of a disorder requires both person-based features (i.e., symptoms) and some level of interference in the individual's life (see also Chavira et al., 2002). It is certainly possible for an individual with a very high level of social anxiety to become extremely successful, to build a solid social niche, and to be perfectly satisfied with his or her life. Such an individual would not be considered to have a disorder such as social phobia, despite perhaps showing many of the symptoms of people with social phobia. According to Rapee and Spence (2004), life interference due to social anxiety is not only strongly related to severity of the symptoms but is also influenced by several other factors, including the person's age, sex, and cultural background. Thus, it is likely that the dramatic increase in diagnosis of disorders such as social phobia and depression during adolescence may be influenced by a marked increase in life interference caused by social anxiety during this stage of development.

Almost by definition, many life experiences that become especially important during adolescence are affected by social anxiety. During adolescence, a marked increase in the importance of peers is accompanied by a decrease in influence and dependence on parents (Furman & Buhrmester, 1992). Children who are socially anxious frequently have difficulty making friends and are known to have a smaller number of friends than their more confident counterparts (Greco & Morris, 2005; La Greca & Moore, 2005). Hence, high levels of social anxiety are likely to limit opportunities for peer relationships and subsequent peer acceptance and influence. Around this same period, romantic and sexual relationships become paramount (La Greca & Prinstein, 1999). Social anxiety is known to interfere with romantic interactions, and studies have shown that socially anxious individuals have fewer romantic relationships, are more likely to marry their first partner, and are less likely to have a regular partner (Caspi, Elder, & Bem, 1988).

Finally, entry into adolescence and high school usually signals an increase in expectations and demands for good performance and future career aspirations. People with high levels of social anxiety have been shown to have more limited career choices and aspirations (Phillips & Bruch, 1988), which in turn likely result in marked distress and interference.

Relationship to Specific Disorders

As described earlier, the dimension of social anxiety in itself is not necessarily diagnostic. However, when combined with life interference and/or significant personal distress, it may be associated with several diagnostic entities. Hence, social anxiety, one of the core fundamental features of anxiety, is likely to be found in people with a wide variety of mental disorders. However, the most closely related conditions include social phobia, selective mutism, generalized anxiety disorder, eating disorders, and major depressive disorder and dysthymia. Each is described briefly below, with a focus on the links with social anxiety.

Social Phobia

"Social phobia," a fear of situations in which one might potentially be scrutinized, is characterized by a strong fear of negative evaluation, and subsequent fear and avoidance of social situations. Hence, the similarity and overlap with the dimension of social anxiety are obvious, and this disorder may be thought of as an essentially pure, high level of social anxiety, as indicated by the somewhat newer term "social anxiety disorder." Some of the most common situations that young people avoid include public speaking, dating, speaking up in groups, answering questions in class, and meeting new children. As described earlier, social phobia may be diagnosed at any age, but it becomes somewhat more common during midadolescence (Cohen et al., 1993). There is evidence for continuity across the lifespan, with social phobia being one of the more stable anxiety disorders (Pine, Cohen, Gurley, Brook, & Ma, 1998; Yonkers, Dyck, & Keller, 2001) and providing a significant risk for later anxiety and depressive disorders (Pine et al., 1998; Stein et al., 2001).

Selective Mutism

Although it is a distinct diagnosis in DSM-IV (American Psychiatric Association, 1994), several authors have argued that selective mutism is better conceptualized as a form of social phobia (Black, 1996). Its characteristic feature is the reduction, and in many cases, total absence of verbal interactions with select, other people. Selectively mute children most commonly interact perfectly with close family but usually do not speak to anyone outside of their comfort area. Typically, this involves a lack of verbal interaction at school and outside the home, with teachers, peers, and unfamiliar others (Black, 1996; Cunningham, McHolm, Boyle, & Patel, 2004). Selective mutism may begin very early but is typically not noticed or considered problematic until the child reaches school age. In most cases selective mutism decreases with age and is less common in older childhood and into adolescence than earlier in life.

Generalized Anxiety Disorder

Above-average levels of social anxiety are associated with most anxiety disorders. However, aside from social phobia, social anxiety is most closely associated with generalized anxiety disorder, which is characterized by chronic worry over a variety of life areas. Typical areas of worry in children include relationships, sports and exam performance, health, and miscellaneous worries (Rapee, Wignall, Hudson, & Schniering, 2000). Children with generalized anxiety disorder are often perfectionistic, expressing great concern at making mistakes, and often seek extensive reassurance over the most seemingly trivial of matters. As can be seen, many of these concerns have a strong social orientation; hence, social anxiety may be a core feature of many children with generalized anxiety. Like social phobia, generalized anxiety disorder may be diagnosed at any age, but it becomes somewhat more common in adolescence (Strauss, Lease, Last, & Francis, 1988).

Eating Disorders

The disorders anorexia nervosa and bulimia nervosa are characterized by a clear focus on body weight and ways of limiting weight gain. Whereas people with anorexia religiously limit their caloric intake, thereby dangerously reducing their body fat, those with bulimia typically lose control and engage in dramatic binges (excessive intake of calories). They then try to compensate for these losses of control in various ways, most commonly through vomiting, use of diuretics, or excessive exercise. Eating disorders are characterized by a close connection between perceived body shape and size, and one's sense of self-worth (Fairburn, Shafran, & Cooper, 1999). It is not uncommon for people with eating disorders to have a low sense of self-worth and to believe that control of their weight is vital to positive evaluation by the self and others (Fairburn et al., 1999). Thus, a high level of social anxiety is a common concomitant of eating disorders. The disorders are rare in childhood and increase in frequency in early adolescence (Hoek & van Hoeken, 2003). There is a clear gender imbalance, with a female:male ratio of around 10:1 (Hoek & van Hoeken, 2003).

Major Depressive Disorder

Major depressive disorder is characterized by a lengthy (at least 2 weeks) period of negative mood—either sad and depressed, or increasingly irritable mood. Associated features include weight and sleep changes, loss of interest, low self-worth, and suicidal thoughts and actions. Major depressive disorder is relatively infrequent in childhood, but its prevalence increases dramatically from around age 14 years (Hankin et al., 1998), especially due to a marked increase in the prevalence of depressive episodes in girls this age and older. Depressive episodes tend to be episodic in nature, although episodes can last for some years. However, it is commonly believed that children who are more vulnerable to episodes of major depression are characterized by features such as poor self-concept, doubts about their abilities, social withdrawal, and negative explanatory styles (Garber, 2005; Jaenicke et al., 1987; Kaslow, Rehm, & Siegel, 1984). Furthermore, the related disorder, dysthymia, is a far more chronic condition that shows many of these features. Hence, the common links with social anxiety are apparent, and depressed children have been shown to score high on measures of social anxiety (Schniering & Rapee, 2002). In addition, socially anxious adolescents are at markedly increased risk of developing a major depressive episode at a later time point (Stein et al., 2001).

Comorbidity and Differential Diagnosis

In the previous section we described several diagnostic categories that share a common link with social anxiety. For some, social anxiety may be considered to lie at the core of the disorder, whereas for others, social anxiety forms one central aspect of it. Nevertheless, this common link means that comorbidity and overlap between the disorders is likely to be high, and indeed it is. The following section briefly describes some of the comorbidity between these disorders and points to some of the defining features. In each case, however, the fact that social anxiety forms such a central aspect of the disorder means that management of social anxiety, as we describe later in this chapter, should be a major component of any treatment package for the presenting disorder.

Social Phobia and Selective Mutism

As described earlier, many authors argue that selective mutism can be conceptualized as a form of social phobia (Black, 1996). In one study, 29 out of 30 children with selective mutism also met criteria for either social phobia or avoidant disorder of childhood (Black & Uhde, 1995). Distinguishing between the two disorders in classic cases is not overly difficult, because most selectively mute children are characterized by the far more specific feature of complete lack of verbal interaction with others. However, marked overlap often occurs, with many children showing both a reticence to speak in several situations and many other features of a high level of social anxiety. Nevertheless, from a clinical perspective, a clear distinction is probably not important, because treatment programs for selective mutism and social anxiety are extremely similar (cf. McHolm, Cunningham, & Vanier, 2005; Rapee, Spence, Cobham, & Wignall, 2000).

Social Phobia and Depression

As expected, overlap between these disorders (as between all anxiety disorders and depression) is high (Brady & Kendall, 1992; Lewinsohn, Zinbarg, Seeley, Lewinsohn, & Sack, 1997). Research has shown that up to 55% of adolescents with social phobia meet criteria for major depression, whereas around 20% of adolescents with major depression meet criteria for social phobia (Last, Strauss, & Francis, 1987). Nevertheless, distinguishing between a child with a severe major depressive episode and one with social phobia is not usually too difficult, because the depressive episode represents a marked change from usual functioning and is often accompanied by many clear indications, such as suicidal beliefs, sleep and weight changes, or extreme loss of interest. However, distinction between social phobia and dysthymia, or even low-level, chronic major depression, can be difficult. As mentioned earlier, the large number of shared characteristics means that technical distinction between the disorders is not usually very important in the clinical setting.

Most treatment programs for social phobia and depression share several central features. Where treatment needs to be modified is in cases of low motivation and loss of interest. It is these characteristics of depression that require slightly modified intervention; hence, these are the features that require particular assessment. Similarly, suicide attempts and self-harm behaviors, which are clear features of depression, require specialized intervention; hence, they need to be a particular focus of assessment.

Social Phobia and Generalized Anxiety Disorder

There is marked comorbidity between all of the anxiety disorders, with estimates suggesting that between 20 and 60% of children with one anxiety disorder meet criteria for another (Last et al., 1987; Lewinsohn et al., 1997). Hence, social phobia and generalized anxiety disorder show marked overlap—up to 40% (Last et al., 1987). Diagnostically, whereas social phobia is characterized by a specific fear of social situations, broader concerns across both the social and physical domains characterize generalized anxiety. Thus, distinguishing between classic cases is not difficult. However, because of considerable variation, the most appropriate diagnosis is in many cases almost arbitrary. Clinically, this is irrelevant, because most current treatment programs for childhood anxiety are generic across all of the major anxiety disorders (Barrett, Dadds, & Rapee, 1996; Kendall et al., 1997; Rapee, 2000).

Generalized Anxiety Disorder and Depression

The presenting profiles of people with generalized anxiety and mood disorders, particularly dysthymia, may be very similar. Symptoms such as fatigue, insomnia, weight loss, helplessness, and fearfulness are found with similar frequency in both disorders (Riskind, Hohmann, Beck, & Stewart, 1991). As mentioned earlier, treatment of many of the features of anxiety and mood disorders is very similar; hence, distinguishing between individuals with generalized anxiety and depression is less important clinically. However, again, key features related to motivational aspects and self-harm require more specialized attention and more careful assessment.

Eating Disorders and Depression

Comorbidity between eating disorders and depression is common, with up to 75% of people with bulimia reporting a lifetime history of depression (Hinz & Williamson, 1987). In classic cases, distinguishing between these disorders is not especially difficult. Anorexia, in particular, is characterized by extreme weight loss; bulimia, by clear bingeing and purging cycles; and major depression, by extreme loss of interest, loss of energy, and suicidal thoughts. However, in some cases, especially where the presenting complaint is more physical (e.g., weight loss and low energy), it may be difficult to determine which diagnosis is most appropriate. A focus on the underlying motivation behind the symptoms may help to indicate the best diagnosis. Whereas weight loss in eating disorders is typically motivated by an intention to diet to lose weight and build self-esteem, the same symptom in depression is more likely to be a concomitant of loss of interest and pleasure in eating.

CASE FORMULATION: CONCEPTUAL MODEL OF ASSESSMENT AND TREATMENT

Case Presentation

Hailey and her parents presented to the clinic following a recommendation from Hailey's teacher, who was concerned about her adjustment to a new school. The main concerns identified were Hailey's lack of friendships, inability to speak in the classroom, and the distress she experienced during activities involving performance or sports. Her teacher reported that Hailey never volunteered to speak in class, but that she did give brief, quietly spoken answers if asked a direct question. Hailey appeared very withdrawn at times, spending her breaks either in the school library or reading on her own in the playground. Although Hailey excelled academically, her parents reported that she experienced a lot of distress before tests and spent a lot of time making sure that her work was presented perfectly. Similarly concerned about her appearance, Hailey spent significant amounts of time ensuring that she looked the same as other children. Although interactive and confident at home, when with people she did not know well, with peers, or in crowded situations Hailey was very quiet and did not voluntarily participate. She did become more social as her familiarity with people improved, particularly in one-on-one interactions. She played well with her cousins and initiated play with two neighbors, who were significantly younger.

Hailey (11), the youngest of three children, was reported by her parents to have always been extremely shy. Hailey and her family had recently moved to the area precipitating the change of school. At her old school, Hailey had one friend, who was similarly quiet with whom she would spend break times. If this friend was absent, then Hailey would spend the time alone. Both girls were often teased and excluded by other children. Although Hailey had expressed the wish to maintain their friendship, she always found an excuse to postpone making contact. Her mother reported that she also had been a shy child, although she continued to feel somewhat uncomfortable during social interactions as an adult, she did not feel that it had an impact on her current activities. There was no other history of anxiety in the family.

ASSESSMENT

Functional Behavioral Analysis

A satisfactory assessment process needs to identify the differential diagnosis, the severity of symptoms relative to peers, and the impact of the symptoms on functioning. For planning treatment, it is also essential to assess factors that maintain the symptoms. Over the past decade, significant improvements in the scientific and clinical utility of diagnostic interviews have facilitated differential diagnosis and questionnaire measures of childhood anxiety disorders have enabled peer comparison (Langley, Bergman, & Piacentini, 2002). These newer measures have been shown to closely relate to the experience of impairment (Essau, Muris, & Ederer, 2002) and are sensitive to treatment effects (Muris, Merckelbach, Gadet, Moulaert, & Tierney, 1999; Silverman et al., 1999). Structured approaches to assessment of maintenance factors are also increasingly available.

The variety of questions to be answered, and the complexity and dependence of a young person's world lead to the need for multimethod, multi-informant approaches to assessment. This need is confirmed by research that indicates young people may underreport certain types of symptoms due to their need to be socially desirable (Comer & Kendall, 2004; DiBartolo, Albano, Barlow, & Heimberg, 1998), and that parental reports may be influenced by parents' perceptions of behavior, for example, interpreting anxious avoidance as oppositional behavior, if they think the cause of the behavior is deliberate defiance (Foley et al., 2004). In addition, there is strong evidence that parents have limited knowledge of the internal experiences of their children (Herjanic & Reich, 1982). Minimum standard practice involves the use of separate interview and self-report questionnaires with a child/adolescent and his or her primary caregiver(s). Additional information from teachers, peers, and other significant individuals in the young person's life may be of particular use in determining the severity and impact of symptoms, and maintenance factors.

Assessment Tools

Several reliable and validated structured and semistructured diagnostic interviews are available for use with children and adolescents (Schniering, Hudson, & Rapee, 2000). The Anxiety Disorders Interview Schedule for Children for DSM-IV (ADIS-IV-C; Silverman & Albano, 1996) is unique in that it provides in-depth assessment of individual anxiety disorders, as well as differential diagnoses for other common childhood difficulties. The ADIS-IV-C is a semistructured diagnostic tool with separate interviews for the young person (from age 6 years) and his or her parents. Administration takes 1–3 hours depending on the number of disorders that need to be examined in depth. Research indicates that the interview has fair to excellent reliability and validity in comparison to self-report anxiety measures (Rapee, Barrett, Dadds, & Evans, 1994; Silverman & Nelles, 1988; Silverman, Saavedra, & Pina, 2001), and that it can successfully distinguish between the different forms of anxiety (Tracey, Chorpita, Douban, & Barlow, 1997; Wood, Piacentini, Bergman, McCracken, & Barrios, 2002). The ADIS-IV-C includes specific sections on interpersonal relationships and social phobia.

Two current measures of anxiety, the Spence Children's Anxiety Scale (SCAS; Nauta et al., 2004; Spence, 1998) and the Screen for Child Anxiety Related Emotional Disorders (SCARED; Birmaher et al., 1997) were designed to gauge severity of symptoms specific to individual disorders or types of anxiety. Both measures reliably distinguish between clinically anxious and non-clinical children, and are able to differentiate between anxious children and those with other types of disorders. The measures have also been shown to have validity in differentiating among the different anxiety disorders, although there has been some difficulty with differentiation due to the high comorbidity of anxiety disorders and the overlap of symptoms within these disorders (Schniering et al., 2000). Each of the measures has self-report and parent-report versions that can be completed in 15–30 minutes. The self-report measures are suitable for children from age 8 years; however, younger children may require assistance with reading the questions. Normative data are available for the measures, facilitating comparison to appropriate peer groups, with both gender and age impacting on expected scores. The questionnaires have also shown sensitivity in a variety of cultural settings without major deterioration of psychometrics (Muris, Schmidt, Engelbrecht, & Perold, 2002).

Several measures specific to the symptoms of social phobia have been developed. The Social Anxiety Scale for Children—Revised (SASC-R; La Greca & Stone, 1993) and the Social Phobia and Anxiety Inventory for Children (SPAI-C; Beidel et al., 1995) assess specific aspects of socially anxious symptomatology in situations relevant to children. The SASC-R provides a measure of children's fear of negative evaluation and their social avoidance and distress in both new situations and in general. The SPAI-C measures social fears in multiple settings, focusing on cognitions, behavior, and physiological responses. In addition, the SPAI-C provides information on children's level of fear/distress when with unfamiliar peers, familiar peers, and adults across situations. Both measures have favorable reliability and validity, including the ability to distinguish between children with social phobia and those with other anxiety disorders (Beidel, Turner, Hamlin, & Morris, 2000; Ginsburg, La Greca, & Silverman, 1998).

In addition to assessment of disorder-specific symptoms, thorough assessment of resulting impairment is necessary to determine whether the symptoms amount to a disorder and, if so, the severity of that disorder. Diagnostic interviews based on DSM-IV criteria such as the ADIS-IV-C incorporate assessment of impairment through questioning about interference in various aspects of a child's life (Silverman & Albano, 1996). This information is then used by the clinician to rate the severity of each disorder and is often utilized as a substitute for more formal measurement. More recently, self- and parent-report questionnaire measures of impairment have been developed. The Child and Adolescent Social and Adaptive Functioning Scale (CASAFS; Price, Spence, Sheffield, & Donovan, 2002) allows children ages 10–17 years to rate their current functioning at school, with peers, within their family, and with self-care. The Child Anxiety Impact Scale (CAIS; Langley, Bergman, McCracken, & Piacentini, 2004) is a parent report of the child's functioning in school, home/family, and social domains, with questions that specifically target performance likely to be affected by anxiety. Initial reliability and validity on these measures are promising, with appropriate relationships with internalizing symptom measures in clinical (Langley et al., 2004) and community (Price et al., 2002) populations. These measures can help clinicians to rate impairment for diagnostic purposes and are useful in determining improvement during treatment.

Research on anxiety disorders in children and adolescents has implicated avoidance of feared situations, cognitive processing biases, coping skills, and aspects of parent–child interactions as factors individually or in combination that potentially maintain anxiety (Barrett, Rapee, Dadds, & Ryan, 1996; Manassis, Hudson, Webb, & Albano, 2004; Spence, Donovan, & Brechman-Toussaint, 1999). During a child's initial evaluation it is useful to assess these maintaining factors and other areas that may need to be targeted during treatment. Although there are no tools that comprehensively assess factors relevant to children with anxiety disorders, several tools can determine the severity of particular categories of symptoms. For example, the Children's Automatic Thoughts Scale (CATS; Schniering & Rapee, 2002) provides a self-report measure of the negative thinking that is typical in anxiety, depression, and anger problems; the Parental Expectancies Scale (Eisen, Spasaro, Brien, Kearney, & Albano, 2004) provides a measure of parents' expectations of their child in life domains such as academics and socialization. These measures may be used to identify the severity of particular maintaining factors, so that they may be monitored during treatment.

Another useful approach for any child with an anxiety disorder is to identify specific, recent situations in which anxiety caused the child great distress and to use these descriptions to increase understanding of antecedents, consequences, and modifying cues for high anxiety. It is important to gain an understanding of the described situation from both the parent's and child's view, because the salient information for each party can differ dramatically. This task may also be a monitoring exercise that parents and (older) children complete between assessment sessions by recording experiences immediately following an anxious event. This information may be used to identify factors that are likely to encourage future expression of anxiety and in turn assists in treatment planning.

The Process of Assessment: Step by Step

Hailey was assessed over two sessions. In the first session, Hailey and her parents were interviewed separately with the ADIS-IV-C, and each completed self-report questionnaires: the SCAS to assess the broad range of anxiety disorder symptoms, the SPAI-C to assess specific social anxiety symptoms, the CATS to assess for cognitive biases, and the CASFAS (child) and CAIS (parents) to assess the interference currently being experienced. In addition, self-report measures of depression and behavioral problems were given for screening purposes.

During the ADIS-IV-C, both Hailey and her parents clearly endorsed all the criteria necessary for a diagnosis of social phobia. Hailey and her parents reported the highest anxiety, avoidance, and distress in situations involving class peers. Hailey was reported to be withdrawn in social situations both at school and with unfamiliar people; however, at home and with people she knew well, Hailey could be interactive and friendly. Although Hailey's parents reported that the teacher thought Hailey was sad much of the time, neither Hailey nor her parents reported symptoms of sadness or depression beyond the concern with social situations. The following dialogue, an excerpt from Hailey's ADIS-IV-C interview, illustrates both formal questions and additional therapist probing in response to Hailey's answers:

THERAPIST: Now I'm going to give you a list of situations. I want to know if you think you get more nervous or scared in these situations than other kids your age do. Answer "yes" only if these situations almost always make you scared or nervous, not if it has just happened once or twice. First just tell me "yes" or "no." (*Continues with list.*)

OK, Hailey, when you say that you're afraid or nervous about joining in on a conversation, how afraid do you feel? Use the thermometer to show me how afraid or nervous you get.

HAILEY: (*Indicates a 7 on the 0- to 8-point scale, Not at all to Very very much.*)

THERAPIST: Do you ever try to stay away from situations where you have to join in a conversation?

HAILEY: Most of the time.

THERAPIST: Can you tell me about times when you can join in?

HAILEY: If it's only one or two girls and I know them really well, that's OK.

THERAPIST: Is there anyone at your new school who you can do that with?

HAILEY: Not really.

In addition to social anxiety, Hailey also endorsed several symptoms in the generalized anxiety disorder section. As illustrated in the excerpt below, careful questioning on the nature of Hailey's reported worries revealed that only her worry about social situations was interfering in her life, whereas other worries she endorsed were age-appropriate. As a consequence an additional diagnosis of generalized anxiety disorder was not considered appropriate.

THERAPIST: Hailey, you just told me that you worry about a lot of things. I'd like to know a bit more about these worries. When you worry about getting your schoolwork done, what do you think will happen if you don't get it finished?

HAILEY: The other kids will think I'm not smart and then they won't like me.

THERAPIST: Do you think anything else will happen?

HAILEY: The kids might laugh at me if I'm last to finish.

THERAPIST: Do you ever worry that you might get in trouble with your teacher if you don't get finished?

HAILEY: No, she's really nice; she only gets mad if kids don't finish because they were mucking around or talking too much.

THERAPIST: Do you worry that you might get a bad grade if you don't get your work finished?

HAILEY: Not much, only tests and projects make grades.

THERAPIST: That's very true. You also said that you worry about your parents' fighting.

HAILEY: Yeah, I don't like it when they fight.

THERAPIST: How often do you think about them fighting?

HAILEY: Sometimes when I'm in bed and I hear an argument.

THERAPIST: How often has that happened since Christmas?

HAILEY: Maybe two times.

THERAPIST: Are there any other times that you worry about them fighting?

HAILEY: Once, when they had a big fight about my uncle coming to stay.

THERAPIST: How much did you worry about that?

HAILEY: Only a bit; it got sorted out and my uncle got to stay.

Results from the self-report questionnaires revealed clinical scores on the Social Phobia subscale of the SCAS and high average scores on the Generalized Anxiety Disorder subscale. Symptoms endorsed as always true included "I worry about what other people think of me," "I feel afraid if I have to talk in front of my class," and "I feel afraid that I will make a fool of myself in front of people." On the CATS Hailey endorsed all of the social threat cognitions, with frequency of thoughts such as "Kids will think I'm stupid," "Other kids are making fun of me," and "I look like an idiot," being particularly problematic. Her score on the depressive cognitions was average for her age. The SPAI-C revealed that Hailey experienced cognitive, behavioral, and physiological symptoms in social situations, and that she found situations involving unfamiliar peers the most anxiety provoking. The interference measures indicated that Hailey's social anxiety had a significant impact at school and in friendships, with only minimal interference at home.

During the second assessment session, Hailey, her parents and the therapist discussed in detail a situation that had recently caused Hailey to become very anxious. They described an incident that had occurred during a visit to the beach. Hailey and her mother were having lunch on the sand when they spotted two class members from Hailey's new school with their parents. Hailey's mother pointed these children out and suggested that Hailey ask if they wanted to go for a swim together, but Hailey refused and soon suggested that they go home. The following partial excerpt is from discussion of what occurred during the incident. During the discussion, the therapist completed a monitoring form that summarized the situation (see Figure 2.1).

THERAPIST: So, Hailey, had you noticed that the girls from your class were also at the beach?

HAILEY: Sort of, I thought I recognized them but wasn't sure.

THERAPIST: What ran through your mind when you realized that it was them?

HAILEY: I hoped they wouldn't notice me.

THERAPIST: What did you think would happen if they did notice you?

HAILEY: I didn't want them to see me in my swim suit. It's the one I had last year, and it wasn't like the ones they had on.

THERAPIST: What happened when your mom suggested asking them to swim with you?

HAILEY: I didn't want to. Those girls aren't my friends, and they don't really like me much.

THERAPIST: Do these girls give you a hard time at school?

HAILEY: No. Emma has said hello to me a couple of times and seems nice. Alice is friends with everyone.

THERAPIST: Is she a friend of yours?

HAILEY: No, I'm not part of her group.

Situation	Thoughts	Behavior
Notice Alice and Emma are at the beach	I hope they won't notice me They'll think this swim suit is silly	Tried to stay out of sight
Mom suggested I ask Alice and Emma to swim	They aren't my friends They will never want to play with me	Asked if we could go home instead

FIGURE 2.1. Assessment monitoring form.

As a final assessment task, the therapist assigned Hailey and her parents a social task to complete during the session. The therapist asked Hailey to go with her parents to the waiting room, and to ask the receptionist for the time, allowing her to observe Hailey's reactions. Hailey expressed hesitation, "Do I have to?" Her father replied, "Its not that hard; just give it a try." Hailey then went with her parents to the waiting room. They sat down together and after a minute Hailey's father prompted her to go ask the time. Hailey made a move, then asked her mother to come with her. When Hailey got to the reception desk, she asked for the time in a very quiet voice. The receptionist replied, "Sorry, sweetie, I couldn't quite hear you." At this point Hailey's mother responded, "We were just wondering what time it is." After the interaction, the therapist asked about both Hailey's and her parents' thought processes during this task.

THERAPIST: You did well, Hailey, giving that a try. What did you think would happen when you asked for the time?

HAILEY: Nothing really. I just thought she'd think I was dumb for asking.

THERAPIST: Sounds like you were a bit worried beforehand. What happened when you went to ask?

HAILEY: She didn't understand what I said.

THERAPIST: What did you think to yourself when that happened?

HAILEY: Now she knows that I'm stupid.

THERAPIST: What did you think, Mom?

MOTHER: She did ask. It wasn't her fault that she couldn't be heard.

THERAPIST: What happened then?

MOTHER: I repeated the question.

THERAPIST: Did Hailey try to ask again?

MOTHER: No, I knew it would be hard for her, so I asked instead.

Link between Assessment and Treatment

The ADIS-IV-C and self-report questionnaires both supported the fact that social situations were difficult for Hailey and indicated that these difficulties might be interfering with Hailey's daily activities, particularly at school and with friends. Using the information gathered during the interview, the situation description, and the in-session social task, the therapist produced the case formulation presented in Figure 2.2. In this formulation, preexisting experiences such as being bullied and moving to a new school, together with having a socially anxious mother and being temperamentally shy, have contributed to Hailey's current presentation. She is sensitive to social threat, expects negative outcomes in social situations, and avoids social situations and attention that

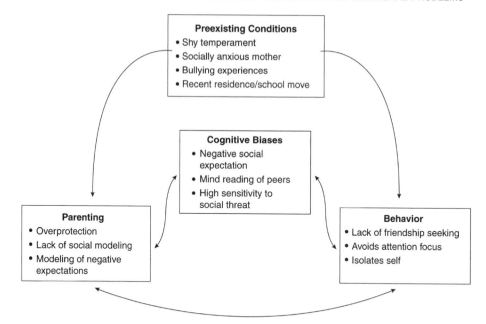

FIGURE 2.2. Case formulation for Hailey.

might otherwise contradict her expectations. In addition, her parents do not participate in many social activities and, in an effort to prevent Hailey's distress, they do not expect Hailey to participate and often complete social tasks for her.

The case formulation suggests that treatment for Hailey's social anxiety should focus on formation of more realistic social expectations, structured skills, and practice in initiating and maintaining interaction with peers, and replace parenting practices that encourage anxious behavior with practices that model the value of social interaction and allow Hailey to complete age-appropriate social tasks independently.

Cognitive-behavioral treatment (CBT) is considered the treatment of choice for children experiencing significant social anxiety. CBT specifically addresses the cognitive processes and behaviors that maintain anxiety, and it has consistently been shown to be effective in reducing symptoms of anxiety in children and adolescents in randomized controlled trials (Barrett, Dadds, et al., 1996; Beidel et al., 2000; Kendall, 1994; see Ollendick & King, 2000). Positive treatment outcomes have been maintained over the long term, with some studies showing maintenance of treatment outcomes as long as 6–7 years after initial treatment (Barrett, Duffy, Dadds, & Rapee, 2001). The results suggest that the skills many children learn in the program can be carried through adolescence and adulthood, assisting the children throughout their lives to be better equipped to cope with anxiety-provoking situations. Because anxiety disorders frequently predate disorders such as depression and substance abuse, anxiety intervention in childhood may lead to prevention of these other disorders (e.g., Hayward et al., 2000; Kendall, Safford, Flannery-Schroeder, & Webb, 2004).

Not all children with social anxiety benefit from the standard 10- to 16-session program. In a recent systematic review, Cartwright-Hatton, Roberts, Chitsabesan, Fothergill, and Harrington (2004) showed that across published randomized clinical trials of childhood anxiety, the remission rate at follow-up was 64%, indicating that roughly one-third of children (including children with disorders other than social phobia) continue to experience significant interference in their lives as a result of anxiety.

A number of variables may impact on the anxious child's outcome in CBT (see Hudson, 2005). For example, preliminary evidence suggests that older children, male children, children with depressive symptoms, children who are less involved in therapy, and children from families with parental psychopathology and family stress may have poorer outcomes in CBT, although results are rarely consistent across studies (e.g., Berman, Weems, Silverman, & Kurtines, 2000; Chu & Kendall, 2004; Crawford & Manassis, 2001). Treatment considerations and adaptations might prove beneficial for these treatment nonresponders (although many of these have yet to be tested through randomized clinical trials), such as treating parental psychopathology, concurrent or prior treatment of comorbid conditions, increased family involvement in treatment, and longer, more intensive treatment and booster sessions.

The evidence about whether to include parents in treatment is still inconclusive. Given the potential role that parents play in the maintenance of child anxiety disorders (e.g., Gar, Hudson, & Rapee, 2005; Ginsburg, La Greca, & Silverman, 1998; Hudson & Rapee, 2001), it makes sense to include parents as a central part of treatment. Consistent with this, a number of studies have compared child-focused treatment to family-focused treatment with positive results (Barrett, Dadds, et al., 1996; Mendlowitz et al., 1999). These studies have indicated that involving families in the treatment may enhance the benefits of the program, particularly for younger children (7- to 10-year-olds) and for girls. In addition, one study has shown preliminary evidence that anxious children with anxious parents do better in treatment when their parents receive concurrent treatment for anxiety (Cobham, Dadds, & Spence, 1998).

Given the suggested importance of the cognitive, behavioral, and parenting factors in the maintenance of Hailey's social anxiety, the therapist considered it appropriate to offer Hailey and her parents a CBT program that would (1) teach Hailey anxiety management skills, (2) help her systematically to reduce her avoidance of social situations, and (3) include her parents directly in the sessions, with the aim of reducing overprotection and increasing appropriate social modeling.

TREATMENT

Preview

The goal of CBT for anxious youth is to provide skills that enable the child and the family to cope more adequately with anxiety-provoking situations. The goal is not to reduce anxiety completely. Rather, the goal is to bring the child's social anxiety to manageable levels, so that the child feels more able to cope with his or her anxiety. Anxiety in social situations is a very normal part of life. It is normal for a child to have some concern, but not excessive or interfering concern, regarding other children's opinions.

Treatment should enable the child to recognize his or her own anxiety by identifying bodily sensations, behaviors, and cognitions that accompany anxiety, and applying certain skills (e.g., cognitive restructuring, problem solving, social skills, assertiveness) to face gradually rather than avoid feared social situations. It is the gradual exposure component of the program that is thought to be most effective in changing the child's fearful expectations and avoidance behaviors. Thus, change is not immediate, but it may start to occur in the latter half of the program, when the child and family have become competent with the gradual exposure techniques. By the end of therapy, the child should be increasingly able to take these steps without the assistance of the therapist and parent.

The skills in the program are taught through verbal instruction, activities, role plays, and modeling. Children are encouraged and rewarded for practice/homework outside the session. Much of the important work is attempted by the child outside the therapy session, in real-life, anxiety-provoking situations that cannot be created in the therapy room. Homework/practice plays a significant part in the program (Hudson & Kendall, 2002) and should be encouraged and rewarded.

Context of Treatment

The "Cool Kids" program was designed as a 10-session treatment for anxious children between the ages of 7 and 16 years, and their parents (Rapee, Wignall, et al., 2000). The treatment materials are not suitable for socially anxious children younger than age 7 given the degree of reading and writing in the program. Having said this, we have successfully treated children as young as 4 years old with the same techniques, but delivered primarily to the parent, with less focus on cognitive restructuring and increased focus on parenting techniques and gradual exposure (Rapee, Kennedy, Ingram, Edwards, & Sweeney, 2005).

At our clinic at Macquarie University in Sydney, Australia, we routinely include parents in treatment of the child's anxiety. We typically spend time with the child alone, with the parent(s) alone, and with the child and parent(s) together. Our treatment usually occurs in a group format with children of similar ages and heterogeneous anxiety problems. Group treatment has been shown in most studies to be equivalent to individual treatment (e.g., Flannery-Schroeder & Kendall, 2000; Barett, 1998). There has been only one study in which children with social anxiety had a poorer outcome in group compared to individual treatment (Manassis et al., 2002); however, this study had only a small number of socially anxious participants (6.4%).

At Macquarie University, we have had favorable results for socially anxious children using the Cool Kids program in a group setting (Rapee, 2000). Some people may argue that for a socially anxious child, a group format may be too overwhelming, and that extreme fear may prevent the child from participating in the therapy and getting the most out of the group. On the contrary, we find that the group format can be an important normalizing process for a socially anxious child. In addition, the group format, if led in a sensitive way, asks for minimal involvement in the first few sessions, with increasing involvement as therapy progresses, thereby serving as inbuilt, gradual exposure to social situations. In a group format, children may be encouraged to keep up with their peers in the homework tasks, and may complete more of the homework tasks than they would if being seen individually.

The treatment program Cool Kids was originally developed for therapy conducted by psychologists in a clinic or mental health setting. Since its original development, the program has been adapted and tested in school (Mifsud & Rapee, 2005) and rural settings (Lyneham & Rapee, 2006) with positive results. The school program is designed to be run by a trained school counselor, who leads a group of around six students in 10 weekly sessions, with two booster sessions and two parent–therapist meetings. The Cool Kids program has been evaluated in the school setting within a low socioeconomic scale population and has shown significant reductions in anxious symptoms (Mifsud & Rapee, 2005). A number of other school-based programs are also available for social anxiety and have shown promise with respect to efficacy (see Lowry-Webster, Barrett, & Dadds, 2001; Fisher, Masia-Warner, & Klein, 2004).

Lyneham and Rapee (2006) adapted the Cool Kids program for use with children who have limited access to mental health services in rural Australia. The program targeted children under the age of 12 and utilized a parent-as-therapist approach. Using a set of child and parent workbooks, the therapist guided parents through readings, activities, and practice tasks that paralleled a standard therapist-led program. A randomized control trial indicated that this bibliotherapy approach was most effective when supplemented with regular telephone consultations between the parent and therapist that focused on applying the program's skills to a child's idiosyncratic fears and worries.

In summary, we encourage a family-focused treatment of the child's anxiety, including both parents and the child in treatment. The treatment may then focus on teaching parents skills to manage their child's (and perhaps their own) anxiety effectively and to provide skills for the child to manage his or her anxiety more effectively. For older children/adolescents, parental involvement in therapy may be reduced to increase adolescents' autonomy and independence. Parents continue to have some involvement in the therapy to ensure that they are familiar with the goals of the program and can provide a supportive, encouraging environment in which the adolescents can develop their skills.

Obstacles to Therapy

A number of obstacles may be present in the treatment of children with social anxiety. One of the major obstacles is actually getting the family to the appropriate services in the first place. Children with anxiety are less likely than children with other psychological problems to present in primary care facilities (Chavira, Stein, Bailey, & Stein, 2004), despite the fact that anxiety is the most prevalent problem in children and adolescents. For children with social anxiety, the main concern is negative evaluation from others. Thus, attending a clinic or a school program that identifies them as "different" or "disordered" is a highly anxiety-provoking situation. We know that parents are also likely to be anxious and may be more likely to avoid social situations and situations in which they may be evaluated. Hence, nonattendance may be a result of social avoidance.

Another issue that hinders treatment seeking is that some parents may not see their child's social anxiety or shyness as a problem. They may interpret the child's behaviors as typical and say things such as "That's just the way he is" or "She'll grow out of it." Socially anxious children are likely to be quiet and shy, and to avoid being the center of their teachers', parents', or peers' attention. Hence, their behaviors and the accompanying distress and interference may slip "under the radar." As mentioned earlier, socially anxious children may have other, more generalized worries as well (as in our case study), such as perfectionistic worries. These children, again, tend to be the quieter children in the classroom as they attempt to avoid getting into trouble and appearing in a bad light. They are likely to go unnoticed. Thus, the low rate of referral may be due in part to the low rate of identification of anxiety problems.

Once in treatment, families or children may resist attending sessions, because it may be difficult to schedule appointments in family members' busy lives. Both parents may not be able to attend the therapy sessions; the parents may not want to pull the child from school or, conversely, the child may not want to be pulled from school and miss entertainment or afterschool activities. These issues require discussion at the assessment. Ultimately, the family needs to be somewhat motivated to attend therapy. If family members cannot attend regularly due to other commitments and stressors, and cannot find a suitable time to attend, they may be encouraged to attend therapy at a later date, when therapy can become a priority. Treatment is not likely to be successful if the family attends irregularly and there is little time (or motivation) for the child and family members to practice their skills between sessions.

To illustrate, the following discussion is between a therapist and two parents, Jo and David, considering treatment for their son, who was experiencing clinically significant anxiety in social situations. The family was considering whether to proceed with treatment: They were about to move, and the mother was experiencing a lot of work-related stress and subsequent financial strain.

THERAPIST: Jo and David, you have a few of options available to you. I see that your child's worries are a concern for you at the moment, but a lot of other issues are making life stressful for you as a family right now. The first option: We could commence a 10-session, weekly program for your son equip him with skills to identify and manage his anxiety and be able to increase his involvement gradually in social situations at school and outside of school. This would involve a commitment from you for 10 sessions, weekly for the first 2 months; then we usually spread out the last two sessions over a couple of weeks. A second option would be to use the self-help manual that we have written for parents. With the book, you could work through the program at your own pace. The third option is to delay the full treatment program for a few months, until the move has happened and things have improved at work. Then you might be able to be more committed to the program, with less stress in your life.

JO: Mmm. Things are pretty stressful right now, and I know I will find it difficult to concentrate on the program with all the stuff that is going on with work and the house. I kind of prefer the third option, but I'm not sure if that's just a cop out and in 3 months' time things won't be any different. David?

DAVID: Yeah, maybe. I could bring him along each week after work, if we wanted to do it now rather than later. But he might be too tired by the time I can get him here. The only day I could do that would be a Thursday. . . .

JO: I would really like to be able to do this with him.

DAVID: Maybe it is best if we just wait until things are a little less stressful. Maybe we should take the self-help book and just read up on the program before we start.

THERAPIST: OK. You can have some time to think about it some more and can call me during the week, if you like. But for now it seems as though your preference is to delay treatment but perhaps do some reading in the meantime. I think this would be a good interim option that may help you move in the right direction with your son's anxiety, even if things are tough at the moment.

Another obstacle to treatment can occur when the child does not believe he or she has a problem with anxiety despite an assessment from parents and outside observers (teachers, clinicians) that indicates the presence of clinically significant social anxiety. A child may state that he is not scared of anything and therefore does not need to attend treatment, as in the following dialogue between a therapist and a 13-year-old, Adam, regarding participation in the program:

ADAM: I don't think I need to be here. You said this was for kids who get scared. That's not me.

THERAPIST: OK. So you don't get scared. Are there times when you might get worried or stressed?

ADAM: I get stressed before exams, but that's normal, right?

THERAPIST: Absolutely. Most kids, in fact adults too, will feel nervous in some situations. Feeling stressed is a really normal reaction when our body thinks something bad might happen, like before an exam. You might be concerned that you will mess up the exam, so naturally you feel worried. Or if you had to give a talk in front of your assembly, you might get butterflies in your stomach.

ADAM: Oh yeah, I wouldn't want to do that.

THERAPIST: So feeling stressed is normal. For some people, though, it can stop them from doing things they like or would want to do. For instance, I recently helped a boy about your age who has a really hard time when he goes to a party. He freezes up and doesn't know what to say to his friends, so he doesn't join in the conversation when he really wants to. He even started saying no to the parties, even though he really wanted to go. This program has really helped him to handle his stress. Are there any difficult situations in your life that you think you could use some help with?

ADAM: Well, I would like to have more friends.

THERAPIST: OK, so you would like to get some help so you could have more friends.

ADAM: I'm kinda quiet too.

THERAPIST: So maybe you would like some help to be more confident.

ADAM: Yeah, I suppose.

In this example, Adam did not identify with the words "scared" or "anxious." Instead, he came up with the word "stressed," so the therapist used this word to help engage the child and attempted to normalize the process of therapy by talking about other children who had experienced anxiety and benefited from treatment. Also, the therapist in this example asked a broader question that helped to engage Adam, by asking if there were *any* situations in his life with which he wanted help. It is important for children to feel that they have some choice in the program and that it is not forced upon them by their parents. Adolescents, in particular, react to this and as a result may not be fully engaged in therapy.

Medication

A number of medications (e.g., fluoxetine, fluvoxamine, and paroxetine) are prescribed for the treatment of childhood social anxiety. Evidence on the efficacy of pharmacological intervention has begun to emerge in the literature (Birmaher et al., 2003; Walkup et al., 2001; Wagner et al., 2004). However, it is generally believed that a CBT approach is the first choice of treatment (Compton et al., 2004). At this stage we do not have evidence from randomized clinical trials regarding the efficacy of CBT and concurrent pharmacological treatment. Future research is needed in this area.

Description of Treatment Components

The specific combination of techniques may vary slightly from clinician to clinician, but the basic techniques that underpin the application of CBT for social anxiety include somatic awareness, cognitive restructuring, problem solving, and gradual behavioral exposure. Family-based programs such as Cool Kids include additional components such as contingency management and parent anxiety management. Children may also benefit from relaxation strategies, such as deep, diaphragmatic breathing and muscle relaxation to help manage their somatic symptoms; thus, a relaxation component is frequently included in the treatment of social anxiety (Rapee, Wignall, et al., 2000). Programs for the treatment of social phobia in adults also include strategies such as attention refocusing and detailed performance feedback (Rapee, 1998). To date, programs for children have not tested the value of these components.

Some children with social anxiety who exhibit social skills deficits may benefit from additional social skills training and/or practice. Many socially anxious children possess the appropriate social skills, but their anxiety may inhibit them from using the skills. In this instance, additional social skills training may not be necessary once the child's anxiety is reduced; other children may require more intensive training. The Cool Kids program has additional social skills and assertiveness modules that may be added for children who require additional training and/or practice. These modules also provide strategies to deal with teasing and bullying, because many socially anxious children are the target of such abuse. Each of these treatment components is reviewed.[1]

Treatment Rationale

The first step in the treatment program is to provide children and families with information to normalize anxiety, such as informing families that anxiety is a normal response accompanied by bodily feelings (physiological symp-

---

[1] For the therapist manuals and child–parent workbooks, see *www.mq.edu.au/muaru.*

toms), thoughts (cognitions), and actions (behaviors). This anxiety interferes with some people's lives and stops them from doing the things they want to do. Thus, treatment targets these three components to help children manage their bodily feelings (through awareness and relaxation), think less anxious thoughts (through cognitive restructuring), and face their fears confidently (through the use of gradual exposure, problem-solving techniques, and social skills training).

Awareness of Bodily Symptoms and Relaxation

The therapist informs the child and parents that when one becomes anxious, changes occur in one's body. Because the body *thinks* it is in danger, these changes prepare the body to handle the situation by increasing the heart rate, quickening the breathing rate, rushing blood to the muscles, and so on. Awareness of these physical symptoms is important, because they serve as a cue or early detection system to "do something" about the anxiety. Techniques such as deep, diaphragmatic breathing and muscle relaxation are often taught as a component in the somatic management of anxiety. Deep breathing is an easy, portable tool for children to utilize. Muscle relaxation may be taught by encouraging children to tense and relax muscle groups sequentially. Relaxation scripts or tapes may be given to children for homework to encourage practice of the technique (see the partial script below, appropriate for middle childhood: see Ollendick & Cerny [1981] for scripts for younger children or see Rapee, Wignall, et al. [2000] for additional scripts). Children are encouraged to practice the somatic management techniques in anxiety-provoking situations.

Relaxation Script

"I want you to get yourself comfortable in your chair, with your feet on the floor and your arms loosely in your lap. Now close your eyes and focus right on the end of your nose. This may be tricky at first, but just try to think about the end of your nose. This will help prepare you for the relaxation and get your mind in focus. Just focus on the tip of your nose. . . .

"Now I want you to focus on your breath. Imagine your breath as it travels in through your nose and down into your lungs, then out through your mouth. You might feel your breath on the back of your throat as it travels down into your lungs. Just imagine this breath as it goes in and out. Now I want you to slow down your breathing just a little bit, and make sure that when you breathe in, your stomach fills out. Make your in-breath go all the way down into your stomach. In . . . Out (let your tummy go back in) . . . In . . . Out . . . In . . . Out.

"Now, as you breath out, I want you to say the word "relax" to yourself. RELAX. You can imagine the word written out, R-E-L-A-X, or you can just imagine the sound of the word. In . . . Out (RELAX). . . . Let your-self feel relaxed as you breathe out. Take a few more breaths until your breathing is comfortable. You might notice that some thoughts creep into your head; that's OK. Just notice the thoughts and come back to my voice. You can imagine that your thoughts are like clouds, and they just pass by in the sky, floating out of view.

"Now we are going to do some muscle relaxation. This will help you learn when your muscles are tense and when they are relaxed. First of all we will start with your hands. Think about your left hand. I want you to bring your left hand out in front of you and make a fist. Try to keep every other part of your body as relaxed as possible and just tense your left hand. Feel the tension in your hand and all the way up your arm. (*Waits for a few seconds.*) Now relax it. Let your hand fall back into your lap. Now concentrate on the feelings in your hand. Notice the difference in the muscles now that the tension is gone. Notice any tingling sensations or feelings of warmth or heaviness. Imagine your arm getting heavier and heavier as you relax it. Keeping your left hand relaxed, think about your right hand."

The same procedure is repeated with the right hand, then the shoulders (by bringing the shoulders up around the ears), face (by making a frown and pursing the lips), stomach (by pulling the stomach in), and legs (by lifting the legs off the floor and tightening the toes). It is important that the child isolate each specific muscle group. Hence, during the tension phase, only the selected muscle group should be tightened, and the child should keep the rest of his or her body relaxed. It is also important that there be sufficient time to relax each muscle, but not so much time that the child gets distracted. During the relaxation, the child should focus on the changes occurring in the muscles when they are tense and relaxed, so the child learns to recognize the tension and relaxation. Most importantly, relaxation is useful when it is practiced regularly. The relaxation can be recorded onto an audiotape to encourage the child–family to use the relaxation regularly.

Cognitive Restructuring

Cognitive restructuring involves first understanding the connection between thoughts and feelings ("The way you think affects the way you feel"). For older children, this process may also involve understanding the impact of thinking errors on feelings and behavior (e.g., always looking for the negatives or mind reading). Second, cognitive restructuring is the process of evaluating or challenging negative thoughts. Children learn to identify their negative thoughts or "self-talk" and make the connection that anxiety is associated with "expecting bad things to happen." Children are instructed to become "detectives" and treat their thoughts as mysteries to be tested and challenged. The "detective" thinking process includes the following steps: (1) identifying the event that is causing concern; (2) identifying the thought behind the feeling; (3) looking for realistic evidence; (4) listing all the alternative things that might happen; and (5) identifying a realistic thought to replace the worried thought. Parents are taught to coach and encourage their children to challenge their own thoughts rather than to provide excessive reassurance when their children have anxious thoughts (e.g., "It's OK. You look fine. No one is going to think you look silly"). Such reassurance only serves to maintain the children's reliance on their parent. Similarly, parents are encouraged not to come up with the evidence for their children, but to ask open-ended questions that allow children to think up evidence on their own. Children are more likely to believe the realistic thought/evidence if they come up with it themselves. Children are encouraged to practice their "detective" or realistic thinking during the week.

Problem Solving

The purpose of problem solving is to help children generate alternative, less avoidant, and more adaptive solutions to a given problem. The aim is to enable children to cope in anxiety-provoking situations without reverting to their usual maladaptive avoidant response. Children are taught to identify a specific problem/situation (e.g., receiving an invitation to a birthday party) and brainstorm possible responses to the problem (e.g., say no to the invitation, go to the party and take a close friend, find out who else is going, go the party for just an hour). In the brainstorming phase, children are encouraged to list all possible responses without evaluating them. Evaluation should occur later, because it hinders the brainstorming process. Once the list is complete, the therapist can encourage the child to consider the advantages and disadvantages associated with each response, and select the most ideal response. Problem-solving skills are most effectively taught by working through a real-life example.

Contingency Management

Contingency management is aimed primarily at parents, but children also need to learn the importance of rewarding courageous behavior. When children engage in exposure to feared situations, rewards are crucial. The therapist models use of appropriate rewards by rewarding the children for contributing during the session and engagement with homework tasks. Parents are also educated about the principles underlying contingent rewards (e.g., when attention is paid to a behavior, the behavior increases), with the aim of encouraging courageous rather than anxious behavior. Often anxious children receive the most parental attention when they are anxious and distressed, hence maintaining the behavior. By paying attention to children's less anxious and more confident behavior, parents can shape courageous behavior. Parents are taught the importance of clear, concrete, specific praise and the use of proportional rewards. Nonmonetary rewards are encouraged, such as spending time with Mom or Dad, choosing the family meal, or staying up later on the weekend.

Parents are encouraged to model courageous behavior. This means identifying situations in which they feel anxious and being able to use the skills to face, rather than avoid, these situations. Some parents who find this very difficult may require additional instructions on specific skills (e.g., cognitive restructuring). Importantly, parents are educated about the "overinvolvement/ overprotection trap" that can affect parents of anxious children; that is, parents might be more likely to do things for their children (e.g., if the child does not want to ask the shopkeeper a question, the parent will do it for him or her). Of course, when parents do this, their children never learn that nothing bad is likely to happen if they do it themselves, or that they can do it on their own. Parents are taught to encourage their children to "fight their own battles" and be more autonomous.

Children are taught that whereas some rewards come from others, they can also reward themselves. The concept of positive self-talk, as a reward, is introduced. For example, children learn how to reward themselves by saying positive things, such as "I did a good job." Rewarding effort and not just a positive outcome is emphasized.

Gradual Exposure

Exposure is considered a key component in the treatment of social anxiety. The rationale of exposure is that one must face the fear to fight it. In exposure, children face fears gradually, working from lesser fears to greater fears. A hierarchy of fears/worries is devised. The feared situations are placed in order of least fearful to most fearful. Stepladders are then created for each fear on the hierarchy: The fear is broken down into simple steps. For example, if a child is fearful that other children will think he or she is stupid for asking a silly question or answering incorrectly, then the therapist first determines what makes the situation more difficult for the child (e.g., asking a question in front of the teacher may be easier than answering a question in front of the whole class, or spelling might be easier than math). The first step on the stepladder might be to ask a spelling question quietly, in front of the teacher only. Each step then becomes increasingly difficult, such as answering a spelling question to which the child knows the answer in front of a few children and asking the teacher a math question. The most difficult step on the hierarchy might to get an answer wrong deliberately in front of the whole class.

The purpose of the stepladder is for children to face their fear and learn (1) that they can cope, (2) that what they thought was going to happen (e.g., look stupid) is not likely, and (3) that even if the worst does happen, they can handle the consequences. Children must successfully face the fear before progressing to the next fear on the hierarchy. Children are encouraged to stay in the feared situation until they learn that "nothing bad happened." Repetition of exposure to the feared situation/stimulus is essential.

Exposure may take many forms, such as imaginal (imagining the feared situation or stimulus), symbolic (using pictures or props), and *in vivo* (actually being in the feared situation or with the feared stimuli). The first exposure is best attempted in the therapy setting and continued by the child for homework between sessions.

Social Skills; Assertiveness; Dealing with Teasing and Bullying

Children who require social skills training are taught specific skills to appear more confident in social situations: confident posture (e.g., not slouching), appropriate tone and volume of voice (e.g., not quiet and in a monotone), and appropriate eye contact (e.g., not always looking away or at the ground). The therapist can demonstrate the appropriate use of these skills before children are given the opportunity to practice. Children are also taught the difference among assertive, passive, and aggressive behaviors through examples and role plays. Practice between sessions is emphasized.

Many children with anxiety also experience problems with being teased and or bullied. Anxious children often become the target of teasing, because they become upset and react in a way that attracts more teasing. Children are taught strategies to respond in a way that instead shows they are confident and not bothered by the teasing. To do this effectively, children need to be competent in the social and assertiveness skills mentioned earlier. The child can develop good "comeback" lines for certain comments and practice them in safe situations. When the bullying becomes violent in any way, we strongly advocate a solid response from parents and from the school that punishes bullying behavior and promotes healthy relationships between peers.

THE PROCESS OF TREATMENT: STEP-BY-STEP GUIDELINES

The following pages outline the session-by-session treatment for Hailey and her family. In the program delivered in an individual format, each session involves Hailey and both her parents.

Session 1

The purpose of Session 1 is to build rapport, provide the treatment rationale, normalize anxiety, introduce the link between thoughts and feelings, and discuss the bodily symptoms associated with anxiety.

Because Hailey is very shy talking to new people, no pressure is put on her to talk in the first session. Instead, to start the session the therapist chooses to play a "get to know you" game with the family, asking family members some non-anxiety-related questions from a card (e.g., "Who takes out the garbage in your house?"). Family members get to ask the therapist

questions from the cards as well. During the game, Hailey begins to participate by answering a couple of questions.

Following the game, the therapist provides the treatment rationale and
informs the family of what to expect throughout the program. Then the therapist spends time with the parents and Hailey separately. During the time with
Hailey's parents, the therapist reiterates the treatment rationale. Hailey's
mother is particularly concerned about "where anxiety comes from," so the
therapist provides some information about the causes of social anxiety and
emphasizes that the causes of anxiety are not as important as what is needed
now to reduce Hailey's anxiety. Importantly, the family needs to know that
the program will help Hailey to face gradually the social situations she has
been avoiding, and assist in changing Hailey's environment to help her
approach rather than avoid these situations. Prompted by the therapist, the
parents generate three specific goals for the treatment program: (1) for Hailey
to be able to ask a friend over to play without getting anxious, (2) for Hailey
to be able to talk in class without getting worried, and (3) for Hailey to take
less time getting ready in the morning. They also add a fourth goal: to be less
frustrated with Hailey when she gets anxious.

During their time alone, the therapist asks Hailey to name three things
she would like to be able to do at the end of the program. Hailey reports that
she would like (1) not to spend her breaks at school on her own; (2) to have a
new friend; and (3) to be able to talk in class without getting worried. The
therapist then introduces the concept of feelings and discusses a range of different feelings, including anxiety and fear. The "worry scale" is introduced: a
0- to 10-point scale that Hailey will use to describe how severe her anxiety/
worry is: 0, *No worry at all*; 10, *The most worry she has ever felt*. The therapist asks Hailey to think about different situations that correspond with different ratings on the worry scale. For example, Hailey says that she feels a "2"
when the teacher asks a question she definitely knows the answer to and an
"8" when she is asked to read in front of the class.

Using the cartoons from the workbook, the therapist introduces a discussion about "thoughts" (see Figure 2.3). The cartoons help Hailey to consider
that different people might have different thoughts in the same situation, and
that certain thoughts are associated with certain feelings. For example, if
Hailey thinks, "The kids are going to laugh at me" when she is giving "news"
in front of the class, then she feels anxious. But if she thinks, "I can't wait to
see Julia's face when I tell her about what I did on the weekend," then Hailey
might feel excited. Hailey picks up on the link between thoughts and feelings
very quickly, so they begin to talk about what happens in Hailey's body when
she feels anxious. The therapist shows Hailey an outline of a body and asks
her to draw the feelings she gets in her body when she has to speak up in class
or talk to someone she does not know. To help Hailey feel less anxious, the
therapist completes a drawing about her own physical feelings when she is
nervous. The therapist and Hailey share their pictures. The therapist normalizes Hailey's bodily feelings (butterflies in her tummy, tense shoulders, and

Situation: You're asked to give a talk in class

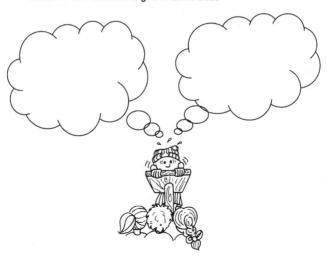

FIGURE 2.3. Thought cartoon. From Lyneham, Abbott, Wignall, and Rapee (2003). Copyright 2003 by Macquarie University Anxiety Research Unit. Reprinted by permission.

shaky legs) and discusses the important role that these sensations have in keeping her alive.

At the end of the session, Hailey shows her parents what she has learned. The therapist gives Hailey a practice task for the week, which is to record daily her thoughts and her feelings (using the worry scale) during situations that occur during the day. The therapist introduces a reward system for Hailey's practice tasks: Each time she completes her practice, she can choose a sticker to put on her book.

Session 2

The purpose of Session 2 is to introduce cognitive restructuring/"detective" thinking. To start the session, the therapist reviews the family's week, as well as Hailey's practice tasks.

Hailey and her family report a stressful weekend. According to Hailey's dad, they had to attend a family function on Sunday, and Hailey had taken a long time to get ready and made the family run late. Her dad reported that Hailey had a tantrum just before they were leaving and did not want to go to the function. Hailey's mom ended up staying at home with Hailey, while the rest of the family went to the function. In her practice task, Hailey reports that she was angry that her dad was rushing her, and that she was feeling worried ("6" on the worry scale) that one of her cousins would make a comment about what she was wearing. Hailey had done a good job of recording her feelings and her thoughts.

The therapist says that they will come back to this situation at the end of the session, after they learn "detective" thinking. Hailey is rewarded for completing her practice.

The therapist introduces cognitive restructuring to the parents alone. The therapist reviews a couple of examples with the parents, using situations in their own lives, and encourages the parents to use these thinking strategies on their own worry and stress. The parents acknowledge that these strategies will be useful in their day-to-day lives, because they both tend to think the worst in difficult situations. Hailey's dad feels that he often gets too stressed by deadlines at work. Hailey's mom identifies that she worries a lot about the kids, particularly Hailey, and also a lot about herself and what other people think of her.

During the child-alone part of the session, the therapist asks Hailey to think of her favorite cartoon/fictional character who is good at solving mysteries or collecting evidence. Hailey chooses Hermione from the Harry Potter novels by J. K. Rowling. Just like Hermione, Hailey is encouraged to look for the truth or the evidence for her thoughts. Using a detective thinking sheet with three columns (Situation, Thoughts, and Evidence), the therapist leads Hailey through her first detective work.

THERAPIST: Sometimes we have thoughts that lead us astray a little, and while we think they might be true at first, if we look for evidence for the thoughts, then they might not be as true as we thought. Hermione is pretty good at looking up facts. We are going to use her brains to help us. Let's take an easy situation to start with. Let's just say you hear a noise downstairs at night time when everyone is in bed. Let's write that in the first column. Let's just say you feel scared, about an 8 on the worry scale. Hailey, what do you think you might be thinking at that time?

HAILEY: That there is a burglar in the house.

THERAPIST: Excellent. If you thought there was a burglar in the house you would be pretty scared right? OK, so let's write that in the second column and get Hermione to help us work out whether this thought is true or not. A first question might be "Do we know for sure?"

HAILEY: No, because we can't see them.

THERAPIST: OK. So the first thought was "it is a burglar." But we don't know for sure, right? What else could the noise be?

HAILEY: It could be Mom getting a drink of water.

THERAPIST: Yes. Or it could be the cat.

HAILEY: Or it could be the wind knocking something over, or the roof making a funny noise.

THERAPIST: OK. So there are heaps of things that the noise could be. Another question you could ask yourself is "Have I heard this noise before, and if so, what happened?"

HAILEY: Yeah, 'cause I hear noises a lot when I am lying awake at night.

THERAPIST: And what are the noises from?

HAILEY: Usually just the house making funny sounds, or sometimes it is a noise outside.

THERAPIST: What other questions do you think Hermione might ask to work out what the noise is?

HAILEY: She would go out and check out what the noise is.

THERAPIST: She probably would, wouldn't she? I wonder if she would ask herself, "Have we ever had a burglar in our house before?" What would you say if you asked yourself that question?

HAILEY: Never. We've never had a breakin. My cousin did though. They didn't take anything, but my auntie had to get new locks on all the windows.

THERAPIST: OK, so your cousin has had a breakin but you haven't. How likely do you think it is that there would be a burglar in your house then?

HAILEY: Not very likely. Our neighborhood is pretty safe.

THERAPIST: Now we have a lot of evidence about this noise, don't we? We could go and check on the noise, but let's just say we couldn't. We have some good evidence that it is pretty unlikely that it is a burglar, and the noise is most likely something else. So let's think of a "realistic thought" that you could have in this situation?

HAILEY: No one is breaking in. It's just a funny noise.

THERAPIST: And what do you think your worry rating would be if you had this thought?

HAILEY: A zero.

In this example, the therapist uses a less threatening situation to get Hailey started with the detective thinking. Hailey then tries a more difficult situation to practice her new detective skills: answering a question in class. In this situation, the anxious thought is "I will get the question wrong and everyone will laugh." The therapist works through this example with Hailey. First, they work on the evidence for the thought, "I will get it wrong," then separately, "If I get it wrong, everyone will laugh." The therapist gives Hailey lots of prompt questions, such as "What happens when other people in the class get the answer wrong?," "How many times have you got the answer wrong before?", and "What else could happen?" The therapist discusses with Hailey that sometimes it is easy to fall into the trap of mind reading, that is, thinking you know what other people are thinking. The therapist challenges Hailey's belief that she knows what other people are thinking.

At the end of the session, Hailey shows her parents what she has learned, and the family tries one more example. Modeling for the parents, the therapist leads Hailey through her thoughts from the previous Sunday and examines the evidence for her thought that her cousins would comment about what she was wearing. At the end of the exercise, there is some evidence that, yes, maybe her cousin might have said something about what she was wearing, but it was more likely to be a positive than a negative comment. Hailey has brought her worry down from a "6" to a "3." The therapist then briefly explores the "So what?" of the situation, and asks Hailey to think about the following reaction: "Well, so what if my cousin did say something negative about what I was wearing? What would be so bad about that?"

The practice task for the week is to use the detective thinking sheet five times to get as much practice as possible. The parents are also encouraged to complete a realistic thinking sheet on their worries during the week.

Session 3

The purpose of this session is to review the detective thinking skills, to introduce rewards, and to introduce contingency management to the parents. Session 3 is primarily spent with the parents.

For example, Hailey's practice tasks are reviewed and discussed. Hailey has been able to use her detective thinking during the week. At times she has struggled to come up with more than a couple of pieces of evidence, so the therapist helps Hailey think of more evidence to write down. The family reports a very stressful week. Hailey had a test during the week and panicked the night before, because she had trouble understanding one of the test topics. Hailey had an argument with her parents, because she could not understand what they were saying to her. Her parents tried to use the detective thinking with her, telling Hailey that she always did well and it was only a test. The parents report that the realistic thinking "just didn't work." The therapist works through this example with Hailey's parents, reminding them that at first it is much easier to practice the detective skills after or before rather than "during" the situation. The therapist encourages them not to provide the evidence for Hailey, but to prompt her with the questions and sit down together to work on the sheet in a more systematic way.

During the session with the parents, the therapist reviews the principles of contingency management. Both parents admit that they find it extremely difficult to be consistent with Hailey at home. Hailey's mother identifies with Hailey's feelings and reports that she is easy on Hailey and does not make her do the things she does not want to do. Her dad, on the other hand, reports that he gets really frustrated with her and cannot understand why she is worried. The parents admit that this pattern leads to a lot tension between them as a couple, and they often argue about how to respond to Hailey. The therapist suggests that this way of responding usually means that Hailey avoids the situation. During this session, the therapist encourages the parents to decide together how to resolve issues with Hailey. The problem-solving technique is introduced at this point as a way to assist Hailey's parents to work as a united front. The therapist encourages them to work toward a solution that will help Hailey approach rather than avoid the situation. Both parents report that they tend to do more for Hailey than for their other children, because she is the youngest and is more touchy and sensitive. The therapist discusses with the family the pros and cons of encouraging Hailey to be more independent.

During this session, the therapist also encourages both parents to continue using their realistic thinking sheets, so that they can model courageous behavior. Hailey's mother talks about the difficulty she experiences in social situations and how she, like Hailey, would prefer to stay at home. The therapist encourages Hailey's mother to use the strategies she has been learning to face her own social fears in the coming weeks.

The use of rewards is introduced both with Hailey and her parents in this session. During her time with Hailey, the therapist encourages her to praise herself for times when she tries hard in a test or is brave in answering even the easiest of questions. The family also discusses a series of rewards that Hailey could use later in the program, such as choosing what to eat for dinner, having her favorite dessert, going to the movies with her dad, going on a shopping trip to buy a new top with her mom (and no sibling), and, being able to stay up as late as her older siblings.

The practice task for this week is for Hailey to record times when she rewards herself. The therapist sets a practice task for Hailey's parents that involves using the problem-solving techniques to resolve a difficult situation during the week with Hailey.

Session 4

The purpose of this session is to introduce gradual exposure and to review the practice tasks.

Hailey forgot to do her practice task during the week, so the therapist and Hailey complete the practice in session. No reward is given. Hailey's parents report some success with the problem-solving technique and that they were able to respond more consistently to Hailey when she became upset about her homework during the week. They also started up a new family system for the chores, using the strategies that had been discussed.

The therapist introduces the concept of gradual exposure by using a role-play example. She pretends she is scared of heights and has been invited to a friend's birthday party on the top floor of a skyscraper in the city. She really wants to go but is too scared. The therapist asks the family to help her. Hailey suggests that she use her detective thinking. The therapist encourages Hailey's suggestion, then asks whether there is anything else she could do. Together the family members suggest that the therapist practice going up and down in the elevators of smaller buildings before the party as practice for the skyscraper.

I find these things really hard to do	Asking a question in class
	Answering a question in class
	Talking to someone I don't know
	Taking a test
	Joining in with other kids at lunch
I find these things hard to do	Reading aloud
	Asking my friend from my old school to come over
	Joining in with other kids at recess
	Getting an answer wrong
	Having messy homework
I find these things make me a little worried	Answering questions that I know the answer to
	Asking a friend over to play
	Buying something at the shop

FIGURE 2.4. Hailey's fears and worries list. Reprinted with permission from Lyneham, Abbott, Wignall, and Rapee (2003). Copyright 2003 by Ronald M. Rapee. Reprinted by permission.

Using this example, the therapist talks about the principles of gradual exposure and begins to develop a list of fears for Hailey (see Figure 2.4). From this list the therapist and the family choose something relatively easy on this list to begin developing the first stepladder: "Buying something at the shop." The therapist asks Hailey and her parents a number of questions to help determine what makes "buying something at the shop" easier rather than harder, so that Hailey can manipulate the steps easily. Hailey reports that the large shopping center is scarier than the corner shop. Having her mom there with her makes it easier, as does having the right change and going when it is not busy, and not having to ask for help. Figure 2.5 shows Hailey's exposure stepladder. At the end of the session, the family decides to complete up to Step 4 by the next session.

Step 1. Go to the corner store with Mom to buy milk, when it is not busy with the right change.
Reward: Choose what to have for dinner that night.

Achieved
☐

Step 2. Go the corner store to buy bread, when it is not busy with the right change, while Mom waits at the back of the store.
Reward: Choose what to have for dessert that night.

Achieved
☐

Step 3. Go to the corner store with a $5 bill to buy milk/bread on a busy day, while Mom waits in the car.
Reward: Choose what to have for dessert that night.

Achieved
☐

Step 4. Go to the corner store with Mom and ask if they sell my favorite chocolate.
Reward: My favorite chocolate.

Achieved
☐

Step 5. Go to the mall with Mom on a quiet day, and buy a drink from a shop with a $5 bill.
Reward: Choice of drink.

Achieved
☐

Step 6. Go to the mall with Mom on a quiet day, and go into the supermarket and ask the shopkeeper if they sell my favorite chocolate.
Reward: My favorite chocolate.

Achieved
☐

Step 7. Go to the mall and go into the supermarket while Mom waits outside and buy a magazine.
Reward: My choice of magazine.

Achieved
☐

Step 8. Go to the mall and go into a store on my own with a budget, choose a top, and ask the shop assistant if they have my size.
Reward: Buy the top.

Achieved
☐

FIGURE 2.5. Exposure stepladder: "Buying something from the shop."

Sessions 5–9

The purpose of these sessions is to continue working on gradual exposure. Additionally, in Sessions 7 and 8, the therapist works with the child on assertiveness strategies, and dealing with teasing and bullying. Each week the therapist reviews the stepladder tasks set the previous week.

Hailey is making good progress with her "buying something from the shop" stepladder and adds another step at the end of the ladder, in which she is required to buy something from the shop and not have the correct change. In this exposure task, Hailey is able to face her fear that she will not have the exact amount of money. Before completing this task, the therapist and Hailey come up with a plan to help Hailey feel less anxious when the shopkeeper tells her she does not have the correct change.

In Session 5, the family starts work on a second stepladder: "Answering questions in class." With this stepladder, Hailey starts with "Answering questions that I know" and works up to being able to "Deliberately answer the question incorrectly." The purpose of these steps is to help Hailey realize that it is OK to get the answer wrong. By the end of Session 9, Hailey is working through a number of stepladders, including "Joining in with other children," "Getting ready more quickly," "Taking tests," "Reading aloud," "Asking a friend over," and "Having messy homework."

During these latter sessions, the therapist and Hailey continue to work on detective thinking. In particular, they work on challenging Hailey's core beliefs that people will be mean to her and that she is unlikable. Using the detective sheets, Hailey is able to generate evidence that she is a likable person, and even if someone does not like her, it is not the end of the world.

In Sessions 7–9, the therapist introduces assertiveness training. Hailey is quite able to use appropriate social skills when she is not anxious, but she becomes less confident and less able to use her skills in anxiety-provoking situations. The therapist discusses with Hailey the difference between assertive, passive, and aggressive behavior. Hailey and the therapist act out different scenarios illustrating assertive, passive, and aggressive responses. Hailey identifies that she almost always acts in a passive way (except with her siblings), because she does not want people to think she is mean. The therapist suggests that by being assertive, Hailey could challenge this thought and in the process be more likely to have people like and respect her, and to have her own needs met rather than always making sure others' needs are met. The therapist and Hailey develop another stepladder for being assertive (see Figure 2.6).

Although teasing is no longer a big issue for Hailey, the therapist works with her to develop strategies to deal with teasing in the future. Using role plays in which the therapist first models an appropriate response, Hailey is able to act out assertive responses to the teasing, with the intent of letting the bully know she does not care about what the kids are saying.

During the second half of the program, it becomes increasingly important for Hailey's mom also to develop a hierarchy regarding her own social fears. The therapist assists Hailey's mother in work on a series of stepladders to increase her confidence in social situations. Some of the steps include starting conversations with family members at family gatherings, not spending all the time in the kitchen at parties/functions, inviting people over for dinner, asking an old friend out for coffee, confronting a colleague at work, and talking face-to-face rather than e-mailing the boss with an issue about work hours. In fact, Hailey and her mother work on the assertiveness stepladder together.

Session 10

The purpose of Session 10 is to review the strategies learned throughout the program, discuss relapse prevention, review goals, and set future objectives.

Step 1. Go out to a pizza restaurant with the family and ask if we can have half a pizza with mushrooms and half without.
Reward: Choose the pizza.

Achieved
☐

Step 2. Go to the store with Mom and try on several clothes without buying anything.
Reward: One point toward going to the movies with Dad (5 points for a movie).

Achieved
☐

Step 3. Ask a girl at school if you could borrow a CD that you like.
Reward: One point toward going to the movies with Dad.

Achieved
☐

Step 4. Tell my parents if I didn't like part of the dinner.
Reward: Choose dessert.

Achieved
☐

Step 5. When talking with Gina, tell her what I think of the band she is talking about, even if I don't like them.
Reward: One point toward going to the movies with Dad.

Achieved
☐

Step 6. Go to a restaurant and send back something that I ordered.
Reward: One point toward going to the movies with Dad.

Achieved
☐

Step 7. Go into a clothes shop and ask to put something on hold and then go back half an hour later saying that I have decided against it.
Reward: One point toward going to the movies with Dad.

Achieved
☐

Step 8. Return something (e.g., clothes, CD) at the store.
Reward: Buy something different.

Achieved
☐

FIGURE 2.6. "Being assertive."

Hailey and her parents report that Hailey has achieved the goals they set out to achieve in Session 1. Hailey reports that she still feels a little anxious doing these things, but much less so. The family discusses future stepladders that Hailey might work on, including answering the phone. They also feel that Hailey needs to continue working on the last few steps of some of the stepladders.

The therapist gives a number of new scenarios to the family members and asks that they develop a treatment plan if the situations arise in the future. For example, the therapist asks Hailey to imagine that school camp is coming up and she feels really nervous. What would she do? Or what if she started feeling scared whenever she got into an elevator? What would she do?

The purpose of these scenarios is to review the skills the family members have learned and to encourage them to apply these skills to future, unknown scenarios. During this process, the therapist encourages Hailey first to come up with answers, without the help of her parents.

CONCLUSION

This chapter has provided an overview of the nature, assessment, and treatment of children with social anxiety. Using a cognitive-behavioral approach as the first line of attack, therapists can help children and their parents to feel more equipped to handle anxiety-provoking situations. As indicated in the literature, such intervention can go a long way in preventing future distress and increasing the child's ability to cope with stressful situations. By approaching rather than avoiding social situations, socially anxious children learn that their negative expectations are unlikely to occur, and even if the consequences are negative, they are able to cope.

Children for whom social situations continue to be problematic may need to continue treatment to achieve more progress on their hierarchy of fears. A number of obstacles to treatment may need to be addressed before they achieve progress. In the case study we presented, for example, Hailey's progress might not have been as rapid if her mother's anxiety had not been targeted. In addition, the inclusion of the parents in this program allowed the therapist to address the parent's inconsistency in the sessions. Without this change, Hailey might have continued to escape anxiety-provoking situations. This family began to work on increasing Hailey's independence in other ways as well. These factors are likely to ensure that Hailey's progress during treatment is maintained over the long term.

REFERENCES

American Psychiatric Association. (1994). *Diagnostic and statistical manual of mental disorders* (4th ed.). Washington, DC: Author.

Asendorpf, J. B. (1990). Beyond social withdrawal: Shyness, unsociability, and peer avoidance. *Human Development, 33,* 250–259.

Barrett, P. M. (1998). Evaluation of cognitive-behavioral group treatments for childhood anxiety disorders. *Journal of Clinical Child Psychology, 27,* 459–468.

Barrett, P. M., Dadds, M. R., & Rapee, R. M. (1996). Family treatment of childhood anxiety: A controlled trial. *Journal of Consulting and Clinical Psychology, 64,* 333–342.

Barrett, P. M., Duffy, A. L., Dadds, M. R., & Rapee, R. M. (2001). Cognitive-behavioral treatment of anxiety disorders in children: Long-term (6-year) follow-up. *Journal of Consulting and Clinical Psychology, 69,* 135–141.

Barrett, P. M., Rapee, R. M., Dadds, M. M., & Ryan, S. M. (1996). Family enhancement of cognitive style in anxious and aggressive children. *Journal of Abnormal Child Psychology, 24*(2), 187–203.

Beidel, D. C., Turner, S. M., & Dancu, C. V. (1985). Physiological, cognitive and behavioral aspects of social anxiety. *Behaviour Research and Therapy, 23,* 109–117.

Beidel, D. C., Turner, S. M., Hamlin, K., & Morris, T. L. (2000). The Social Phobia and Anxiety Inventory for Children: External and discriminative validity. *Behavior Therapy, 31*(1), 75–87.

Beidel, D. C., Turner, S. M., & Morris, T. L. (1995). A new inventory to assess childhood social anxiety and phobia: The Social Phobia and Anxiety Inventory for Children. *Psychological Assessment, 7*(1), 73–79.

Beidel, D. C., Turner, S. M., & Morris, T. L. (2000). Behavioral treatment of childhood social phobia. *Journal of Consulting and Clinical Psychology, 68,* 1072–1080.

Berman, S. L., Weems, C. F., Silverman, W. K., & Kurtines, W. M. (2000). Predictors of outcome in exposure-based cognitive and behavioral treatments for phobic and anxiety disorders in children. *Behavior Therapy, 31,* 713–731.

Birmaher, B., Axelson, D. A., Monk, K., Kalas, C., Clark, D. B., Ehmann, M., et al. (2003). Fluoxetine for the treatment of childhood anxiety disorders. *Journal of the American Academy of Child and Adolescent Psychiatry, 42,* 415–423.

Birmaher, B., Khetarpal, S., Brent, D., Cully, M., Balach, L., Kaufman, J., et al. (1997). The Screen for Child Anxiety Related Emotional Disorders (SCARED): Scale construction and psychometric characteristics. *Journal of the American Academy of Child and Adolescent Psychiatry, 36*(4), 545–553.

Black, B. (1996). Social anxiety and selective mutism. In L. J. Dickstein, M. B. Riba, and J. M. Oldham (Eds.), *Review of psychiatry* (Vol. 15, pp. 469–495). Washington, DC: American Psychiatric Press.

Black, B., & Uhde, T. W. (1995). Psychiatric characteristics of children with selective mutism: A pilot study. *Journal of the American Academy of Child and Adolescent Psychiatry, 34*(7), 847–856.

Bogels, S. M., & Lamers, C. T. J. (2002). The causal role of self-awareness in blushing-anxious, socially-anxious, and social phobic individuals. *Behaviour Research and Therapy, 40*(12), 1367–1384.

Brady, E. U., & Kendall, P. C. (1992). Comorbidity of anxiety and depression in children and adolescents. *Psychological Bulletin, 111,* 244–255.

Briggs, S. R. (1988). Shyness: Introversion or neuroticism? *Journal of Research in Personality, 22,* 290–307.

Bruch, M. A., & Cheek, J. M. (1995). Developmental factors in childhood and adolescent shyness. In R. G. Heimberg, M. R. Liebowitz, D. A. Hope, & F. R. Schneier (Eds.), *Social phobia: Diagnosis, assessment, and treatment* (pp. 163–184). New York: Guilford Press.

Buss, A. H. (1980). *Self-consciousness and social anxiety.* San Francisco: Freeman.

Buss, A. H., & Plomin, R. (1984). *Temperament: Early developing personality traits.* Hillsdale, NJ: Erlbaum.

Campbell, M. A., & Rapee, R. M. (1994). The nature of feared outcome representations in children. *Journal of Abnormal Child Psychology, 22*(1), 99–111.

Cartwright-Hatton, S., Roberts, C., Chitsabesan, P., Fothergill, C., & Harrington, R. (2004). Systematic review of the efficacy of cognitive behaviour therapies for childhood and adolescent anxiety disorders. *British Journal of Clinical Psychology, 43,* 421–436.

Caspi, A., Elder, G. H., Jr., & Bem, D. J. (1988). Moving away from the world: Life-course patterns of shy children. *Developmental Psychology, 24,* 824–831.

Chavira, D. A., Stein, M. B., Bailey, K., & Stein, M. T. (2004). Child anxiety in primary care: Prevalent but untreated. *Depression and Anxiety, 20,* 155–164.

Chavira, D. A., Stein, M. B., & Malcarne, V. L. (2002). Scrutinizing the relationship between shyness and social phobia. *Journal of Anxiety Disorders, 16,* 585–598.

Chu, B. C., & Kendall, P. C. (2004). Positive association of child involvement and treatment outcome within a manual-based cognitive-behavioral treatment for children with anxiety. *Journal of Consulting and Clinical Psychology, 72,* 821–829.

Cobham, V. E., Dadds, M. R., & Spence, S. H. (1998). The role of parental anxiety in the treatment of childhood anxiety. *Journal of Consulting and Clinical Psychology, 66,* 893–905.

Cohen, P., Cohen, J., & Brook, J. (1993). An epidemiological study of disorders in late childhood and adolescence: II. Persistence of disorders. *Journal of Child Psychology and Psychiatry, 34*(6), 869–877.

Comer, J. S., & Kendall, P. C. (2004). A symptom-level examination of parent–child agreement in the diagnosis of anxious youths. *Journal of the American Academy of Child and Adolescent Psychiatry, 43*(7), 878–886.

Compton, S. N., March, J. S., Brent, D., Albano, A. M., Weersing, R., & Curry, J. (2004). Cognitive-behavioral psychotherapy for anxiety and depressive disorders in children and adolescents: An evidence-based medicine review. *Journal of the American Academy of Child and Adolescent Psychiatry, 43*(8), 930–959.

Crawford, A. M., & Manassis, K. (2001). Familial predictors of treatment outcome in childhood anxiety disorders. *Journal of the American Academy of Child and Adolescent Psychiatry, 40,* 1182–1189.

Cunningham, C. E., McHolm, A., Boyle, M. H., & Patel, S. (2004). Behavioral and emotional adjustment, family functioning, academic performance, and social relationships in children with selective mutism. *Journal of Child Psychology and Psychiatry, 45,* 1–10.

DiBartolo, P. M., Albano, A. M., Barlow, D. H., & Heimberg, R. G. (1998). Cross-informant agreement in the assessment of social phobia in youth. *Journal of Abnormal Child Psychology, 26*(3), 213–220.

Eisen, A. R., Spasaro, S. A., Brien, L. K., Kearney, C. A., & Albano, A. M. (2004). Parental expectancies and childhood anxiety disorders: Psychometric properties of the Parental Expectancies Scale. *Journal of Anxiety Disorders, 18*(2), 89–109.

Essau, C. A., Muris, P., & Ederer, E. M. (2002). Reliability and validity of the Spence Children's Anxiety Scale and the Screen for Child Anxiety Related Emotional Disorders in German children. *Journal of Behavior Therapy and Experimental Psychiatry, 33*(1), 1–18.

Fairburn, C. G., Shafran, R., & Cooper, Z. (1999). A cognitive behavioural theory of anorexia nervosa. *Behaviour and Research Therapy, 37*(1), 1–13.

Fisher, P. H., Masia-Warner, C., & Klein, R. G. (2004). Skills for social and academic success: A school-based intervention for social anxiety disorder in adolescents. *Clinical Child and Family Psychology Review, 7,* 241–249.

Flannery-Schroeder, E., & Kendall, P. C. (2000). Group and individual cognitive-behavioral treatments for youth with anxiety disorders: A randomized clinical trial. *Cognitive Therapy and Research, 24,* 251–278.

Foley, D., Rutter, M., Pickles, A., Angold, A., Maes, H., Silberg, J., et al. (2004). Informant disagreement for separation anxiety disorder. *Journal of the American Academy of Child and Adolescent Psychiatry, 43*(4), 452–460.

Furman, W., & Buhrmester, D. (1992). Age and sex differences in perceptions of networks of personal relationships. *Child Development, 63,* 103–115.

Gar, N. S., Hudson, J. L., & Rapee, R. M. (2005). Family factors and the development of anxiety disorders. In *Psychopathology and the family* (pp. 125–145). Oxford, UK: Elsevier.

Garber, J. (2005). Depression and the family. In J. L. Hudson & R. M. Rapee (Eds.), *Psychopathology and the family* (pp. 225–280). Oxford, UK: Elsevier.

Ginsburg, G. S., La Greca, A. M., & Silverman, W. K. (1998). Social anxiety in children with anxiety disorders: Relation with social and emotional functioning. *Journal of Abnormal Child Psychology, 26*(3), 175–185.

Greco, L. A., & Morris, T. L. (2005). Factors influencing the link between social anxiety and peer acceptance: Contributions of social skills and close friendships during middle childhood. *Behavior Therapy, 36*(2), 197–205.

Hackmann, A., Surawy, C., & Clark, D. M. (1998). Seeing yourself though others' eyes: A study of spontaneously occurring images in social phobia. *Behavioural and Cognitive Psychotherapy, 26*, 3–12.

Hankin, B. L., Abramson, L. Y., Silva, P. A., McGee, R., & Moffitt, T. E. (1998). Development of depression from preadolescence to young adulthood: Emerging gender differences in a 10-year longitudinal study. *Journal of Abnormal Psychology, 107*(1), 128–140.

Harrist, A. W., Zaia, A. F., Bates, J. E., Dodge, K. A., & Pettit, G. S. (1997). Subtypes of social withdrawal in early childhood: Sociometric status and social-cognitive differences across four years. *Child Development, 68*(2), 278–294.

Hayward, C., Varady, S., Albano, A. M., Thienemann, M., Henderson, L., & Schatzberg, A. F. (2000). Cognitive-behavioral group therapy for social phobia in female adolescents: Results of a pilot study. *Journal of the American Academy of Child and Adolescent Psychiatry, 39*, 721–726.

Henderson, L., & Zimbardo, P. (2001). Shyness, social anxiety, and social phobia. In S. G. Hofmann & P. M. DiBartolo (Eds.), *From social anxiety to social phobia: Multiple perspectives* (pp. 46–64). Needham Heights, MA: Allyn & Bacon.

Herjanic, B., & Reich, W. (1982). Development of a structured psychiatric interview for children: Agreement between child and parent on individual symptoms. *Journal of Abnormal Child Psychology, 10*(3), 307–324.

Hinz, L. D., & Williamson, D. A. (1987). Bulimia and depression: A review of the affective variant hypothesis. *Psychological Bulletin, 102*, 150–158.

Hoek, H. W., & van Hoeken, D. (2003). Review of the prevalence and incidence of eating disorders. *International Journal of Eating Disorders, 34*(4), 383–396.

Hudson, J. L. (2005). Efficacy of cognitive behavioural therapy for children and adolescents with anxiety disorders. *Behaviour Change, 22*(2), 55–70.

Hudson, J. L., & Kendall, P. C. (2002). Showing you can do it: The use of homework assignments in cognitive behavioral treatment for child and adolescent anxiety disorders. *Journal of Clinical Psychology, 58*, 525–534.

Hudson, J. L., & Rapee, R. M. (2001). Parent–child interactions and the anxiety disorders: An observational analysis. *Behaviour Research and Therapy, 39*, 1411–1427.

Hudson, J. L., & Rapee, R. M. (2004). From anxious temperament to disorder: An etiological model of generalized anxiety disorder. In R. G. Heimberg, C. L. Turk, & D. S. Mennin (Eds.), *Generalized anxiety disorder: Advances in research and practice.* New York: Guilford Press.

Jaenicke, C., Hammen, C., Zupan, B., Hiroto, D., Gordon, D., Adrian, C., et al. (1987). Cognitive vulnerability in children at risk for depression. *Journal of Abnormal Child Psychology, 15,* 559–572.

Kagan, J., Reznick, J. S., Clarke, C., Snidman, N., & Garcia-Coll, C. (1984). Behavioral inhibition to the unfamiliar. *Child Development, 55,* 2212–2225.

Kagan, J., Reznick, J. S., & Snidman, N. (1987). The physiology and psychology of behavioral inhibition in children. *Child Development, 58,* 1459–1473.

Kaslow, N. J., Rehm, L. P., & Siegel, A. W. (1984). Social-cognitive and cognitive correlates of depression in children. *Journal of Abnormal Child Psychology, 12,* 605–620.

Kendall, P. C. (1994). Treating anxiety disorders in children: Results of a randomized clinical trial. *Journal of Consulting and Clinical Psychology, 62,* 100–110.

Kendall, P. C., Flannery-Schroeder, E., Panichelli-Mindel, S. M., Southam-Gerow, M., Henin, A., & Warman, M. (1997). Therapy for youths with anxiety disorders: A second randomized clinical trial. *Journal of Consulting and Clinical Psychology, 65,* 366–380.

Kendall, P. C., Safford, S., Flannery-Schroeder, E., & Webb, A. (2004). Child anxiety treatment: Outcomes in adolescence and impact on substance use and depression at 7.4-year follow-up. *Journal of Consulting and Clinical Psychology, 72,* 276–287.

Kim, J., Rapee, R. M., Oh, K. J., & Moon, H-S. (2007). *Pathways from social withdrawal during adolescence to maladjustment in young adulthood: Cross-cultural comparisons in Australian and South Korean students.* Manuscript submitted for publication.

La Greca, A. M., Dandes, S., Wick, P., Shaw, K., & Stone, W. L. (1988). Development of the Social Anxiety Scale for Children: Reliability and concurrent validity. *Journal of Clinical Child Psychology, 17,* 84–91.

La Greca, A. M., & Moore, H. H. (2005). Adolescent peer relations, friendships, and romantic relationships: Do they predict social anxiety and depression? *Journal of Clinical Child and Adolescent Psychology, 34*(1), 49–61.

La Greca, A. M., & Prinstein, M. J. (1999). The peer group. In W. K. Silverman & T. H. Ollendick (Eds.), *Developmental issues in the clinical treatment of children and adolescents* (pp. 171–198). Needham Heights, MA: Allyn & Bacon.

La Greca, A. M., & Stone, W. L. (1993). Social Anxiety Scale for Children—Revised: Factor structure and concurrent validity. *Journal of Clinical Child Psychology, 22*(1), 17–27.

Langley, A. K., Bergman, R., McCracken, J., & Piacentini, J. C. (2004). Impairment in childhood anxiety disorders: Preliminary examination of the Child Anxiety Impact Scale—Parent Version. *Journal of Child and Adolescent Psychopharmacology, 14*(1), 105–114.

Langley, A. K., Bergman, R., & Piacentini, J. C. (2002). Assessment of childhood anxiety. *International Review of Psychiatry, 14*(2), 102–113.

Last, C. G., Strauss, C. C., & Francis, G. (1987). Comorbidity among childhood anxiety disorders. *Journal of Nervous and Mental Disease, 175,* 726–730.

Lewinsohn, P. M., Zinbarg, R., Seeley, J. R., Lewinsohn, M., & Sack, W. H. (1997). Lifetime comorbidity among anxiety disorders and between anxiety disorders and other mental disorders in adolescents. *Journal of Anxiety Disorders, 11*(4), 377–394.

Lovibond, P. F., & Rapee, R. M. (1993). The representation of feared outcomes. *Behaviour Research and Therapy, 31,* 595–608.

Lowry-Webster, H. M., Barrett, P. M., & Dadds, M. R. (2001). A universal prevention trial of anxiety and depressive symptomatology in childhood: Preliminary data from an Australian study. *Behaviour Change, 18,* 36–50.

Lyneham, H. J., Abbott, M. J., Wignall, A., & Rapee, R. M. (2003). *The Cool Kids Program—Children's Workbook.* Sydney, Australia: MUARU, Macquarie University.

Lyneham, H. J., & Rapee, R. M. (2005). Evaluation and treatment of anxiety disorders in the general pediatric population: A clinician's guide. *Child and Adolescent Psychiatric Clinics of North America, 14,* 845–861.

Lyneham, H. J., & Rapee, R. M. (2006). Evaluation of therapist-supported parent-implemented CBT for anxiety disorders in rural children. *Behaviour Research and Therapy, 44,* 1287–1300.

Manassis, K., Hudson, J. L., Webb, A., & Albano, A. M. (2004). Beyond behavioral inhibition: Etiological factors in childhood anxiety. *Cognitive and Behavioral Practice, 11*(1), 3–12.

Manassis, K., Mendlowitz, S. L., Scapillato, D., Avery, D., Fiksenbaum, L., Freire, M., et al. (2002). Group and individual cognitive-behavioral therapy for childhood anxiety disorders: A randomized trial. *Journal of the American Academy of Child and Adolescent Psychiatry, 41,* 1423–1430.

McHolm, A. E., Cunningham, C. E., & Vanier, M. K. (2005). *Helping your child with selective mutism: Practical steps to overcome a fear of speaking.* Oakland, CA: New Harbinger.

Mendlowitz, S. L., Manassis, K., Bradley, S., Scapillato, D., Miezitis, S., & Shaw, B. F. (1999). Cognitive-behavioral group treatments in childhood anxiety disorders: The role of parental involvement. *Journal of the American Academy of Child and Adolescent Psychiatry, 38,* 1223–1229.

Mifsud, C., & Rapee, R. M. (2005). Early intervention for childhood anxiety in a school setting: Outcomes for an economically disadvantaged population. *Journal of the American Academy of Child and Adolescent Psychiatry, 44,* 996–1004.

Muris, P., Merckelbach, H., Gadet, B., Moulaert, V., & Tierney, S. (1999). Sensitivity for treatment effects of the Screen for Child Anxiety Related Emotional Disorders. *Journal of Psychopathology and Behavioral Assessment, 21*(4), 323–335.

Muris, P., Schmidt, H., Engelbrecht, P., & Perold, M. (2002). DSM-IV-defined anxiety disorder symptoms in South African children. *Journal of American Academy of Child and Adolescent Psychiatry, 41,* 1360–1368.

Nauta, M. H., Scholing, A., Rapee, R. M., Abbott, M., Spence, S. H., & Waters, A. (2004). A parent-report measure of children's anxiety: Psychometric properties and comparison with child-report in a clinic and normal sample. *Behaviour Research and Therapy, 42*(7), 813–839.

Ollendick, T. H., & Cerny, J. A. (1981). *Clinical behavior therapy with children.* New York: Plenum Press.

Ollendick, T. H., & King, N. J. (2000). Empirically supported treatments for children and adolescents. In P. L. Kendall (Ed.), *Child and adolescent therapy: Cognitive Behavioral Procedures* (pp. 386–425). New York: Guilford Press.

Otto, M. W., Pollack, M. H., Maki, K. M., Gould, R. A., Worthington, J. J., Smoller, J. W., et al. (2001). Childhood history of anxiety disorders among adults with social phobia: Rates, correlates, and comparisons with patients with panic disorder. *Depression and Anxiety, 14,* 209–213.

Phillips, S. D., & Bruch, M. A. (1988). Shyness and dysfunction in career development. *Journal of Counseling Psychology, 35,* 159–165.

Pine, D. S., Cohen, P., Gurley, D., Brook, J., & Ma, Y. (1998). The risk for early-adulthood anxiety and depressive disorders in adolescents with anxiety and depressive disorders. *Archives of General Psychiatry, 55,* 56–64.

Price, C. S., Spence, S. H., Sheffield, J., & Donovan, C. (2002). The development and psychometric properties of a measure of social and adaptive functioning for children and adolescents. *Journal of Clinical Child and Adolescent Psychology, 31*(1), 111–122.

Prior, M. (1992). Childhood temperament. *Journal of Child Psychology and Psychiatry, 33,* 249–279.

Rapee, R. M. (1998). *Overcoming shyness and social phobia: A step-by-step guide.* Northvale, NJ: Aronson.

Rapee, R. M. (2000). Group treatment of children with anxiety disorders: Outcome and predictors of treatment response. *Australian Journal of Psychology, 52*(3), 125–129.

Rapee, R. M. (2002). The development and modification of temperamental risk for anxiety disorders: Prevention of a lifetime of anxiety? *Biological Psychiatry, 52,* 947–957.

Rapee, R. M., & Abbott, M. J. (2006). Mental representation of observable attributes in people with social phobia. *Journal of Behavior Therapy and Experimental Psychiatry, 37,* 113–126.

Rapee, R. M., Barrett, P. M., Dadds, M. R., & Evans, L. (1994). Reliability of the DSM-III-R childhood anxiety disorders using structured interview: Interrater and parent–child agreement. *Journal of the American Academy of Child and Adolescent Psychiatry, 33*(7), 984–992.

Rapee, R. M., & Heimberg, R. G. (1997). A cognitive-behavioral model of anxiety in social phobia. *Behaviour Research and Therapy, 35,* 741–756.

Rapee, R. M., Kennedy, S., Ingram, M., Edwards, S. L., & Sweeney, L. (2005). Prevention and early intervention of anxiety disorders in inhibited preschool children. *Journal of Consulting and Clinical Psychology, 73*(3), 488–497.

Rapee, R. M., & Spence, S. H. (2004). The etiology of social phobia: Empirical evidence and an initial model. *Clinical Psychology Review, 24,* 737–767.

Rapee, R. M., Spence, S. H., Cobham, V. E., & Wignall, A. (2000). *Helping your anxious child: A step-by-step guide for parents.* Oakland, CA: New Harbinger.

Rapee, R. M., Wignall, A., Hudson, J. L., & Schniering, C. A. (2000). *Treating anxious children: An evidence based approach.* Oakland, CA: New Harbinger.

Riskind, J. H., Hohmann, A. A., Beck, A. T., & Stewart, B. (1991). The relation of generalized anxiety disorder to depression in general and dysthymic disorder in particular. In R. M. Rapee & D. H. Barlow (Eds.), *Chronic anxiety: Generalized anxiety disorder and mixed anxiety–depression* (pp. 153–171). New York: Guilford Press.

Rubin, K. H., & Asendorpf, J. B. (1993). Social withdrawal, inhibition, and shyness in childhood: Conceptual and definitional issues. In K. H. Rubin & J. B. Asendorpf (Eds.), *Social withdrawal, inhibition, and shyness in children* (pp. 3–17). Hillsdale, NJ: Erlbaum.

Sanson, A., Pedlow, R., Cann, W., Prior, M., & Oberklaid, F. (1996). Shyness ratings: Stability and correlates in early childhood. *International Journal of Behavioral Development, 19*(4), 705–724.

Schniering, C. A., Hudson, J. L., & Rapee, R. M. (2000). Issues in the diagnosis and assessment of anxiety disorders in children and adolescents. *Clinical Psychology Review, 20*(4), 453–478.

Schniering, C. A., & Rapee, R. M. (2002). Development and validation of a measure of children's automatic thoughts: The Children's Automatic Thoughts Scale. *Behaviour Research and Therapy, 40*(9), 1091–1109.

Silverman, W. K., & Albano, A. M. (1996). *The Anxiety Disorders Interview Schedule for DSM-IV: Child and Parent Versions.* San Antonio, TX: Psychological Corporation.

Silverman, W. K., Kurtines, W. M., Ginsburg, G. S., Weems, C. F., Lumpkin, P. W., & Carmichael, D. H. (1999). Treating anxiety disorders in children with group cognitive-behavioral therapy: A randomized clinical trial. *Journal of Consulting and Clinical Psychology, 67*(6), 995–1003.

Silverman, W. K., & Nelles, W. B. (1988). The Anxiety Disorders Interview Schedule for Children. *Journal of the American Academy of Child and Adolescent Psychiatry, 27*(6), 772–778.

Silverman, W. K., Saavedra, L. M., & Pina, A. A. (2001). Test–retest reliability of anxiety symptoms and diagnoses with Anxiety Disorders Interview Schedule for DSM-IV: Child and Parent Versions. *Journal of the American Academy of Child and Adolescent Psychiatry, 40*(8), 937–944.

Spence, S. H. (1997). Structure of anxiety symptoms among children: A confirmatory factor-analytic study. *Journal of Abnormal Psychology, 106*, 280–297.

Spence, S. H. (1998). A measure of anxiety symptoms among children. *Behaviour Research and Therapy, 36*(5), 545–566.

Spence, S. H., Donovan, C., & Brechman-Toussaint, M. (1999). Social skills, social outcomes, and cognitive features of childhood social phobia. *Journal of Abnormal Psychology, 108*(2), 211–221.

Spence, S. H., Rapee, R. M., McDonald, C., & Ingram, M. (2001). The structure of anxiety symptoms among preschoolers. *Behaviour Research and Therapy, 39*, 1293–1316.

Stein, M. B., Fuetsch, M., Muller, N., Hofler, M., Lieb, R., & Wittchen, H.-U. (2001). Social anxiety disorder and the risk of depression: A prospective community study of adolescents and young adults. *Archives of General Psychiatry, 58*(3), 251–256.

Strauss, C. C., & Last, C. G. (1993). Social and simple phobias in children. *Journal of Anxiety Disorders, 7*, 141–152.

Strauss, C. C., Lease, C. A., Last, C. G., & Francis, G. (1988). Overanxious disorder: An examination of developmental differences. *Journal of Abnormal Child Psychology, 16*, 433–443.

Thomas, A., & Chess, S. (1977). *Temperament and development.* New York: Brunner/Mazel.

Tracey, S. A., Chorpita, B. F., Douban, J., & Barlow, D. H. (1997). Empirical evaluation of DSM-IV generalized anxiety disorder criteria in children and adolescents. *Journal of Clinical Child Psychology, 26*(4), 404–414.

Wagner, K. D., Berard, R., Stein, M., Wetherhold, E., Carpenter, D. J., Perera, P., et al. (2004). A multicenter, randomized, double-blind, placebo-controlled trial of paroxetine in children and adolescents with social anxiety disorder. *Archives of General Psychiatry, 61*, 1153–1162.

Walkup, J. T., Labellarte, M. J., Riddle, M. A., Pine, D. S., Greenhill, L., Klein, R., et al. (2001). Fluvoxamine for the treatment of anxiety disorders in children and adolescents. *New England Journal of Medicine, 344*, 1279–1285.

Wallace, S. T., & Alden, L. E. (1991). A comparison of social standards and perceived ability in anxious and nonanxious men. *Cognitive Therapy and Research, 15*, 237–254.

Wilson, J. K., & Rapee, R. M. (2006). Self-concept certainty in social phobia. *Behaviour Research and Therapy, 44*, 113–136.

Wood, J. J., Piacentini, J. C., Bergman, R., McCracken, J., & Barrios, V. (2002). Concurrent validity of the anxiety disorders section of the Anxiety Disorders Interview Schedule for DSM-IV: Child and Parent Versions. *Journal of Clinical Child and Adolescent Psychology, 31*(3), 335–342.

Yonkers, K. A., Dyck, I. R., & Keller, M. B. (2001). An eight-year longitudinal comparison of clinical course and characteristics of social phobia among men and women. *Psychiatric Services, 52*(5), 637–643.

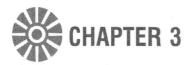

CHAPTER 3

Obsessive Thoughts

Fugen Neziroglu, Merry McVey-Noble,
Sony Khemlani-Patel, and Jose A. Yaryura-Tobias

Obsessive–compulsive spectrum disorders in childhood, once considered rare, are becoming increasingly common and warrant greater attention for several reasons. First, suffering is often widespread and can disrupt a child's social–emotional well-being, peer and family relationships, and academic success. Second is the recognition that childhood suffering often leads to adult disorders. Thus, early intervention has preventive implications as well as provision of immediate relief. Third, despite recent advances in the field, our knowledge base remains limited regarding spectrum disorders such as hypochondriasis (HC) and body dysmorphic disorder (BDD). As such, most clinicians are not well versed in the treatment of these disorders. Now for the first time, the authors, pioneers in the field, help us understand the nature of obsessive thoughts in general and within the context of obsessive–compulsive disorder (OCD), HC, and BDD. Through the case of "Kelli," qualified practitioners will learn how to identify more accurately and effectively manage these debilitating conditions.—A. R. E.

INTRODUCTION

The recognition that children and adolescents may experience obsessive–compulsive symptoms clinically differently than do adults has led to pediatric research in obsessive–compulsive disorder (OCD; for a review see Abramowitz, Whiteside, & Deacon, 2005). Similarly, OCD spectrum disorders such as hypochondriasis (HC) and body dysmorphic disorder (BDD) in children have a distinct symptom presentation compared to their adult counterparts. In this chapter, we present key symptom dimensions that are pertinent to these disorders and discuss how these symptoms manifest themselves. This aids in differential diagnosis of OCD spectrum disorders among themselves and in comparison to other, non-obsessive–compulsive spectrum disorder. The key symptom dimensions that we discuss are obsessions, doubting, compulsions and phobic avoidance behaviors, overvalued ideas/unrealistic thoughts, and shifting, all of which we believe are crucial to obsessive–compulsive spectrum disorders. This chapter covers these symptom dimensions, differential diagnosis, assessment, and treatment. Step-by-step evidence-based guidelines on how to diagnosis, assess, and treat a child presenting with OCD, HC, and BDD are presented.

Symptom Dimensions

Obsessions

Obsessions take the form of thoughts, images, and impulses. Obsessions have certain qualities, such as intrusiveness, persistence, pervasiveness, and repetitiveness, that are distressing and unacceptable. The content is usually inappropriate and inconsistent with the person's personality, moral values, and ideals. Some researchers have proposed that intrusions are the heart of the psychopathology of OCD (Rachman & De Silva, 1978; Salkovskis, 1985), whereas others purport that intrusiveness is just one quality of an obsession (Yaryura-Tobias & Neziroglu, 1997). Rachman and De Silva (1978) reported that the intrusive thoughts reported by almost 90% of a nonclinical population were indistinguishable from obsessional thoughts in content, although they were less frequent and less intense compared to thoughts of patients with OCD. It is unclear whether specific beliefs or core beliefs were assessed in this study, and a distinction needs to be made between the two types of beliefs. The cognitive models assume that obsessions derive from normal intrusive thoughts, thus making an individual's interpretation of these thoughts the distinguishing factor that separates obsessions from normal intrusive thoughts. Salkovskis (1985) indicated that individuals with OCD just attach meaning to the intrusive thought and give it importance.

A cognitive-behavioral analysis classifies obsessions as thoughts that belong within the category of beliefs specific to OCD (i.e., "I believe the doorknob in the public bathroom is contaminated by others"; "I believe I must have a good thought to enter my bedroom") and those that are general and found in other anxiety disorders (i.e., "Being vigilant to our environment is necessary at all times"; "We have control over having good and bad things happen"). The latter, which is called a core belief, refers to an individual's basic beliefs about the self and the world. Cognitive theory of obsessions states that intrusive thoughts or images are appraised; that is, they are interpreted. How one appraises a thought or image is based on learned assumptions from earlier experience. Assumptions or core beliefs are more general than appraisals of particular events and are held across contexts. Salkovskis suggested that the unique feature of obsessional problems lies not in the occurrence of ideas of danger or threat, although this by definition is necessary, but in the motivation of the compulsive component of the problem. Neutralizing appears to be always present in obsessional problems. The cognitive theory of obsessional problems accounts for neutralizing by specifying that the occurrence and/or content of intrusions is interpreted (appraised) as indicating that the person may be responsible for harm to him- or herself or others. Salkovskis proposed that intrusions develop into obsessions only when intrusions are appraised as posing a threat for which the individual is personally responsible. The goal of therapy is to give the persons an alternative for how they appraise, or attach meaning to, their obsessions.

The Obsessive Compulsive Cognitions Working Group (OCCWG; 1997, 2001) identified six general belief domains (i.e., perfectionism, intolerance of uncertainty, overestimation of threat, overinflated sense of responsibility, overimportance of thoughts, and need to control thoughts). In therapy these are the underlying assumptions about the specific beliefs that need to be targeted.

From a purely behavioral perspective, obsessions are either targeted directly by exposing the individual to the specific disastrous consequences or automatically extinguished through repeated exposure to the thought or image. Obsessions are believed to extinguish over time if the individual is exposed to the underlying beliefs, images, and impulses. A cognitive shift occurs, and this shift may in fact be a change in the appraisal of the obsessions. As stated earlier, Yaryura-Tobias and Neziroglu (1997) purport that intrusions are only one quality of obsessions; thus, obsessions are distinguishable from everyday thoughts that individuals entertain. We believe that individuals with obsessions do not in fact want to give importance to their thoughts. The thoughts themselves become important only because they are always there and the individual cannot easily entertain other, nonobsessional thoughts. In addition, the individual with an obsession does not want to control the thought except in the sense of getting rid of it. As we discuss obsessions in various disorders it will become clear that obsessions present themselves differently mainly in content, not necessarily in form.

Doubting

Doubting is a variant of an obsession. There are obsessions that do not involve doubting, such as horrific images or impulses, repetitious songs, thought action fusion or magical thinking, and so forth. Doubting refers to hesitancy, uncertainty, and indecisiveness regarding ones thoughts and actions. In doubting, judgment is withheld, because the person is uncertain of the truth of his or her belief, or the reality of an event. Often doubting involves hesitancy around making a decision or rendering a judgment. Doubting may take on many different forms, from reviewing conversations to deciding whether one has offended a person, or in making decisions about what to wear, whether something should be thrown out, whether to make a phone call, whether a physical symptoms is a sign of a particular illness, whether someone understood exactly what one is trying to say, or whether to attend a particular event, and so forth. These are all forms of doubting that involve making a decision and the hesitancy surrounding it. In the case of doubting, even if a decision is made, its correctness is doubted. Thus, the person thinks through all the possibilities over and over again. Sometimes it is easier to let someone else make the decision, but usually the person even doubts the accuracy of someone else's decision. Doubting may be the consequence of wanting not to make a mistake, not to be held responsible for an incorrect decision, the belief that one cannot cope with the consequences of an improper decision, and/or wanting to be perfect.

Legrand Du Salle (1830–1886) renamed obsessive disorder as *folie de doute avec delire de toucher* (insanity of doubting with disorder of touching). Although the German school conceptualized obsession (*Vorstellungen*) as a disorder of thinking, the French viewed it as *delire emotif*, an emotional disorder. Currently obsessions, compulsions, and doubting may be viewed as encompassing both thoughts and emotions, in that the thoughts have an affective component. As we shall see, doubting occurs in many disorders, and we discuss its presentation in some of them.

Compulsions and Phobic Avoidance Behaviors

Compulsions are active avoidance behaviors that are performed to diminish anxiety. They are negatively reinforcing in that they do decrease negative affect. For cognitivists, compulsions or neutralizing behaviors are conceptualized as efforts to remove intrusions and to prevent any perceived harmful consequences. Salkovskis (1985) advanced two main reasons why compulsions become persistent and excessive. First, they are reinforced by immediate distress reduction; second, they prevent the person from learning that his or her appraisals are unrealistic (e.g., that if one touches the doorknob, then he or she will not die). He states that compulsions can strengthen a person's perceived responsibility by removing the disastrous consequences, so that the person believes that he or she is responsible for the positive outcome. Responsibility interpretations lead the person to try to avert harm in several ways (i.e., by focusing on control of mental activity), including attempts to be sure of the accuracy of one's memory, to take into account all factors in one's decisions, to prevent the occurrence of unacceptable material, and to ensure that an outcome has been achieved even though the achievement may be imperceptible, such as washing one's hand sufficiently to remove contamination. Thus when a person appraises intrusions as posing a threat for which he or she is personally responsible, the person becomes distressed and attempts to remove the intrusions and to prevent their perceived consequences. This increases the frequency of intrusions. Thus, intrusions become persistent and distressing, and escalate into obsessions (Taylor, 2002).

Salkovskis et al. (2000) reported on studies that investigated responsibility assumptions and appraisals in patients with OCD, patients with other anxiety disorders, and healthy controls. They noted that obsessional patients were more likely than nonobsessionals to endorse general responsibility beliefs and assumptions, and to make responsibility-related appraisals of intrusive thoughts of possible harm. Also they noted a relationship between responsibility cognitions and the occurrence of compulsive behavior and neutralizing. Patients with OCD differed from both healthy controls and patients with other anxiety disorders. Other studies had previously demonstrated that a decrease in perceived responsibility is followed by a decreased in discomfort and a decline in compulsions (Lopatka & Rachman, 1995; Shafran, 1997). Salkovskis and Forrester (2002) contended that all six belief domains mentioned under obsessions and established by the OCCWG (1997, 2001) relate to responsibility. In summary, the cognitive explanation of the maintenance of compulsions boils down to decreasing one's overinflated sense of responsibility.

Could there be other explanations for the maintenance of compulsions? Mowrer (1947) described a two-factor model of fear and avoidance behavior in anxiety disorders. He suggested that fear is acquired through classical conditioning and maintained by operant conditioning. This theory was later applied by Dollard and Miller (1950) to the acquisition of OCD. Through classical conditioning a neutral stimulus paired with an unconditioned stimulus (UCS) acquires the same properties as the UCS, thus eliciting anxiety. The second stage comprises a negative reinforcement paradigm, in which one learns new responses to decrease one's anxiety in the presence of the conditioned (neutral) stimulus (CS). These learned responses are termed "avoidance" or "escape" responses. They remove anxiety and are therefore negatively reinforcing. A compulsive checker may associate an electrical appliance (CS) with death (UCS; starting a fire) and feel anxiety (unconditioned response [UCR] and conditioned response [CR]) in the presence of a stove. The checking behavior is negatively reinforced because it removes anxiety.

Regardless of which explanation one adopts for maintenance of compulsions their symptoms presentation is apparent in several disorders, and specifically in the ones discussed in this chapter: OCD, BDD, and HC. How they manifest themselves in each disorder is discussed later.

Phobic avoidance behaviors manifest themselves in a variety of ways, from simple avoidance or escape to more complex avoidance behaviors. All avoidance behaviors are attempts at evading negative emotions. A person may simply avoid a particular person, animal, object, or place, as in simple phobias, or escape from any one of those stimuli if unexpectedly confronted. This is referred to as "passive avoidance," because the individual merely avoids the antecedent event that gives rise to the fear, or any negative emotion. Another way to engage in avoidance behaviors is to remove the negative feelings by engaging in some behavior, such as compulsions. Besides compulsions, individuals may engage in some action that results in the removal of the distress. This is called "active avoidance," because the person actually engages in a behavior rather than merely avoiding the source of a negative feeling. In behavior terms, it is known as "negative reinforcement," because the behavior reinforces by removing a negative feeling or distress. Both passive and active avoidance behaviors are noted in OCD, BDD, and HC. They are discussed later in the chapter.

Overvalued Ideas/Unrealistic Thoughts

"Overvalued ideation" refers to the intensity or strength of conviction in a belief. Kozak and Foa (1994) have suggested that overvalued ideas are on a continuum between rational thought and delusions. We propose that overvalued ideas do not fluctuate spontaneously, but are fixed and possibly modifiable only if challenged. Wernicke (1906) stated that overvalued ideas are drawn from the periphery and are resistant to modification. He suggested that they involve misattribution due to lack of insight, which is governed by affect. Others, such as Jaspers (1913), viewed overvalued ideas as challengeable, transient, isolated, and bound to personality and situation. Overvalued ideas are distinctly different from "poor insight," a specifier used in the DSM. "Insight" refers to a gradation of personal awareness into one's disorder, giving rise to disorder-specific beliefs. The term "overvalued ideas" refers more to the reasonableness, sensibleness, accuracy, and strength of a belief. High overvalued ideas are common in the obsessive–compulsive spectrum disorders such as BDD and HC, and in hoarders (McKay, Neziroglu, & Yaryura-Tobias, 1997; Neziroglu, McKay, & Yaryura-Tobias, 2000; Neziroglu & Khemlani-Patel, 2005; Neziroglu, Peterson, Yaryura-Tobias, & Weissman, 2007). Overvalued ideation as a symptom dimension is very important because of its predictive value in treatment (Neziroglu, Stevens, McKay, & Yaryura-Tobias, 2001).

Shifting

The ability to shift from one topic to another, or from one action to another, is a symptom dimension that is often not discussed. If mentioned with regard to perseveration, then it is often noted to occur within the pervasive developmental disorders. However, the inability to shift is a characteristic found in OCD, BDD, and HC, but not, for example, in generalized anxiety disorder (GAD). Perhaps this inability is due to the importance given to thoughts, so that subsequent attention is focused exclusively on trying to control the thought. We examine the role of shifting within a variety of disorders.

Relationship of Symptom Dimensions to Specific Disorders

Obsessions, compulsions, or phobic avoidance behaviors, overvalued ideas, and shifting are all symptom dimensions involved in various degrees in OCD, BDD, and HC. We compare GAD briefly on some of these dimensions as well, because of its similarity to OCD. The worry or preoccupation component of

GAD is often aligned with obsessions. We take each symptom dimension as it relates to the specific disorder.

In OCD, almost 90% of patients have both obsessions and compulsions, with approximately two-thirds reporting more than one obsession (Foa & Kozak, 1995). Although it is rare for a person to have a compulsion without an obsession, we do see it in children, and there are few adults who engage in motor acts such as hand washing without knowing why. On the other hand, about 20–25% of people have pure obsessions without compulsions. Doubting, a form of obsession, is quite common and involves the question "What if . . . Happened?; "What if I am gay?"; "What if I am a sinner?"; "What if I actually contaminated myself?"; "What if I left the stove on?"; etc. Compulsions are deliberate acts to undo an obsession. They may become automatic and habitual over time. Most patients can tell a compulsion from a noncompulsion by their sense of needing to perform an act (feeling an urge to do it). Because the compulsion reduces the anxiety, it maintains the compulsion.

In BDD, obsessions occur over an imagined bodily defect, and/or if the defect is present, then it is very minimal and the person's rumination is excessive. Individuals with BDD may spend hours obsessing over whether they have smooth complexions, or whether their faces are red or have pimples. They may also doubt that their appearance has changed since the last time they looked at it. Obsessions may last from an hour to whole day. Avoidance behaviors take the form of seeking reassurance about their appearance, camouflaging their defects, avoiding or constantly checking mirrors, excessive grooming, and avoidance of various situations, lighting, people, and so on.

In HC, obsessions revolve around whether particular physical symptoms are signs of an illness. Individuals with HC are hypervigilant to their bodily cues, and obsess over what they feel and whether they have other sensations; review what they have read or heard about these physical symptoms in the past; and spend hours in rumination over having a particular illness. They obsess over being ill, dying, being left alone, being isolated, unloved, and so on, because of this imagined illness. To reduce anxiety, they seek reassurance, read about the illness, try to figure out whether their symptoms correspond to the illness, go to doctors, expose themselves to numerous medical tests, and in some cases even undergo various procedures. These are all avoidance behaviors that in the long run usually does not reduce the anxiety. They continue in a never-ending process of doubting their health.

In all three disorders, OCD, BDD and HC, the beliefs may be overvalued; however, overvalued ideation tends to be greater in BDD and HC. Perhaps this is the reason that treatment is also more difficult. As for shifting, the ability to go on to another thought or action readily, persons with each of the three disorders experience difficulty in specific areas relative to the disorder. In other words, patients do not usually have a problem with discussing topics unrelated to their obsessions or changing from one behavior to another that is unrelated to their compulsions. They differ from patients who worry a lot, such as those with GAD, who worry about one topic after another. The "what if" applies to numerous situations, places, and people rather than to one specific area.

Prevalence and Onset

The prevalence rate for OCD is 2.5%; for BDD, it is 0.7 to 13% (Otto et al., 2001); for HC, 4.2 to 13.8% (Noyes et al., 1993), and for GAD, 4 to 6% (Robins & Regier, 1991). The rates may vary at times depending on the sample size and population. It is interesting that for OCD and GAD the age of onset is less than 25 years of age, whereas for BDD onset is during adolescence and the disorder peaks in the 40s and 50s.

Comorbidity

Major depression, phobias, GAD, eating disorders, obsessive–compulsive personality disorder, avoidant personality disorder, and Tourette syndrome are comorbid with OCD (American Psychiatric Association, 2000). Approximately 30% of individuals with BDD also have OCD, although BDD is also comorbid with major depression (80%), social phobia (36%), substance abuse (27%), and delusional disorder (27%) (Phillips & Diaz, 1997). Anxiety, depressive, and somatoform disorders, as well as physical pain are usually comorbid with HC (American Psychiatric Association, 2000). Major depression and other anxiety disorders, substance abuse, or physical illness such as irritable bowel syndrome are the major comorbid conditions with GAD (Hoehn-Saire & McLeod, 1991).

A large-scale study of an adult and child clinical sample recorded comorbidity of several disorders in children with OCD (Fireman, Koran, Leventhal, & Jacobson, 2001). Approximately 75% of the child sample exhibited at least one comorbid psychiatric disorder. Results indicate that 34% of the child sample had comorbid attention-deficit/hyperactivity disorder (ADHD), and 33% had major depression. Tourette syndrome was found in 18% of the sample. In another study, approximately 60% of patients with OCD had a lifetime history of tics (Leonard et al., 1992).

Course

OCD is known to begin in adolescence or early adulthood. However, males modally experience the disorder earlier than females. Males' average age range is from 6 to 15 years of age, whereas for women the average range is 20–29 years. Normally the onset is a gradual process, but there have been cases of rapid onset. Most individuals display a chronic waxing and waning of symptoms that appear to be related to stress levels. Approximately 15% of individuals with OCD have an eventual decline in social and occupational performance (American Psychiatric Association, 2000).

The course for BDD, HC, and GAD is less known. It appears that symptoms wax and wane, and are usually chronic unless treated. The authors have noted that in their BDD population symptoms tend to get worse over time, often leading untreated individuals to become homebound.

Genetic Factors

Recent research indicates that genes may play a role in the development of OCD in some cases. OCD does tend to be a familial disorder. Someone with OCD has a 25% chance of having a blood relative who has it (Carson, Butcher, & Mineka, 2000). There is no current evidence for a genetic basis to BDD and HC. Although clearly there is a familial connection within anxiety disorders, the earlier GAD studies appear inconclusive. However, twin studies have indicated some genetic contribution to the progression of GAD (American Psychiatric Association, 2000).

Differential Diagnosis

Some symptoms are common to BDD, OCD, HC, and GAD, such as preoccupation and attentiveness in some areas of concern sometimes to the exclusion of others. In differentiating one diagnosis from another, the therapist must pay attention to the predominant symptom presentation. Once a primary diagnosis is made, the therapist must make associations to other conditions that generally coexist (are comorbid) with that diagnosis. For example, if the individual were diagnosed with OCD, then one would go through the list of common obsessive–compulsive spectrum disorders (i.e., BDD, HC, Tourette syndrome, and trichotillomania). If BDD is diagnosed along the way, then one might look for social phobia, because of its high incidence of comorbidity with BDD. In a patient with Tourette syndrome, one would look for comorbid attention deficit disorder (ADD) or ADHD. Of course, this only allows one to diagnose comorbid conditions, not to differentiate among symptoms or diagnoses.

Differential diagnosis is necessary when symptoms are not clear cut and there are similarities. For example, often one needs to differentiate among OCD, somatic type; somatization disorder; and HC. For example, obsessions about health are quite common. Here is an example of differential diagnosis when the therapist encounters a patient with health obsessions. Is the individual afraid of contracting an illness if he or she touches something, or walks past someone with a particular illness? Does the individual think he or she has a particular illness because of some specific physical symptom? Does the individual constantly complain about physical symptoms? Does the person experience physical symptoms and fear imminent death? If the answer to the first question is yes, then the person may be diagnosed with OCD. If the answer to the second question is yes, then he or she probably has HC. A yes answer to the third question probably indicates somatization disorder. If the answer to the fourth question is yes, then he or she may be experiencing panic disorder. Let us look at why.

In the first scenario, the individual obsesses about getting something in the future and performs either active or passive behaviors to avoid the item or situation and ward off the possibility of contracting something. In the second situation, the individual actually misinterprets a physical symptom as a sign of a serious medical condition (e.g., "I have a headache; therefore, I must have a tumor"). In the third situation, the person experiences many physical symptoms and is hypervigilant to those symptoms. In the fourth case, the person has physical symptoms and interprets them to be a sign of immediate (panic disorder) rather than future (hypochondriasis) danger.

Our decision tree (see Figure 3.1) indicates that once obsessions and compulsions are established one has a diagnostic choice of OCD, BDD, HC, eating disorders, Tourette syndrome, and possibly GAD. The content of obsessions and compulsions differ in each of the disorders, with the exception of GAD, which may involve only obsessions/worrying, and Tourette syndrome, which may include compulsions but not obsessions. In OCD, typical obsessions revolve around the belief that something bad will happen to one's parents or oneself. A child may repeat phrases or ask for reassurance to prevent harm. The therapist observes whether the child has tics, twitches, and/or sniffing (not due to a cold) to determine whether he or she has Tourette syndrome. If the therapist observes grimacing, then he or she should ask about vocal tics.

If OCD symptoms appear suddenly, as if overnight, then it is prudent to consider the presence of OCD induced by streptococcal infection, called

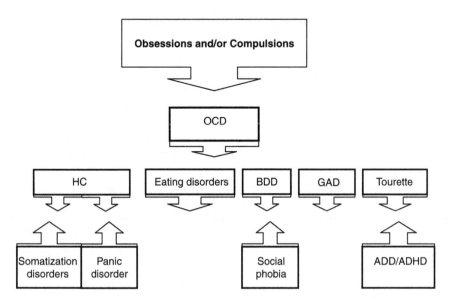

FIGURE 3.1. Decision tree.

PANDAS (pediatric autoimmune neuropsychiatric disorder associated with streptococcal infections), which is still a controversial issue. It is hypothesized that antibodies to Group A beta-hemolytic streptococcal infection (GABHS) may affect the basal ganglia in the brain, leading to the sudden onset of OCD symptoms and/or vocal and motor tics associated with Tourette syndrome (Swedo, Leonard, & Garvey, 1998). Others symptoms associated with PANDAS include emotional lability, irritability, sensory hypersensitivity, oppositional/defiant symptoms, and ADHD symptoms such as hyperactivity–impulsivity and distractibility. If OCD and/or tics appear abruptly, or if there is an exacerbation of either disorder, along with some of the aforementioned symptoms, then it may be prudent to refer the patient to a pediatric neurologist, an infectious disease specialist, or a psychiatrist/psychopharmacologist with specialized experience in this area. Specific blood titers are thought to identify the presence of PANDAS, such as the antistreptolysin O (ASO) and the antistreptococcal DNAse B titers (see Figures 3.1 and 3.2 for decision trees to facilitate differential diagnosis).

CASE FORMULATION:
CONCEPTUAL MODEL OF ASSESSMENT AND TREATMENT

Case Presentation

Kelli, a 10-year-old Caucasian girl, was referred for cognitive and behavioral therapy by her neurologist, who had been treating her since the age of 5 for ADHD (combined type). Though Kelli had not experienced ongoing academic problems as a result of her ADHD diagnosis since her treatment with psychostimulants began in the first grade, she began to display some ADHD symptoms. In the past month and a half, her teachers reported several times that Kelli seemed distracted and inattentive, and was not participating in class (would not get up to write on the board, and was leaving class several times per period). When Kelli's mother, Mrs. M., brought her in for a consultation with her neurologist, the doctor increased her psychostimulant medication, thinking a recent growth spurt might have necessitated a medication adjustment, and scheduled a follow-up appointment for the next month.

At the time of the neurological follow-up, Kelli stated that she was feeling anxious. Though Mrs. M. had attributed her daughter's increase in anxiety to the increased dose of psychostimulant medication, her neurologist noticed that Kelli's hands were raw and red, and questioned her. Kelli stated that she had been engaging in excessive hand washing and that she was afraid to touch certain objects, people, and even her dog. The neurologist also noticed that Kelli had lost approximately 6 pounds in the last month. Kelli's mother noted that her daughter had been eating much less, often stating that she was not hungry when her mother commented about the uneaten food in her lunchbox. Mrs. M. had attributed this to the increase in Kelli's medication, but when the

I. Anxiety as a symptom
   A. Do you feel nervous, scared, or afraid a lot?
   B. Do you have worries or scary thoughts?
   C. Do you have scary or nervous feelings in your body?

If the child endorses anxiety symptoms, go through the differential diagnostic questions for anxiety disorders in children first (using the ADIS-IV—Child Version).

If the ADIS-IV reveals symptoms consistent with OCD, pursue more specific questioning using the OCS decision tree below.

II. Obsessive–Compulsive Spectrum Disorders
   A. Do you have sticky thoughts that you just can't get out of your brain? (Obsessions)
      1. Do they pop into your head?
      2. Do they scare or worry you?
      3. Are they about things that you know are not real, or that are unlikely to happen, even if they upset you a lot?
      4. Do you have trouble getting them out of your head?
      5. Do you have one or two worries or do you worry about lots of different things everyday? (suggests GAD)
   B. Do you do or think certain things to try and make those sticky thoughts go away? (Compulsions)
      1. Do they make your worry go away or quiet down right away?
      2. Do you do them over and over again?
      3. Do you doubt that you did them and then redo them?

If the individual endorses obsessions and compulsions, as measured by criteria A and B above, then probe for the specific types of worries to make an accurate differential diagnosis.

III. Do you worry about your body?
   A. Do you worry about the way you look?
      1. Do you have sticky thoughts that a part of your body is ugly or deformed looking?
      2. Do you look in the mirror a lot or try to stay away from mirrors?
      3. Do you try to hide your "defect" by wearing certain clothes or hats?

        Yes to Questions 1, 2, and 3 suggests BDD

      4. Do you have sticky thoughts that you are fat, even though other people say you're thin?
      5. Do you not eat to get rid of that thought?
      6. Do you feel like you need to exercise to get rid of that thought?

        Yes to Questions 4, 5, and 6 suggests anorexia nervosa

(continued)

FIGURE 3.2. Differential diagnosis decision tree.

B. Do you worry about your health?
   1. Do you experience lots of intense physical symptoms that come on quickly, and worry that they may lead to immediate death, are a sign of going crazy, or losing control? *(suggests panic disorder)*
   2. Do you worry that you might get sick or catch a disease? *(suggests OCD)*
      a. Do you worry about catching a disease from touching something?
      b. Do you worry about catching a disease from sick people?
      c. Do you worry that if you don't do a certain action, you may get sick?
   3. Do you worry that you have a disease? *(suggests HC)*
      a. If you get an ache, pain, or other physical symptoms, do you worry that it is a sign of a disease?
      b. Do you check your body a lot? (temperature, glands, breathing, etc.)
   4. Do you have a lot of aches, pains, and physical complaints (e.g., headaches, stomach pain, etc.)? *(suggests somatization disorder)*

FIGURE 3.2. *(continued)*

neurologist questioned Kelli, she admitted to specifically avoiding a variety of foods. Kelli's neurologist made provisional diagnoses of OCD and an eating disorder, and referred Kelli for cognitive-behavioral therapy.

At the initial consultation, Kelli stated that she was very nervous and did not want to discuss her fears, because she thought that the evaluating psychologist would think she was "stupid and crazy." This issue was quickly and effectively resolved when the consulting psychologist stated that Kelli had to be at least somewhat intelligent to worry and think as much as she did, and that truly "crazy" people were generally unaware of their own mental status. Kelli also said that she had read about OCD with her mother online and insisted that she was not afraid of germs and did not think she was fat or that she had an eating disorder. The consulting psychologist stated that Kelli, in fact, might be right and said that no determinations would be made until Kelli's symptoms had been thoroughly explored.

When asked about how she had been feeling, Kelli said she had been very "nervous." She said she could not keep her mind on her schoolwork and that she had been "daydreaming a lot." When asked about the content of her "daydreams," whether they were fun, interesting, weird or worrisome, Kelli stated that she was worrying a lot and felt that her mind was like "e-mail with no spam filter." Basically, she was having a variety of intrusive, anxiety-provoking thoughts. However, she was reluctant to provide the specific content of these intrusions.

To encourage her, the examiner ran through several categories of the "Top 10 Things Kids Worry About": (1) death and disasters (e.g., parents, siblings, or self will die in fires, plane crashes, car accidents), (2) doing or saying something rude, offensive, or inappropriate (e.g., cursing, insulting people, sexual thoughts, "sinning," stealing), (3) doing something dangerous (e.g., harming the self or others), (4) germs or dirt (e.g., not wanting to touch dirty things, hating to have sticky, dirty, or "contaminated hands"), (5) making mistakes or not being perfect (e.g., wanting to get only A's, needing to have perfect hair or to win every game), (6) symmetry (e.g., needing to have things equal on both sides, "evening out" movements or clothing), (7) getting sick (e.g., having and or catching diseases), (8) doing or saying something stupid or embarrassing in front of others, (9) looking ugly, deformed, or fat (e.g., thinking one's nose is too big, one's face is too long, or that one is fat, even if other people say one is), and (10) the right feeling (e.g., thinking that one needs to get the right feeling to move on from one thing to another).

After hearing these options, Kelli was amazed that she recognized her specific worries in the list. She said that she had always worried about death and dying, and since a boy in her fourth grade class had died of a brain tumor the previous year, she had been worrying about getting sick too. At first, she worried mostly about cancer. Every time she had a headache, Kelli began to worry that she had a brain tumor. She said that other physical symptoms, such as dizziness (which occurred once as a result of getting overheated after a tennis match in warm weather) and nausea (which she had during a bout of the stomach flu) also caused her to "get stuck on the brain tumor thing." When this occurred, Kelli said she had started making "question calls" to her older sister's boyfriend's brother, a pediatrician. At first, Mrs. M. said that everybody thought it was very cute that Kelli called Dr. L. Dr. L. himself thought Kelli was just a "really inquisitive little kid." When questioned about these calls during the consultation, however, Kelli admitted that she had been seeking reassurance, which initially had helped her feel a lot less anxious. The problem was, she stated, that she became quickly "addicted" to her calls to Dr. L., which were occurring almost daily at the time of her consultation.

However, since she had experienced seasonal allergies in the fall of fifth grade, Kelli said she had been worrying a lot about having allergies, "not just the seasonal kind, but the serious kind." When questioned about what she meant by "the serious kind" of allergies, Kelli said that when she had looked allergies up on the Internet about 2 months ago, she read about anaphylaxis and became consumed by the idea that she might develop a deadly allergy that resulted in suffocation and eventually death. She became extremely anxious and feared for her life every time she had a stuffy nose, watery eyes, a sore throat, or felt itchy (at which point, she would immediately call Dr. L.). She was sure she was going into shock.

In addition, she had also begun visiting the school nurse every time she experienced one of these symptoms, "just to make sure I wasn't dying." Kelli also began begging her mother to have her checked out by her own pediatrician quite frequently, stating that she wanted to be sure she was not having a severe allergic reaction when she experienced any of these physical sensations. When her mother refused, Kelli became hysterical and very panicky but settled down within an hour or so, because she realized that true anaphylaxis would have killed her by then. Despite this, Kelli frequently requested that her mother give her a Benadryl at bedtime on days she had experienced symptoms she considered to be consistent with impending anaphylaxis.

Kelli also said that part of the reason she had been distracted in school was worry about inhaling chalk dust, so she had tried not to breathe in class, or had breathed through her sleeve. She also indicated that she had avoided writing at the board, because she didn't want chalk dust on her hands. In addition, Kelli said that if her teacher had chalk dust on her hands and touched her, or if a paper the teacher handed back might have chalk dust on it, she immediately washed her hands thoroughly (often several times during class).

Kelli also stated that this fear had gotten so "out of control" that she was "checking" her breathing all day long, by taking big deep breaths to make sure her airways were not constricted. She also checked the color of her nailbeds for cyanosis, her face for signs of visible swelling, and swallowed "constantly" to make sure that she could still do so. Hence, although it was originally assumed that she was just inattentive and distractible in class as a result of her ADHD, Kelli was preoccupied with intrusive thoughts and actually avoided doing work so she would not have to accept it back. Pretending she had lost her place in the lesson was a strategy that Kelli admitted she had developed to avoid having to go up to the chalkboard as well.

Kelli stated that at home she had avoided touching her mother, or anything her mother had touched, because Mrs. M. was also a teacher. In addition to her obsession about a deadly allergy to chalk, Kelli stated that she had recently become concerned that she might have a similar allergy to her dog. This was particularly disturbing to her, because her dog was "her favorite person in the world," and she had avoided touching or cuddling with him for the past 3 weeks. Additionally, she engaged in frequent and vigorous hand washing when near him, especially before eating, or if she had the urge to touch her face or mouth. Kelli said that this was "the worst" part of her fear of anaphylaxis.

When questioned about her recent eating disturbances, Kelli emphatically insisted that she did not think that she was fat. In fact, she was worried that she was too skinny. The consulting psychologist asked what foods she was avoiding, and basically it appeared that Kelli was avoiding all dairy products and red meat. When asked why she seemed to be avoiding all cow-related products, Kelli sheepishly admitted that she was terrified of mad cow disease (bovine spongiform encephalopathy [BSE]). When asked what she knew about this disease, she stated that she had heard on the news that "it can make you confused and weak." She also thought that it made cows go crazy and then die. Kelli stated that whenever she felt confused in class, or weak after tennis, she had a panic attack and would then feel like she was going crazy, which intensified her fear even further, because she thought her symptoms might be related to having eaten contaminated beef or dairy products. Because she had made this spurious association between these symptoms occurring as a result of consuming dairy or beef products, Kelli not only avoided these food groups but had also begun to check food labels compulsively (even when she knew there was no milk or beef in the product) before consuming any foodstuff.

Kelli also avoided eating any unpackaged food, which was most of the food her mother prepared for her, because she could not be 100% sure of the ingredients.

Kelli had seen on the news that no cases of BSE had been identified in the United States, but this still gave her no comfort. She stated that every time she was preparing to eat, the thought "What if my food has Mad Cow in it?" seized her. She was often so anxious as a result of this thought that she completely lost her appetite. At lunch, Kelli could not bring herself to eat anything unpackaged (e.g., her sandwich, fruit, carrots), and she spent so much time checking the ingredients of her chips or cookies that she simply ran out of time. She was also afraid of eating foods that might have been placed next to dairy products or red meat. In the supermarket she closely watched to see whether someone who handled meat would touch other products. She then believed that the other products had gotten contaminated. She also stated that her fear of mad cow disease was worse at school, because she was so anxious about the chalk allergy fear.

Finally, Kelli also sometimes worried about her appearance, which contributed to her distraction in class, because she was seated near a window and spent a fair amount of time checking her reflection when she began to worry that she looked too thin. This was why, she said, she had become so annoyed when it was suggested that she might have an eating disorder.

Kelli, a petite girl, was lean and muscular due to her involvement in competitive tennis. She said she had never really worried about her size or shape until "the talk" about puberty and sexuality in the beginning of the school year. At that point she began to notice that some of her peers were developing more womanly shapes and became aware of her thin, less mature body.

Two months later, Kelli said that she had developed the irresistible urge to look in every reflective surface to see whether she was still "skinny and young looking." She reported that though she knew it would not happen over the course of a day, or even a week, she believed she might suddenly burst into puberty, attaining the curvy, feminine shape she wished she had. Kelli had also been mirror checking in the bathroom after she washed her hands, and she admitted to having layered her clothing to appear larger than she was. She said she was very self-conscious, especially in demand situations when "everyone" might be looking at her (i.e., raising her hand in class or standing at the blackboard). She was very concerned about her recent weight loss but felt "more afraid of mad cow than of looking skinny."

Kelli's mother stated that she had had no idea that her daughter had been worrying so much about so many things. She also seemed relieved, because the symptoms her daughter endorsed put her worrisome behaviors in context. Mrs. M. said that Kelli had always endorsed fears of her parents dying, and had asked many reassurance-seeking questions before they flew, went on cruises, or drove in bad weather. Mrs. M. also reported that anxiety disorders ran in her family, that she had contended with panic attacks and a "brief brush" with agoraphobia postpartum, and that her mother had had many "phobias." In addition, she indicated that unbeknownst to Kelli, her eldest daughter was being treated for anorexia nervosa, though she was currently away at college.

Kelli and her mother were informed that Kelli had both OCD and HC, which is a variant of OCD that involves specific obsessions about illness and death, and related compulsions. Her misinterpretation of physical symptoms such as a stuffy nose, watery eyes, and a sore throat as signs of anaphylactic shock led to the diagnosis of HC. Her avoidance behaviors specific to HC were seeking reassurance from her pediatrician, checking the Internet for information, taking precautionary Benadryl, breathing through her sleeve to avoid breathing chalk dust, and not writing on the blackboard. She had previously experienced HC when she misinterpreted her headaches, dizziness, and nausea as signs of a brain tumor. Her OCD symptoms were more related to her fear of getting mad cow disease. Kelli had both contamination fears and somatic obsessions. She believed red meat and dairy products were contaminated and should be avoided at all costs. She obsessed about getting the disease and engaged in both passive and active avoidance behaviors to keep herself safe. Preoccupation with her appearance and compensatory behaviors seemed to indicate an additional diagnosis of BDD. These diagnoses effectively accounted for Kelli's obsessive thinking and compulsive behaviors, high anxiety, and behavioral avoidances. In addition, what initially appeared to be an exacerbation of ADHD symptoms turned out to be inattention, distractibility, and preoccupation related to the intrusive obsessions resulting from HC and BDD. She did not have an eating disorder.

Assessment

Clinical Interviews

Of all the instruments available to a clinician, a valuable component of the functional behavioral analysis is a thorough clinical interview. This is especially salient when working with children, especially those with some of the more atypical symptom presentations that may not be adequately detected or identified by available assessment instruments. It is important to ask children direct questions about their thoughts, feelings, and behaviors. In addition, parents and teachers can help clinicians hone in on relevant symptom clusters to make the accurate diagnosis leading to appropriate and effective treatment.

When conducting a thorough clinical interview, particularly with children, it is important to pose questions directly in terms that they can easily understand. Often, clinicians assume (incorrectly) that children lack the awareness and/or vocabulary to articulate their specific obsessions or compulsions, and how they affect their lives. In our clinical experience, children as young as 3 years of age (albeit bright, verbally precocious 3-year-olds) are capable of identifying and expressing felt anxiety, depression, and anger, as well as describing intrusive and obsessional thoughts, and repetitive or compulsive behaviors.

A clinician who hopes to get accurate information during a consultation interview must ask questions in terms that are appropriate to children's developmental level to help them express their emotional and cognitive experiences. For example, when a therapist questions young children, it is helpful to ask about anxiety using terms such as feeling "nervous," "frightened," "scared," or "worried." When attempting to identify whether the child is experiencing obsessions, the therapist can describe obsessional thinking (i.e., "thoughts that you can't stop thinking even if you try"), or discuss obsessional thoughts as "sticky thoughts" or "worries." Even qualities of obsessions, such as intrusiveness, can be simplified (e.g., "pop-in thoughts").

Similarly, compulsions can be described to children (as "redo's" and "repeats," of particular behaviors), so that they can improve their symptom reporting. Also, when a clinician describes the relief that comes with having completed a compulsion, and the quick, rebounding urge to do it all over again, children who in fact experience this phenomenon seem to recognize immediately their particular compulsive behaviors, as the following dialogue illustrates:

THERAPIST: Everybody, kids and grown-ups too, feels nervous, scared, or worried sometimes. Do you ever feel that way?

CHILD: Yeah, I have a massive worry about chicken pox. That I could get it. That I could die.

THERAPIST: Do you worry about chicken pox a lot?

CHILD: Yeah, like every second.

THERAPIST: There are some worry thoughts that we call "sticky thoughts." No matter what, your brain keeps getting stuck on them. Does your Chicken Pox thought do that? (*Assesses for ability to shift to another thought.*)

CHILD: Yes! I keep saying to my brain, "Shut up!" It never listens to me.

THERAPIST: That's not your fault. I can teach you some cool ways to get your brain to shut up. Right now, though, can you tell me what you do to make the chicken pox "sticky thought" go away?

CHILD: Umm, I wash my hands a lot. I try never to touch anything that I see people with pimples or people who are coughing touching. I look at my arms a lot to see if I got any pimples or pox.

THERAPIST: You know what? I think you have a worry bully. Some people have these worries in their heads, like your "sticky thought." But they're not just regular old worries. The worries make them do things and promise that they'll go away if they do them, but they lie. The worry bullies make all the rules and then just keep messing with you.

Once obsessions, compulsions, anxiety, and other emotional experiences have either been confirmed or ruled out, clinicians can begin to pinpoint the specific thoughts and behaviors (as well as their frequency, intensity, and duration) that lead to the child's functional impairments. In addition, this is generally the point at which the consulting clinician begins to evaluate the specific content, theme, and functionality of both the obsessions and compulsions to develop a more specific diagnosis within the obsessive–compulsive spectrum (OCS).

Some clinicians question the purpose of distinguishing among the OCS disorders, especially in children and adolescents. However, accurate diagnosis can help the treating professional to address the underlying, or core, fears that tend to differ by disorder. When a clinician taps into a core fear specific to a particular disorder, treatment goes beyond addressing the fears to which children readily admit and may assist the clinician in asking very specific questions to help children express fears that they might not have been able to articulate or to admit having. Well-directed questions based on an accurate diagnosis help children to express themselves and the rationale behind their behaviors better and may improve both the treatment process and treatment efficacy.

PARENT INTERVIEWS

During the clinical interview, it is also important to ask parents about their observations of and experiences with their child's behaviors. Attempting to obtain a chronology of the genesis of their child's fear, in addition to any symptoms that the child has endorsed, may help to round out the clinician's view of the child's disorder. Parents can often shed light on their child's avoidances that may have become so entrenched that even the child may not realize it. In addition, parents can also provide important information about how they (or other members of the family) react to their child's fear-related behaviors, articulated thoughts, and feelings. This can further assist the clinician in understanding how significant others' responses may reinforce certain aspects of a child's fear.

The clinician should ask parents to allow children to explain, in their own words, what they have been thinking, feeling, and doing. He or she then asks the parents whether they have observed what is the same or different. If a parent's views or observations differ significantly from the child's, it is advisable to spend some time alone with the parent to obtain more information (this can also be achieved with a follow-up phone call to query some of the responses from the initial consultation). In addition, it is also important to assess for parent and family psychopathology both directly, by asking about certain behaviors, fears, avoidances, and so on; and indirectly, by taking detailed family medical and psychiatric histories.

It can also be very enlightening for treatment professionals to interview children's significant others, such as siblings, or other extended family members with whom they may spend a significant portion of their time. The more information that we obtain regarding a child's functioning in multiple domains and from varying perspectives, the more complete our clinical picture going into treatment.

TEACHER INTERVIEWS

When dealing with school-age children, especially those who endorse symptom interference with daily academic routines, it is very helpful to interview teachers. Teachers are able to observe children in relation to their peers, which may allow them to identify specific abnormal behaviors that families may overlook simply because they are used to them, or because they lack a normal reference sample of age-matched peers. Some children's symptoms exacerbate in the classroom; other children's symptoms decrease, depending on the perceived stress related to the classroom environment.

Instead of simply asking teachers about specific compulsions that children and their parents endorse, treatment professionals may gain more information by asking about any high-frequency behaviors in which the child engages, in addition to any out-of-the-ordinary, avoidant, or inattentive behaviors (which, as demonstrated in the case presentation, may be mistaken for the distractibility associated with anxiety). A child's symptom manifestation in school may be unique to the environment, or it may be similar to what is described in the home.

SEMISTRUCTURED INTERVIEWS

In addition to clinical interviewing, when possible it is best to employ the use of a structured or semistructured interview schedule to arrive at an accurate DSM-IV diagnosis in either adults or children. With specific regard to the assessment and diagnosis of anxiety disorders in children, we find that the Anxiety Disorders Interview Schedule for DSM-IV, Parent and Child versions (ADIS-IV-C/P; Silverman & Albano, 1996) is a well-constructed and effective diagnostic instrument. However, when considering OCS disorders (disorders that share in common the core features of obsessions and compulsions; e.g., HC, BDD, and anorexia nervosa), the ADIS-IV-C is not designed to detect subtle differences in the type of obsessions and compulsions that allow for accurate diagnosis. In addition, it does not allow one to make a diagnosis of BDD or HC, because they are not classified as anxiety disorders.

Self-Report Measures

Self-report measures may also be effective tools in assisting clinicians to assess for symptoms of anxiety disorders in children and adolescents. We often use instruments such as the Children's Yale–Brown Obsessive Compulsive Scale (CY-BOCS; Scahill et al., 1997), the Fear Survey Schedule for Children—Revised (FSSC-R; Ollendick, 1983), and the State–Trait Anxiety Inventory for Children (STAIC; Spielberger, 1973). Although these scales quite effectively assist clinicians in identifying specific symptoms of either particular anxiety disorders (e.g., OCD), or specific physiological experiences of anxiety, as in the STAIC, they are not necessarily designed to aid clinicians in the accurate assessment of the OCS disorders. Of note, the STAIC may be quite helpful in assisting a clinician to identify the anxiety-based physiological cues that a child might be misinterpreting signs and symptoms of grave physical illness or impending death, as in HC.

With regard to the more cognitive and behavioral symptoms associated with the anxiety disorders in general, one checklist, the Screen for Child Anxiety Related Emotional Disorders—Revised (SCARED-R; Muris, Dreesen, Bogels, Weckx, & van Melick, 2004) tends to be an effective tool in distinguishing among the childhood-onset anxiety disorders. In addition to evaluating for the physiological symptoms of anxiety (e.g., as in the STAIC), the SCARED-R addresses anxiety-related thinking, behaviors, and emotional experiences, and is helpful in identifying symptom clusters that can improve the accuracy of differential diagnosis among children and adolescents. Despite these unique and positive qualities of the SCARED-R, it is designed to address the anxiety disorders, not the OCS disorders.

Less specific rating scales that have value in assessing symptoms of generalized anxiety, depression, inattention, oppositional behavior, and somatic complaints include the Child Behavior Checklist (CBCL; Achenbach, 1991), the Behavior Assessment System for Children–2 (BASC-2, Child, Parent, and Teacher versions), the Revised Conners Parent Rating Scale (CPRS-R; Conners, Sitarenios, Parker, & Epstein, 1998), the Revised Behavior Problem Checklist (RBPC; Quay & Peterson, 1993), as well as the DSM-IV based interview, the Child and Adolescent Psychopathology Scale (CAPS; Lahey et al., 2004).

Given their general nature, if relied on too heavily, OCS disorders may either be misdiagnosed as OCD, GAD, or panic disorder (especially in the case of HC as a result of overattention to physiological cues), or overlooked altogether. Despite their lack of diagnostic specificity, these scales permit clinicians to obtain information from children, their parents, and teachers that might not have been possible during the clinical interview. In addition, these measures also give clinicians the ability to document "clinically significant" changes resulting from treatment outcome.

Of the OCS disorders, probably the least researched diagnostic category with regard to childhood onset is the somatoform disorders, such as BDD and HC. A developing literature over the past two decades (Williams & Hirsch, 1988; Fritz, Fritsch, & Hagino, 1997; Phillips, 2000; Albertini & Phillips, 2003; Phillips & Castle, 2002; Wright & Asmundson, 2003; Hertzig & Farber, 2003) is beginning to recognize and acknowledge that children and adolescents too can be profoundly affected by these diagnostic categories. Of the somatoform disorders that are beginning to attract some long-deserved attention with regard to children and adolescents, HC and BDD appear to be right on the tip of the research community's proverbial brain.

Although the developing corpus of literature on childhood somatoform disorders has encouraged clinicians to assess directly for disorders within this category (Fritz et al., 1997; Phillips & Castle, 2002; Williams & Hirsch, 1988), until recently, only case reports provided clinicians with any diagnostic information on what these disorders might look like in a child or adolescent.

There is generally a paucity of assessment instruments to evaluate symptoms consistent with the latter disorders. One promising tool for clinicians who evaluate children's health anxiety (which arguably is not interchangeable with HC but may be related to it) is the Childhood Illness Attitude Scales (CIAS; Wright et al., 2003). Though not designed specifically to diagnose HC, the 35-item CIAS that evaluates emotional, cognitive, and behavioral responses to pain, health concerns, and illness. It demonstrates good construct-related validity with other measures of childhood fear, depression, and anxiety sensitivity, and may provide structure for a clinician assessing HC in a child or adolescent.

Although no similar instruments exist for the assessment of BDD in children, Phillips (2000) suggests five key questions in arriving at a diagnosis of BDD. Though the questions appear to be geared to adults, we find that they can be adapted easily to assist in evaluating children and adolescents for symptoms of BDD (e.g., "Are you very worried about your appearance in any way? If yes, what is your concern?" can be made more child-friendly by asking, "Do you have any big worries about the way you look? If you do, can you tell me what they are?").

To date, there are few large-scale investigations of BDD in children and adolescents. One study of 33 children and adolescents with BDD (Albertini & Phillips, 2003) provides prevalence of body areas of concern, compulsive behaviors, and types of functional impairment. Though it may help clinicians to understand the presentation of childhood-onset BDD, because of the small size of the sample, it is neither designed nor intended to be used to assess BDD in children or adolescents.

Behavioral Observations and Behavioral Avoidance Tests

The previously discussed assessment techniques share in common the feature that all information is based on self-reports of the child, his or her parents (or other significant others), and teachers. Although essential, the information gleaned from these sources is no substitute for good, old-fashioned behavioral observation. Direct observation of a child in multiple domains of daily functioning allows a clinician to see and record firsthand specific behaviors, their antecedents, and consequences. This allows the treating professional to (1) obtain baseline frequency, intensity, and duration recordings of compulsive and avoidant behaviors; (2) to identify specific triggers for the latter behaviors; (3) to pinpoint responses to these behaviors that reinforce or discourage their repetition; and (4) to compare data collected across domains regarding the behaviors in question.

As clinicians, we recommend that individuals treating children and adolescents perform direct behavioral observations whenever possible. When doing direct behavioral observations, we recommend a minute-to-minute observation technique that tracks the child's overt actions and environmental events every 60 seconds, over the course of at least 90 (and up to 180) minutes per observation session. Although this is time-consuming and labor-intensive for the clinician, it provides a detailed, data-rich slice of the child's life in particular domains of daily functioning (i.e., school, sports, at home).

BEHAVIORAL AVOIDANCE TESTS

Another type of behavioral observation is also extremely valuable in the assessment of children's and adolescents' symptoms. The behavioral avoidance test (BAT), a staple of behavior therapy, is a behavioral observation contrived by the treatment professional to evaluate in a concrete, measurable way (i.e., inches or feet of distance from a fear stimulus) the intensity of a child's fear in response to the presentation of an anxiety-provoking object, person, or situation. So little in the field of psychology is cut and dried, but a BAT yields real numbers. It is also a tool that may be employed to track treatment in progress over time (symptom improvement may be measured by reductions in behavioral avoidance).

Another advantage of BATs is that they are simple and inexpensive to perform, they can be repeated often, and they can be performed by parents. Children can take part in recording their own BAT data, which brings them into the therapeutic process as active participants even as they are facing their fears.

Empirical investigation of home-based BATs in assessing treatment efficacy in children and adolescents with OCD (Barrett, Healy, & March, 2003) suggests that BATs are sensitive and accurate measures of behavioral avoidance and distress. It is our experience that BATs may be similarly effective in the assessment of the latter variables in OCS disorders and may be valuable tools in both pretreatment assessment of symptoms and treatment as measures of effectiveness of treatment strategies.

A sample of how to explain and solicit a child's participation in a BAT is as follows:

THERAPIST: OK, so we know you stay away from your baby brother, because he's kind of germy and you feel like he could give you chicken pox by touching you, right?

CHILD: Yeah. I know he can't really, but I'm really afraid he could touch me with his spitty hand and give me the pox.

THERAPIST: So, a way we figure out just how afraid people are of things is by looking at how far away they stay from them. Like, if I'm afraid of sharks, do you think I would pet a shark or let it hang out with me in my bath?

CHILD: No. That would be dumb.

THERAPIST: Right. So, Mom will stand over there with your brother, and I'd like you take some steps toward him, so I can measure how afraid or uncomfortable you are with each step you take closer to him. Go as far away from him as you have to, until you don't feel afraid anymore. Now, take steps toward him, until you feel a little afraid or uncomfortable, then put a piece of tape on the floor by your sneaker.

CHILD: OK, I'm a little afraid. I'll put my tape here.

THERAPIST: Excellent. Now come a little closer to him until you feel medium fear, then stop and put your tape there. (*Repeats this same procedure until the child has reached maximum fear and is as close as he or she is willing to get to the avoided person.*)

SELF- (AND OTHER-) MONITORING

Data gleaned by a clinician from direct behavioral observations and BATs, once analyzed, likely reveal specific behaviors that occur reliably in response to particular trigger events (i.e., compulsions and avoidance behaviors). At this point, checklists constructed by the treatment professional assist the child, parents, and teacher to engage in monitoring these specific behaviors. This is a valuable tool, again in the assessment phase prior to treatment, to get a more extended sample of the frequency of these behaviors over the course of days or weeks. However, self-monitoring exercises are another way to get children directly involved in their treatment, by putting them in charge of keeping track of their behaviors. Also, some behaviors may reduce in frequency simply as a result of increased awareness due to self-monitoring. In addition, self-monitoring is another method that allows an individual to track the reduction of specific behaviors over the course of treatment. We encourage clinicians to have children, their parents, and teachers (if applicable) keep track of compulsive and avoidant behaviors, using charts that we develop from data collected during behavioral observations.

When asking children, their parents, and their teachers to monitor certain behaviors, it is important to explain that the task is simply to identify a frequency count of the actions explicitly described. The goal of this exercise is to obtain a tally of certain observable behaviors, not to reinforce or discourage them in any way. So it is sometimes helpful to articulate to those doing the behavioral recording that nobody gets more credit for the "assignment" by doing extra work.

Link between Assessment and Treatment

As discussed throughout the assessment portion of this chapter, information gleaned from the child, parent, and teacher interviews; behavioral observations and BAT's; and self-report and self-monitoring measures all contribute to the development of tailored, individualized treatment protocols for children and adolescents. There are several different aspects of the treatment process in which assessment data may be valuable.

Based on the initial consultation, treatment professionals likely have begun to compile a list of the child or adolescent patient's obsessions, supporting rigid or irrational thoughts, compulsions, and avoidant behaviors. Thus, by honing in on specific information being provided by the child or adolescent and his or her close others, the clinician begins to ask differential diagnostic questions and is more likely to arrive at an accurate diagnosis. Though the right label alone is not correlated with effective treatment, accurately classifying disorders helps us to understand their nuances. For example, an individual treating HC might focus more on a child's fear of being ill, feeling sick, and eventually dying, gearing exposures to particular "pathogenic" people and situations, as well as inducing some of the "symptoms" (or physiological phenomena that the child might fear), while preventing compulsive behaviors such as body checking and medical reassurance seeking. However, a clinician treating OCD with somatic obsessions, in which the fear is more focused on simply having particular symptoms, might focus more on exposure to feared situations, while preventing the individual from discussing or checking for particular symptoms. Similarly, a treatment professional dealing with BDD might focus more on the client's fear of being disfigured, flawed, and imperfect, creating exposures that emphasize the defect in public situations, while preventing mirror checking and camouflaging, in addition to dealing with the ensuing feelings of anxiety and disgust. The same clinician might deal with anorexia nervosa, which is phenomenologically similar, by having the client consume feared foods, while resisting compensatory exercise and compulsive weigh-ins. Our adage is that if you can name it properly, then you can tame it effectively.

Data obtained from various self-report measures may also assist clinicians in this endeavor. For example, item examination of checklists (e.g., CY-BOCS, SCARED-R, or CIAS) can provide the treating clinician with information regarding feared situations, obsessions, and compulsions beyond that provided by the child or parents during the initial consultation.

In addition, by discussing the chronology and development of the particular disorder, activating events and others' responses (e.g., parents, siblings, and teachers) to the child's articulated fears and resultant behaviors, can shed significant light on how the symptoms began, evolved, and have been maintained. In our case presentation, Kelli's fear of illness began when a child her age died from a malignant brain tumor. However, her current obsessions were more linked to her bout with allergies and fear of mad cow disease (which was a hot topic in current events).

This basic information about trigger events, people, and situations, as well as specific responses to these, may also help the treating clinician to develop the basic foundation of the hierarchy. Obtaining baseline measures of the frequency, intensity, and duration of specific compulsive behaviors, combined with data based on direct behavioral observations and planned BATs, tends to flesh out the hierarchy, providing a solid framework for developing exposure with response prevention (ERP) exercises and rational disputations of irrational thoughts.

The latter methods also help the clinician to understand how others' responses may be reinforcing particular maladaptive behaviors, so that he or she can develop parent and teacher training sessions to improve responses to compulsions and behavioral avoidance at home and in school. Often parents, siblings, and teachers, in an attempt to help the identified child feel better, may directly reinforce or even participate in compulsions. Though they may not recognize their role in the maintenance of symptoms, this can be directly observed, then targeted with psychoeducation and behavioral coaching.

Finally, frequent reassessment of symptoms using self-report measures such as checklists, as well as performing BATs, and obtaining subjective units of distress (SUD) ratings for hierarchy items that have been addressed, allows the clinician to evaluate the child's progress in treatment. Empirical support for the use of BATs in measuring treatment-related changes in children and adolescents with OCD (Barrett et al., 2003) suggests that BATs may also be a sensitive and effective measure for assessing treatment progress in children with OCS disorders.

Direct behavioral observation is also a tool by which to gauge treatment responses in various settings, and can help the clinician hone in on areas that need to be addressed, especially if treatment is not progressing as expected based on what the family, the child, or teachers are reporting. Sometimes an individual close to the child may be reinforcing a particular behavior without even knowing it, despite following the prescribed treatment protocol closely in other ways. When in doubt, we recommend that clinicians make a site visit to observe for themselves what environmental contingencies might be reinforcing particular maladaptive behaviors. For example, one of our child clients with HC seemed to be experiencing an unexplained symptom exacerbation in school. The teacher said that she was following the plan for dealing with the child's reassurance seeking to the letter of the law and could not identify the source of trouble. However, during a school observation, the clinician identified that the child had been asking for hall passes, during which she had been making trips to the school nurse. This made little sense, because the school nurse had also been trained in how to handle the child's requests for having her pupils, skin, and glands checked; temperature taken; and so on. The psychologist who visited the nurse's office met the substitute nurse, who had been filling in while the regular school nurse was out with an injury. Though well-intentioned, she had been giving into the child's bids for escalating reassurance. Our opinion is that you may not know unless you go.

Treatment

Overview

Our treatment philosophy is based on a biopsychosocial model. We attempt to evaluate and conceptualize each case with regard to these three dimensions and recognize that there is a reciprocal relationship between them. These factors may account for the etiology of the disorder and/or impact the progression and prognosis of it. We attempt to consider these factors from the first intake evaluation and throughout the treatment process, from case conceptu-alization to treatment prognosis to treatment planning.

Our first consideration are biological factors, including (1) family history of mental illness; (2) medical conditions that may contribute to the illness; (3) developmental history, including maternal prenatal history, complications at birth, and age of developmental milestones; (4) presence of diseases that may lead to psychological disorders; and (5) current medications and previous response to pharmacological agents. A thorough assessment of biological fac-tors allows for appropriate treatment planning. For example, if the child pres-ents with certain symptoms that cannot be accounted for by psychological diagnosis alone, then treatment may involve enlisting other professionals, such as psychiatrists/psychopharmacologists, pediatricians, and neurologists, for a complete diagnosis. Our philosophy is to develop a treatment team for the individual child that may involve multiple agencies and professionals, in con-junction with our psychological intervention.

The child's psychological functioning involves assessing not only the symptoms of the particular disorder but also the presence of commonly occur-ring comorbid disorders, as well as other psychological factors such as intel-lectual abilities and personality traits. This may involve conducting personal-ity, neuropsychological, and/or academic assessments to evaluate properly the child's intellectual abilities, visual processing skills, personality tests, attention and concentration, academic achievement, abstract reasoning abilities, and memory functioning—all of which may potentially interfere with treatment progress and prognosis. We recommend the appropriate assessments for a variety of circumstances, including an undiagnosed learning disability, poten-tial neurological impairment, as well as ADHD.

The contribution of sociocultural factors, including both the person's individual social environment and the larger cultural context in which he or she lives is also an important component of case conceptualization. This involves assessing factors such as the child's family relationships, school envi-ronment, and extracurricular activities to determine how these may contribute to the child's disorder and progress. It is important to assess whether the child can return to optimal functioning in his or her sociocultural environment.

Context of Treatment

As clinicians, we are aware that there are many individual differences, and that motivational levels may vary. We have encountered some adolescents who independently researched treatment options and subsequently requested that their parents schedule an appointment, whereas other children sit silently in our offices session after session. As we stated earlier, it is important to con-sider a number of variables when designing a treatment plan, such as the moti-vation level of the patient, family relationships and response to the illness, and even one's style as a therapist. For example, treatment for a resistant child may involve multiple sessions of rapport and motivation building before implementation of specific behavioral techniques. Treatment for a child with comorbid depression may involve addressing depression before one addresses the targeted disorder. Treatment for a child whose parents are enabling every compulsion may involve multiple parent training sessions before progress is experienced. Furthermore, the OCS disorders can impact almost every activity in which the child engages, requiring the therapist to be involved in every aspect of the child's life. This may mean speaking to a patient's soccer coach, guidance counselor, and psychiatrist to develop a comprehensive treatment plan. In this section, we hope to offer guidelines on coping with all of these factors when treating a child with an OCS disorder.

Encountering a resistant/noncompliant patient or a patient who is not demonstrating an expected level of improvement is one of the most stressful aspects of being a therapist. A variety of individual variables may become obstacles in treatment. The most common variables include (1) depression and other comorbid diagnoses; (2) high, overvalued ideation; (3) lack of education regarding the diagnosis or treatment; (4) comorbid personality disorders; and (5) unrealistic patient expectations. Family variables may also impact the treatment process, such as (1) parenting style, (2) parental reaction to the disorder, and (3) psychiatric diagnoses of other family members. Therapist/therapeutic environmental factors also need to be considered when a patient is not progressing. These include (1) therapist style, (2) anxiety in the therapeutic environment, and (3) pacing of sessions and homework.

Variables Affecting Treatment

COMORBIDITY

The presence of multiple comorbid conditions can complicate the clinical picture. Certain diagnoses, such as depression, may impact motivation levels and consistent follow through on treatment recommendations. Based on comorbidity statistics, the typical child or adolescent patient is likely to demonstrate another anxiety, depressive, behavioral, or tic disorder in addition to the targeted OCS condition.

It is best to address first the disorder that is creating the most distress for the patient. If, however, certain symptoms interfere with the patient's ability to attend session regularly or participate in treatment but are not necessarily the patient's primary goal, then these symptoms may need to be addressed first regardless of other factors or opinions. Comorbid depression traditionally has been viewed as one important variable impacting treatment outcome. Individuals with comorbid severe depression do not experience between- or within-session habituation during ERP (Foa, 1979). If initial assessment yields moderate to severe comorbid depression, it is important either to target those symptoms exclusively for a number of sessions or concurrently with treatment of the OCS disorder. Traditional cognitive therapy, behavioral assignments to increase participation in pleasurable activities, behavioral activation, and a psychopharmacological consultation for antidepressant medication all may be in order.

OVERVALUED IDEATION

As we mentioned previously, overvalued ideation may be an important variable impacting treatment outcome. Overvalued ideation, in our experience, does not tend to shift from day to day; rather, it is fixed and does not change unless directly targeted in treatment. A proper assessment of the child's strength of conviction in the belief helps to determine the pace of treatment. Patients are quite reluctant to engage in ERP when their beliefs are strong; thus, cognitive therapy to lower the strength of the belief is necessary. In fact, children are less likely to recognize their behaviors as excessive or unreasonable compared to adults (Wagner, 2003). Psychoeducation of OCS disorders, with special emphasis on the neurobiological framework, is an integral part of the treatment process to address highly overvalued ideation. Cognitive therapy, in the case of higher overvalued ideation, should be consistently utilized in every session and may involve strategies such as constructive self-talk and cognitive restructuring (March & Mulle, 1998). Although the Overvalued Ideas Scale (OVIS; Neziroglu, McKay, Yaryura-Tobias, Stevens, & Todaro, 1999) was developed for adults, the wording may be modified to give the therapist some idea of the child's strength of belief. This is quite important, because the OVIS has been demonstrated to predict adult treatment outcome (Neziroglu et al., 2001).

Identifying the child's overly negative or positive self-statements before, during, and after exposure and homework assignments may improve compliance. Teaching the child to have realistic appraisals of anxiety and the ability to cope help the child follow through on exposure exercises and decrease avoidance behaviors. For example, teaching Kelli to say "This is hard, but I can do it," rather than "I won't be able to handle the anxiety if I eat that roast beef sandwich," helped her engage in exposure exercises. Self-talk can also may be utilized to "talk back to the OCD" (March & Mulle, 1998) by saying things like "You're a bully and I don't have to listen to you." Identifying OCD as an external entity also helps children increase their insight level (March & Mulle, 1998).

Cognitive restructuring should be utilized to challenge directly the child's faulty beliefs, such as overestimation of risk ("It's definitely going to happen") and overestimation regarding responsibility for the outcome ("And it'll definitely occur because of something I did"). Challenging Kelli's belief that she will definitely get mad cow disease from that particular sandwich involves identifying the exact probability of that outcome occurring in the first place (What are the chances of getting mad cow disease?). The use of pie charts to determine all the possible factors that could be responsible for the outcome is another cognitive restructuring strategy (March & Mulle, 1998) aside from dialogues in which the therapist challenges the beliefs. For example, identifying all the possible reasons why "everyone" was looking at Kelli in class helped to challenge the BDD belief that others were noticing her "skinny and young-looking" body.

FAMILY VARIABLES

Researchers in the field of OCD have realized the impact of family variables in treatment outcome and have begun devoting time to address the issue (for a review of literature, see Steketee & Van Noppen, 2003). Research has shown that families of patients with OCD tend to respond in either antagonistic or accommodating ways. Families of children with OCD also demonstrate low levels of emotional support, warmth, and closeness (Valleni-Basile et al., 1995), as well as high expressed emotion, specifically defined as high levels of criticism, hostility, and/or overinvolvement (Hibbs et al., 1991). Up to 75% of family members accommodate the OCD by participating in rituals, modifying personal or family routines, providing reassurance, and/or taking over house-hold and other duties for the patient (Calvocoressi et al., 1995, 1999). One study found that family members of patients with OCD tend to make less use of positive problem solving, and parents are less likely to reward independence in their children (Barrett, Short, & Healy, 2002). Accommodation (Amir, Freshman, & Foa, 2000) and high expressed emotion (Steketee, 1993; Steketee & Van Noppen, 2003) may impact treatment outcome, although more research is necessary to make definitive conclusions.

The inability of parents to cope effectively with the disorder is likely to lead to significant marital discord and increase overall family tension, impacting all members of the household. In fact, in one study of 225 family members of adult patients with OCD found that up to 80% of patients reported that the illness was disruptive in the personal lives of family members (Cooper, 1996).

Psychoeducation and family involvement in cognitive-behavioral therapy (CBT) for patients, adults, and children alike are becoming an integral component of effective treatment. One study demonstrated that a structured treatment protocol involving parent and sibling psychoeducation and coaching on how to manage the child's OCD led to positive results in both individual and group formats (Barrett, Healy-Farrell, & March, 2004). In adults, when family members were involved in family intervention groups, patients responded better to CBT for OCD (Grunes, Neziroglu, & McKay, 2001).

Although less research has investigated family variables in HC, GAD, and BDD, it is reasonable to conclude that parent training in most childhood diagnoses is a valuable treatment goal. Our treatment protocol consists of regular involvement of family members in the child's treatment, either in separate appointments or for 15 minutes at the end of sessions. We frequently bring the family in to demonstrate exactly how to coach the child when he or she is having an obsession, how to coach him or her through a therapeutic homework exercise, and so on. Parents are often unsure how to be supportive without inadvertently giving in to a child's compulsive reassurance seeking. This involves showing parents how to express their support and to validate their child's anxiety level but be firm in not engaging in the ritual with their child.

Parents who are on the accommodating end of the continuum may make cosmetic surgery or repeated dermatological appointments for their child, sit in the bathroom and assist with every step of the ritualistic grooming, or allow their child repeatedly to miss school because of anxiety. Reminding parents that the philosophy of behavior therapy is habituation to anxiety rather than avoidance of any situation that creates anxiety is beneficial. We often provide parents with scripted responses to their child's request for aid in a compulsion. For example, the therapist coached Kelli's mother on how to respond to Kelli's questions by saying, "I know how difficult this is for you and I know how badly you want the answer to that question, but it sounds like the worry monster/bully is trying to trick us into having this conversation again. Remember, he's like a mean and selfish bully who will just demand more and more of our time if we listen to him. So, can we try to ignore his questions for a little while and see if he'll get bored with us?" The goal initially is to delay engaging in the compulsions systematically, in the hope that Kelli's anxiety decreases naturally.

Parents who have an antagonistic style in response to the OCD may punish their child for engaging in a ritual, accuse the child of faking anxiety, and/ or may not believe that their child's behavior is a result of a psychiatric illness. In this case, parent training involves a significant amount of psychoeducation about the biological basis of the disorder, including provision of reading material, so that the parents understand that their child's condition is as real as diabetes or cancer. The style of the therapist is an important variable, because an overly judgmental or didactic style may be offensive to the parents. It is usually more effective if the therapist frequently validates the parents' anxiety and frustration at having to cope with a child with a disorder, such as saying that it must be very confusing for them to watch their child demonstrate irrational beliefs and behaviors in some situations and seem rational in other situations, with the result that the child appears completely dysfunctional in some situations and excels in others. Furthermore, the child's responses may not seem to follow conventional logic, because certain things that cause significant anxiety in one situation may not do so in others. For example, a child with contamination OCD may be able to touch a faucet in a public bathroom at a crowded baseball stadium but not his or her own family bathroom faucet because he or she once passed by the bathroom as his or her brother was urinating and did not hear him washing his hands. Drawing on the parents' strengths and positive attributes rather than appearing judgmental and disapproving of their behavior leads to a more positive therapeutic alliance, with obvious benefits for the child's recovery.

Another important family variable to consider is the presence of psychological diagnoses in the parents. Because studies have shown that similar disorders run in families, it is common to come across a parent with the same or a similar diagnosis as one's patient (Yaryura-Tobias, Grunes, Walz, & Neziroglu, 2000). Often parents have not gotten treatment for their own illness. This can compromise the parents' ability to play the role of a cotherapist/coach outside of the session. In this case, we do attempt to recommend individual treatment for the parent once rapport has been established. Often, only one parent aids in treatment process.

THERAPIST/THERAPY VARIABLES

Often a patient with an OCS disorder may seem resistant to attending a session because a particular aspect of the therapeutic environment is anxiety provoking. For example, a patient with BDD may be anxious about the bright lighting in the office or a crowded waiting room. Similarly, a patient with OCD may be unable to leave home for a lengthy period of time for fear of needing to use a public restroom, or he or she may find the waiting room too "dirty," and so on. These types of factors may be addressed easily and rectified once they are identified. If a patient appears visibly uncomfortable during the session, the therapist simply asks if any aspect of the setting is making them anxious. Children and adolescents may not be able to articulate the cause of their discomfort, and providing the examples mentioned earlier may decrease their discomfort.

Setting the appropriate pacing for exposure exercises and assigning a reasonable level of therapy homework are also key factors in treating OCS disorders. We have observed that because exposure exercises for children are typically done in game format, it takes children longer to reach their peak anxiety and to habituate during the session time. This means that in a typical, 45-minute therapy session, a patient may leave the session at the height of his or her anxiety; consequently, the child may resist coming back week after week, believing that he or she has to leave every session extremely anxious and upset. Scheduling longer sessions for particularly challenging exposures may be beneficial.

The standard suggestion in behavior therapy is to develop exposure exercises with a great deal of input from the patient. This also applies to children and adolescents. Often parents set arbitrary deadlines for treatment and want their child to be better in time for summer camp or for the new school year, and so on. It is important to pace treatment with your patient's, rather than his or her parent's, expectations.

Therapists working with OCS disorders sometimes find it a challenge to find the right balance between respecting the patient's right to say no and pushing the patient to engage in exposure exercises. It is prudent to proceed slowly in the beginning stages of treatment to develop a strong therapeutic relationship. Individuals vary in their ability to predict their anxiety level accurately during exposures, so if a child consistently overestimates how anxious he or she will be during a particular exercise but does well with some encouragement, then it is probably safe to push him or her a bit harder than a child who has a very low tolerance for anxiety and does not habituate quickly.

We find that children and adolescents are usually impatient to experience some relief from their symptoms, so pacing treatment to meet this expectation is also important. It is usually beneficial for this reason to minimize the amount of cognitive therapy in the session. Children and adolescents may find it harder to sit and simply "talk" about their obsessions. Behavioral exercises hold their attention and keep them more engaged in sessions than does disputing their irrational beliefs. We find that devoting a small amount of time each session to cognitive therapy is sufficient.

The use of humor and creativity is often overlooked in the behavioral treatment literature, but it is worth some attention, because it may lead to increased compliance. Engaging in behavioral treatment can be a daunting experience for patients; they willingly attend session after session, with the knowledge that the goal is to create anxiety to achieve symptom relief. For example, we often write scripts that patients may use for flooding between sessions. Incorporating humor into the script creatively by writing it as a newspaper article or headline in which the patient's disastrous consequences are mentioned in a humorous way helps the patient to comply and to participate more readily in treatment homework assignments.

INTENSIVE TREATMENT

Early research investigating ERP effectiveness demonstrated that intensive treatment is more effective than weekly sessions (Franklin & Foa, 2002). Whenever feasible, we recommend that patients who are experiencing moderate to severe symptoms and are functionally impaired begin with more than one session a week. Our general guideline is based on the average number of hours the patient engages in rituals and the degree of impairment in life domains. If an individual has stopped attending school and engages in rituals for 6 hours a day, then weekly sessions will obviously be ineffective. However, if the child continues to maintain grades, participate in extracurricular activities, and symptoms occupy 2 hours a day, weekly sessions will suffice. Multiple sessions a week lead more quickly to relief of symptoms, especially if scheduled in the beginning stages of treatment, and have the added benefit of providing the family and the child with hope and belief in the treatment process.

DISORDER IN MULTIPLE SETTINGS

As mentioned earlier, symptoms of OCD, BDD, GAD, and HC may be evident in the child's activities throughout the day in a variety of settings that extend from school hours to extracurricular activities after school. Dealing with a child in all of these areas may seem overwhelming to a therapist, especially when multiple adults may be responding in different ways to the child's symptoms. The job of the therapist may at times be to act as head coach and provide these key individuals with specific guidelines. At times we have typed up a step-by-step approach for people in the child's life to follow, including how to respond to a request for reassurance, what to do when the child is unable to engage in a required activity, and how to coach the child through an anxiety-provoking trigger. Each adult in the child's life may experience different aspects of the disorder, because different settings may involve different types of triggers and behavioral manifestations of the disorder. In the case of Kelli, both speaking to the pediatrician and contacting the school regularly were extremely helpful. The school kept us abreast of the amount of food Kelli was eating during lunch and whether she was able to sit through class. Helping to develop a behavioral reward system for Kelli's class attendance was also necessary.

Components of Therapy

Very few studies have systematically investigated the outcome of CBT for children with anxiety and OCS disorders. Available research indicates that CBT is efficacious. In one open trial of CBT for children and adolescents with OCD, 9 out of 15 children showed at least a 50% reduction in symptoms, and 6 children were asymptomatic (March, Mulle, & Herbel, 1994). In a 12-week open trial of CBT for children ages 8–17 years, with no concomitant pharmacotherapy, 62% of patients demonstrated at least a 50% improvement in OCD symptom severity (Benazon, Ager, & Rosenberg, 2002). In this randomized controlled trial for pediatric OCD, results indicated that CBT alone, sertraline alone, and the combined treatment all were efficacious in addressing OCD. Combined treatment was superior to CBT alone or sertraline alone. Remission rates were approximately 54% for combined treatment, 39% (not statistically different) for CBT alone, and 21.4% for sertraline alone (Pediatric OCD Treatment Team [POTS], 2004). CBT alone and CBT in combination with family-based therapy have been shown to be effective for adolescents with GAD, social phobia, and separation anxiety disorder (Siqueland, Rynn, & Diamond, 2005). Group CBT is also effective with parental involvement (Fischer, Himle, & Hanna, 1998; Martin & Thienemann, 2005). Behavioral therapy in game format has also been effective (Moritz, 1998). A review of advances made in adult and pediatric OCD research from 1995 to 2005 is discussed by Neziroglu, Henriksen, and Yaryura-Tobias (2006).

THE PROCESS OF TREATMENT: STEP-BY-STEP GUIDELINES

Preview

The first four sessions are traditionally for the purpose of rapport building, information gathering, treatment planning, and psychoeducation. However, some treatment can be snuck into the session. For example, if a child is seeking reassurance in a session, then we can explain how reassurance seeking may reduce the obsession immediately but eventually make it much worse. As the child agrees to do a behavioral experiment to delay reassurance, we can begin to observe his or her anxiety increase, then plateau, and finally plummet when he or she engages in response prevention. We demonstrate how anxiety may be reduced by having the child try response prevention techniques, such as "talking back," when worries become overwhelming, and approach anxiety in a humorous, over-the-top way. Modeling these methods for the child is often helpful. If anxiety reduction is achieved during the session both the child and the parents gain confidence in the strategies being employed.

The first four sessions of treatment also allow us to begin working with the parents and child to develop the framework for future treatment. After the consultation appointment, we develop a plan of action, including a determination of the frequency of treatment, which is largely based on the severity of the disorder. Scheduling the first few sessions within a short space of time is helpful, so that specific exposure and response prevention exercises may be started sooner. Patients, and especially parents, are eager to experience a change sooner rather than later, especially because part of the first four sessions is spent setting the stage for future sessions. During this time, it is especially important to get the child and parents actively involved in all aspects of treatment (i.e., hierarchy construction, self-monitoring, thinking of examples of times they faced fears and the results), so that their motivation does not wane.

Session 1

The two primary goals of Kelli's first treatment session are (1) to establish rapport with Kelli and her mother, and (2) to provide psychoeducation about OCD, BDD and HC, linking them to the other OCS disorders. The objective is to have Kelli and her mother leave this session understanding Kelli's symptoms. It is important also to help them to understand that obsessions, like a runaway train of worry in the brain, can only go on as long as it has a constant fuel supply, and that compulsions fuel the obsessions. Making specific links to the symptoms associated with HC and BDD, and their particular obsessions and compulsions, helps to make this even clearer.

Once this has been established, the "enemy" is clear, and the foundation for future dialogues about fighting this enemy has been laid. It is also important to reinforce the concept that people in Kelli's life, including Kelli, are members of the same team fighting together.

THERAPIST: I know that the last time I met you we talked a lot about the worries you've been having. We gave them names, too; "obsessive–compulsive disorder," "hypochondriasis," and "body dysmorphic disorder," or OCD, HC, and BDD. Let's talk a little more about what they are how they're bullying you around and messing things up in your life, so we can figure out how to kick their butts. OK?

KELLI: OK. I just want you to know that I'm really scared, because I don't want to die or be ugly. I know I have anxiety, but sometimes it feels real and I just can't fight it.

THERAPIST: I know you're scared. Most kids and adults we work with are scared...in the beginning. Then we teach them how to fight. Do you really think that your treatment involves dying or being ugly? We'd be out of business if that's how we treated people's anxiety. I know we talked about facing fears last time, but that doesn't mean they come true.

KELLI: You have a point. I just don't get how OCD, HC, and BDD are all about fears. People do get sick and die. And some people are really ugly.

THERAPIST: Yeah, that's true. But do you think everyone who gets sick or is ugly worries about it, or spends their whole life trying really hard not to be that way? Did you ever see a really ugly person?

KELLI: Yeah. My lunch lady is kind of gross. She has this sick mole and it has hairs and stuff growing out of it. Ugh. I can't believe she leaves the house. I'd so not ever leave my room if I looked like that.

THERAPIST: The fact that you've seen her means she's not so worried about it. Usually, people worry about things that they're afraid will happen, not what's really happening. OCD, HC, and BDD are all about anxiety and worries. Did you know that OCD, HC, and BDD are actually related to each other, like first cousins?

KELLI: Oh, awesome. I have a family of disorders living in my head?

THERAPIST: No, just cousins. Here's how it works: certain people have the sticky worry thoughts we talked about last time I saw you, called "obsessions." Then they try to make them go away by doing certain things over and over again. Those actions or thoughts are called "compulsions." There are a whole bunch of different illnesses that all have something important in common, so we grouped them together. We call them the "obsessive–compulsive spectrum disorders." HC and BDD are both body-related and have obsessions and compulsions in common. HC makes you worry that you have something really physically wrong with your body and that you will die, and OCD makes you think that you will get some type of illness unless you either avoid certain things, like red meat, or you better do something to make it better, like wash your hands. It is your BDD that makes you think that something's wrong with the way you look. Got it? It seems like a lot, but really they are all pretty much the same thing.

KELLI: I get it. But why do I have to have these worries? What's wrong with my brain?

THERAPIST: Scientists who have done lots of studies on people with anxiety and obsessive thoughts believe that a brain chemical called serotonin may be involved. Serotonin is a very busy chemical that helps balance a lot of different emotions and behaviors, including worries, anxiety, depression, and repeating actions. When there isn't enough serotonin in our brain, certain worries and thoughts get stuck in our head and we can't get them out. It's like our brain keeps telling us that there is something dangerous out there when there isn't. Our brain gives off a fear message when there's no real danger. It's like a broken smoke alarm that keeps ringing even though there's no fire. Do you understand?

KELLI: All right. I got it. So because of my low serotonin, I worry a lot about things that other people don't always think about.

THERAPIST: Exactly. And your obsessions are obnoxious, and they keep popping into your head uninvited. They usually say things like "What if . . . ?" and "How do you know that . . . ?" They make you doubt what you know, and that makes you more nervous. Rude, right?

KELLI: Very rude.

THERAPIST: Obsessions are like spoiled brats who bother you and bother you, screaming at you and making your really anxious. And like brats, they make demands. The problem is that doing a compulsion is like giving into your obsession, like giving it a cookie. It makes it happy for a while, then it starts crying again and you have to keep giving it cookies, which makes it grow. Then it gets big enough to start pushing you around and bullying you by making you more and more worried.

KELLI: You said that the things I do over and over make my unwanted obsessions stay longer? You mean things like reading the ingredients on my food a lot or washing my hands?

THERAPIST: That's correct. We call all of those actions "compulsions," and all compulsions fuel obsessions. If you want an obsession to go away, you need to quit giving it cookies. Obsessions are the bullies that demand your lunch money. If you give a bully your lunch money, what happens?

KELLI: Then he keeps bugging you for money every day.

THERAPIST: Absolutely, he may go away and stop bothering you for a little while, but then he just comes back looking for more. OCD, HC, and BDD are like that. So what do you think works when a bully is bothering you?

KELLI: My mom says to ignore him, tell him to go away or not give him what he is asking for.

THERAPIST: We're going to do the same thing with your worry thoughts. We're going to learn to talk back to your worries and learn that doing the opposite of what the bully tells you to do will eventually make him go away. It sounds like your mom knows what she is talking about. We are going to need her and your dad's help to fight the bully.

KELLI: So what can I do now to stop giving it my lunch money?

THERAPIST: Is there anything that you could probably not give into, but sometimes do, because it feels easier in the moment? Because that would be perfect for a little experiment.

KELLI: Yeah, sometimes I don't eat chicken, because I wonder if a chicken and a cow hung out together on a farm and that the chicken could have gotten mad cow.

THERAPIST: OK, but don't expect to feel awesome the second you eat chicken. You might feel really nervous for a while, because your OCD is such a major brat and is so used to getting its way. If you get nervous, remind yourself that you just punched your OCD and it's punching back. Do not avoid eating the foods that are around it, do not wash your hands, do not check the Internet for symptoms of mad cow disease and how one gets it. Let your mom know when you're fighting your bully, so she can be extra supportive and help you get through it by hanging out and talking or playing a game with you until the urge to check or seek reassurance passes. OK? Also, you can totally call me or e-mail me if you have any questions or need a hand. OK?

KELLI: OK, cool.

THERAPIST: So the first thing we have to do is to give the bully a name. Let's come up with two names, one for the bully that bothers you about diseases and another for the bully that bothers you about your appearance.

KELLI: I don't know.

THERAPIST: That's OK. Maybe you can do that for me this week, before our next appointment.

Session 2

The goals of this session are to introduce the concept of CBT and to review the material presented in Session 1, as illustrated by the following dialogue:

THERAPIST: So, did you name the bullies we talked about last week?

KELLI: Yeah, Dumb and Butt. Funny, right? Hey! I ate chicken. I was really nervous like you said, but then I didn't do any of my checking.

THERAPIST: That is great. You saw how your anxiety rose up and then fell down when you didn't give into it. So, remember how we talked about the family of illnesses that all have anxiety, worry thoughts, and repeating behaviors in common? Do you have any questions?

KELLI: No.

THERAPIST: Today I'd like to keep teaching you how we're going to help you beat up the bully. The first rule is that you are the boss, not the bully. He can threaten you or try to trick you, but you're going to boss him back, OK? The second rule is that you are stronger than the bully, even if it doesn't always feel that way. The third rule is that if you do the opposite of what he wants, he will eventually get bored with you and give up. When you first learn to do the opposite of what he bosses you to do, it may sometimes feel worse before it feels better, like after you ate chicken. He did what a bully does when you first say "No!" to him. He acted like a punk and tried to intimidate you. But you didn't give in, you kept right on fighting.

KELLI: For a little while, when I was nervous, I kept feeling like an idiot, like I made a mistake and he was just mocking me, saying, "Oh, you ate chicken and it hung out with cows, and now you're going to get mad cow, because you tried to fight me."

THERAPIST: Exactly, he will try lots of ways to get your lunch money before he gives up. This may make you feel more anxious at first, but you know that giving in will make him come back for more. The way you carried out your experiment is what we'll be doing together. It's a treatment called "exposure and response prevention." This kind of therapy really works to fight back worries. We will be working together to face the situations that make you nervous, and that your bully tells you to stay away from. That is called "exposure." And we will practice not doing the repeating and checking behaviors, and that's called "response prevention."

KELLI: Eating chicken wasn't that hard. I chose it because I do it sometimes. But my other stuff, the stuff I never do, is going to be really, really hard. I can't do that.

THERAPIST: I know it seems that way, but we will make a list together of all the things that make you nervous. We will start with the things that make you feel the least anxious and work our way up to the hard stuff. Once you've done the easy stuff, you'll feel much better, and the hard stuff won't seem so hard anymore. We'll just work as slow or as fast as you can, OK? And we'll make a deal now. Whatever you do, we'll all do with you.

KELLI: Seriously?

THERAPIST: Seriously. Hey, I'd like you to start making notes each day on what you worry about, and what you're doing when you started to worry, and what you did in response to the worry. It doesn't matter if you can't fight it; this is just to find out how often you worry, what you're worrying about, and what you're doing when you're worried. And keep enjoying your chicken.

Homework

Ask the child to record the date, time, and situation in which he or she engaged in a compulsive behavior and the obsession/worries that preceded that compulsion. It may be unreasonable to ask for a daily record for a week, but 2 to 3 days is sufficient to collect the necessary data for treatment planning (see Figure 3.3).

Date and time	What was I doing?	What were my worry thoughts?	What did I do about it? (repeating behaviors)
EX: March 16, 2007	Playing basketball outside and saw a dog	Oh no, what if he has rabies and bites me!	Ran inside and took a shower and asked my mom if she thought I was safe.

FIGURE 3.3. Self-monitoring of compulsions

Other components of treatment include psychoeducation, in which the child is taught that anticipatory anxiety is worse than the actual experience, and that facing fears is the only way to overcome them. Meeting with parents separately and with the children to reinforce the same language of "bossing back the bully" should also be a part of the initial sessions. Children at this point may ask questions about exactly what to expect in future sessions. It is important to refrain from giving too many examples of exposure exercises, which would certainly be too frightening for Kelli at this point in treatment. Hearing about specific exercises to confront feared or avoided situations may lead to a child's refusal to attend future sessions.

Points of Resistance

Addressing the child's and parents' questions about the time line of treatment is appropriate during the first two sessions. Giving a child or adolescent an exact time line of treatment may backfire at some point, when the proposed deadline approaches and he or she is still in treatment. It is more appropriate to say that most people feel better relatively soon if they work hard, and to explain that CBT was designed to be a shorter-term, goal-oriented treatment approach. Providing patients with an overall treatment plan to decrease frequency of sessions as they improve is also rewarding in most circumstances. Being more specific with parents is reasonable and may in fact prevent undue pressure on the child to improve before some artificial deadline, such as summer camp or a family vacation. At this point, reiterating that CBT teaches skills to cope with the disorders but is not a cure also helps parents set realistic expectations of the process and of their child.

It is also important to continue building the rapport that is such an integral component of ERP. Asking a patient to engage in some very anxiety-provoking situations requires his or her trust that nothing truly bad will happen. For a patient to comply and trust a therapist, a strong relationship is necessary.

Sessions 3 and 4

The goals are to develop hierarchies for OCD, HC, and BDD, as well as to review the information provided in the first two sessions (see Figures 3.4 and 3.5).

Every therapist has his or her own style for eliciting items for a hierarchy. Essentially, by the third session, many clinicians have already heard sufficient details about symptoms to have a good understanding of the kinds of situations to include in a hierarchy. Patients will report difficulty engaging in particular tasks, or express fear or disgust when the therapist mention certain situations. It is helpful to keep a list of potential hierarchy items throughout the consultation and initial stages of treatment. One concrete strategy in eliciting

100 Eating a steak
90 Eating a burger at a restaurant
80 Eating a taco at a restaurant
80 Drinking milk
75 Eating a burger prepared at home
60 Eating Jell-O™
50 Eating something with milk in it
40 Eating something with gelatin
30 Eating something that had been close to the milk in the refrigerator
20 Getting something out of the refrigerator that was close to the milk

FIGURE 3.4. Kelli's hierarchy for OCD.

hierarchy items is called the "typical day," in which the therapist asks the patient to serve as a guide through a typical day, from the very first waking moment until he or she falls asleep. As the patient narrate his or her day, the therapist is cognizant of any descriptions of tasks and behaviors that appear to be related to the disorder. This technique also helps patients recall seemingly "minor" compulsions or fears that they may not think to mention otherwise. Therapists can get very detailed information about showers and bedtime rituals, recording each step of the process, so that changes and exposure items can be designed later. Similarly, observing the child in the home environment or school setting may provide a tremendous amount of information that the therapist cannot observe within the confines of a therapy office setting.

Once the therapist has a good understanding of the patient's fear, it is easier to hypothesize other items that may need to be included in his hierarchy. Ranking the items from least to most anxiety provoking may be difficult for children and adolescents, because they are being asked to imagine how anxious they would feel in a hypothesized situation. Sometimes writing each item on a separate piece of paper and allowing the child to shuffle the papers around to order them from least to most anxiety producing is a more concrete and tangible exercise.

THERAPIST: Kelli, do you remember how we talked about fighting back the bully by doing the opposite of what he tells you to do? Today we are going to make a list of all the places, things, people, and situations that make you feel nervous when you do them, or things you just can't do at all. This list is called a "hierarchy." So, you mentioned to me that eating something that is not in a package is difficult, correct?

KELLI: That's correct. I can't eat anything like that, because there's no label to read, so I can't make sure there's no cow-related products in there.

THERAPIST: OK, so the first thing we should list is that. Is it easier to eat things your mom makes than to eat in restaurants?

HC

100   Breathing in chalk dust
100   Feeling shortness of breath
 90   Touching chalk
 90   Seeing nails looking grayish or bluish
 90   Touching dog and then lip (without washing hands)
 80   Touching face, including nostrils, after touching dog
      (without washing hands)
 80   Eating after touching a handed back paper
      (without washing hands)
 75   Feeling congested
 75   Not going to nurse when not feeling well
 70   Touching her teachers or her mom (until after Mom's shower)
 70   Touching her dog
 70   Standing near a teacher or her mom (until after Mom's shower)
 70   Not checking breathing
 60   Seeing a hive
 60   Not calling Dr. L. when feeling sick
 55   Not checking for facial swelling
 50   Feeling itchy
 50   Eyes looking puffy
 50   Not checking swallowing
 50   Not reading about anaphylaxis on the Internet
 40   Not breathing through sleeve
 30   Sitting in class for the whole duration
 20   Writing a letter on the blackboard

BDD

100   Swimming in the community pool
 95   Wearing only one layer of clothing to school
 90   Wearing shorts and a T-shirt to school
 80   Writing at the blackboard in school while others watch
 70   Going to school with a "young" hairstyle like a ponytail
 60   Wearing T-shirts with logos on them
 50   Leaving for school without checking appearance in the mirror
 40   Leaving home without asking Mom how she looks
 30   Going to a store with one layer of clothing
 20   Raising hand in class

FIGURE 3.5. Kelli's hierarchies for HC and BDD.

KELLI: Yes. Restaurants are really hard, because I really don't know where the food came from. But I watch my mom cook and ask her a million times what she put into the food.

THERAPIST: So, we should list those two things separately: "things that my mom makes" and "food in a restaurant." I'm also going to write down eating "things Mom makes without me watching her or asking questions." It is also hard for you to eat anything that's meat or dairy, right? I guess we should write down milkshakes and cheeseburgers on our list of scary situations, right?

KELLI: Yuck. You're not going to make me eat those things, are you? Because I never will!

THERAPIST: Don't worry. I will never force you do anything you don't want to do. But you know that OCD, HC, and BDD give you false alarm danger messages, right? The only way to fight back and prove that nothing bad will truly happen is to try and face those fears. I will never suggest that you do something I would not do, either. So, whatever you do, I do also. As you can see, for now, I am just putting aside your BDD until we get through the OCD and HC fears. Then we will tackle your BDD.

KELLI: OK, but I'm still not eating a cheeseburger.

THERAPIST: I understand. So let's add some other items to your list. How about being near chalk?

Homework

The therapist makes a copy of the hierarchies and asks the child to add items as the week progresses. Hierarchy items are elicited by generating hypothetical situations for the patient. Once the list is complete, the therapist asks the patient to put the situations in order from least to most anxiety provoking, then assign a number from 1 to 100, with 100 representing the highest anxiety the patient can imagine. Many patients just tell the therapist that everything is an anxiety level of 100. In this case, it is easier to take two items on the list and have the patient decide which is scarier. Then the next item is presented for comparison to the first two, and so on.

First a hierarchy was generated for OCD and HC, and then for BDD. Selecting items with an SUD rating of about 30–50 allows Kelli to experience more anxiety than she did with her own experiment, while gaining mastery of the concepts of exposure and response prevention. Using humor in the process of exposure is a helpful way to get kids relaxed and invested in the process, and to assist them in really talking up their fears to flood them, while helping them feel in control. It is also important to have children articulate exactly what they fear will happen if they face their avoided stimulus, so that they can be fully exposed to all of the relevant cues. If a clinician is unaware of the specific consequences a child fears, the exposure may not be maximally effective.

Points of Resistance

At this stage of therapy, children may become fearful of doing in-office ERP. One good way to deal with this type of resistance is always to be willing to compromise. If a child says that he or she is not ready to face even a mild to moderate hierarchy item (e.g., SUD = 30), the therapist does not give up. He or she compromises by asking what the child will do (e.g., making up a silly story about the worry, drawing it, or even just talking about it all can be preliminary steps to help child and adolescent patients who resist ERP when it is initially presented).

Session 5

The goal here is to help Kelli choose and fully articulate a moderately anxiety-provoking hierarchy item to practice in-session ERP.

THERAPIST: OK, Kelli. Let's go through your OCD hierarchy, since that's the stuff that bothers you the most, and pick out a couple of fears with a rating of 30–50. Then, we'll decide together how to handle facing them, OK?

KELLI: OK. What can we pick?

THERAPIST: You rated not checking a package for cow products as a 30, eating a food that's not packaged that could have cow products in it as a 40, and eating something you didn't watch your mom make as a 40, too. You rated eating something with gelatin in it as a 50. Which one of these would you like to pick to work on here today?

KELLI: Wait. No. I'm chickening out. I can't do anything. (*crying*) Please don't think I'm a total baby. I just can't do it. The chicken was easy, that's why I picked it, but all these things seem like 100's now.

THERAPIST: Hey, you're not a baby. This stuff is hard. Let's just talk about your fear of mad cow for a minute. OK? Hey, do you even know what mad cow really is? What do you think it will do to you?

KELLI: First, I think, you get really confused. Then you get weak and can't walk, and then you shake a lot, go nuts, and just die. I can't eat food that might be contaminated by that. I don't want to die.

THERAPIST: I don't exactly have a death wish either. Would I be stupid enough to do something that would get both of us killed? I mean, even if I didn't care at all about you, which is not the case, at least I care about myself.

KELLI: I know. I really do. I'm just so afraid.

THERAPIST: OK, let's just draw what you think a mad cow would look like. I'll do one too. Make it the sickest, most pathetic, and crazy beast you can. (*Both draw some deranged, sick cows—it's even funnier if neither of them can draw*).

THERAPIST: OK, here's mine. What do you think? I'm no artist, but I think my cow looks both totally insane and pretty ill.

KELLI: *(laughing)* Umm, you're right. You're no artist. Your cow looks retarded and like it's trying to dance. Check mine out. Is that not the sickest and looniest cow you've ever seen?

THERAPIST: OK. Where's your SUD level now?

KELLI: It's better. Like a 50. I'm really nervous, but I think I can do it.

THERAPIST: You are so brave. Before we do this, just tell me what you're afraid will happen?

KELLI: That I'll eat it, then start to go crazy like a mad cow. I'll be all dizzy and won't be able to walk, then I'll just go nuts. The worst would be that I could lose bowel control too.

THERAPIST: OK, I'm game. I'm eating my chip. Are you ready to eat yours? Hey, do you feel confused yet? A little shaky maybe? Weak?

KELLI: Oh yeah, I'm shaking all over. I think I'm too confused and weak to answer you.

THERAPIST: Good. You're not letting it bully you. You're not giving in to the doubt. I'm going to ask you to postpone checking for a little while. Let's start with an hour. Do you think you can do that? Also, do not, under any circumstances, wash your hands.

KELLI: Maybe. What if I can't do it for the whole hour?

THERAPIST: Then wait 30 minutes and see how you feel. If you're even a little less nervous, wait another 30 minutes. Put it off for as long as you can, as long as you're less nervous each time. Just keep trying. And Mrs. M., can you help Kelli to resist this by not answering questions and by keeping her busy playing games and having fun, to help her ride out her difficult urges?

MRS. M.: Of course. But what should I do if Kelli asks me a question, then gets upset because I won't answer?

THERAPIST: It's important to tell Kelli that you know she's really nervous, but that she's fighting her bully and you want to help. Remind her that if she ignores him, she'll wear him out, and he'll get tired and leave her alone.

Once ERP is well underway, as in the previous session's example, it is important to stay focused and to move up the hierarchy systematically, even if the child seems enthusiastic. The superordinate goal of treatment from this point forward is steady, dependable progress. If the child is eager to do more, the therapist can design exposures with built in challenges both in the session and as homework. If a child's actual SUDS rating is significantly below what he or she predicted during an exposure, the therapist asks for the child's permission to pump up the level a bit, or encourages the child to do this for him- or herself.

Points of Resistance

In proceeding with a patient up his or her hierarchy, it is essential to make sure that during exposure exercises (in the office and in homework), the patient is practicing total response prevention. Sometimes, in order not to disappoint their parents or the therapist, children may attempt exposures that are too difficult for them. They may cope by doing compulsions covertly (e.g., mental compulsions) or overtly, but privately. It is important to ask about compulsive behaviors, especially if a patient is trying to move too fast. Exposure without response prevention simply increases fear.

Sessions 6–10

The next several sessions are similar to Session 5. Once the patient has moved to items much higher on his or her hierarchy, the therapist may want to stop and have the patient rerate all of the original items to evaluate treatment progress, as well as to identify the direction to take in future sessions. Other initial assessment tools, such as the BAT, may also be repeated for the same purposes. After dealing with all of her mad cow–related hierarchy items, Kelli is now ready to face her worst fears related to anaphylaxis.

Points of Resistance

Sometimes, as people in treatment begin to feel better, they may lose a measure of their initial motivation. Although they may still be experiencing major symptom interference in their daily functioning, they are significantly better than they were at the time of the initial consultation. We often refer to this as the "better enough" feeling that may lead patients to hit a plateau in treatment. They may claim that they can live with their current symptoms, even if they do make life difficult. This is particularly true of children and adolescents, who already have more than enough difficulties dealing with the demands of daily life.

When this occurs, it is important to encourage children at least to maintain the gains that they have fought so hard to achieve. Then, by having them identify things they really want to get out of treatment, the clinician can set up specific ERP exercises to help them achieve these goals and become reinvested and remotivated. Applying cognitive restructuring to some articulated irrational beliefs can also be helpful at this point.

Session 11

The goal is to have Kelli identify her own motivation for continuing to do very difficult exposures, while maintaining her current treatment gains.

THERAPIST: Kelli, I know you told me that you're really starting to feel better, and I'm so glad for that. It's really due to your fighting the bully every day. That can be tiring though.

KELLI: Yeah. I know we're supposed to tackle the biggest stuff on my list, but I'm really feeling pretty OK, and I'm sort of OK with having things the way they are.

THERAPIST: Are you really OK with how they are, or are you just really afraid?

KELLI: Sort of both. Really, the only things on that list that I want are to hug and pet my dog, and to hug my mom whenever I want, not just after her shower at night.

THERAPIST: Those sound like two really big-deal things. I can't imagine how hard it must be for you to not to be able to hug your mom or the dog. What if, for the moment, we just work on those things? After we do that, if you're in the mood to do more, we certainly can. If that's all we do, then at least you'll win back two very important things from your HC.

KELLI: What if this is totally different? What if this is not just an obsession?

THERAPIST: Do you 100% believe that this is real?

KELLI: No, I know it's the same as the mad cow thing. I just feel like it's more real and true, because it scares me even more.

THERAPIST: If I told you a stupid lie, like that you were a ferret, would you believe me?

KELLI: Umm, no. That's totally stupid?

THERAPIST: What if I said it all day and all night?

KELLI: I still know I'm not a ferret.

THERAPIST: What if I screamed it at you and threatened to beat you up unless you agreed with me?

KELLI: I'd be scared and think you were a freak, but I still know I'm a human.

THERAPIST: Then you can also fight your fears of anaphylaxis. They are lies your brain tells you, same as the mad cow stuff.

KELLI: But they feel more real.

THERAPIST: Just because they scare you more doesn't make lies more true, does it?

KELLI: No.

THERAPIST: I know you've felt like you had anaphylaxis many times, right? But how many times have you really had it?

KELLI: Never really, but I felt like my throat was closing, and I was not able to breathe and I couldn't swallow.

THERAPIST: But never so that you needed to go to the hospital or get a shot of an EpiPen or anything right?

KELLI: No. I never had to do that. I guess I'm thinking about it happening all the time, but it's never really happened.

THERAPIST: That's your brain tricking you then.

KELLI: But I feel real nervous, scared.

THERAPIST: Right. So let's make some ERP exercises to do with your mom and your dog.

KELLI: Can I bring in my dog?

THERAPIST: I'd love that. Actually, we could do a lot if he were here. Bring him next time.

To assist children and adolescents in addressing their worst fears, it is often important for a therapist to demonstrate a willingness to go the extra mile. This may mean making a home visit if the trouble is at home, or allowing a patient to bring a pet or family member into the session, when the obsession concerns that person or animal.

Sessions 12–15

The goals of Sessions 12–15 are to have Kelli do ERP with both her dog and her mother, so that she can feel free to touch and hug them without hand washing, calling Dr. L., or going on the Internet to check about the symptoms of anaphylactic shock.

In the first few sessions of treatment, Kelli constructed three separate hierarchies: for OCD, HC, BDD. Kelli's OCD and HC symptoms led to much more anxiety and functional impairment, and were generally more severe than her BDD symptoms. As a result, they were the initial focus of the treatment. However, as Kelli gains mastery over even the most difficult symptoms of her HC related to her fear of anaphylaxis, and OCD symptoms related to mad cow disease, she will be ready to shift gears to deal with her BDD.

The goal of all future sessions is to begin addressing the BDD hierarchy, similar to the approach with OCD and HC. It is important to continue monitoring the reemergence of OCD and HC symptoms. Because BDD was not a major component of Kelli's symptoms, it may have to be put on hold to devote more attention to the HC.

Relapse Prevention

Maintaining treatment gains and helping to decrease the chances of setbacks and/or relapses is a crucial component of treatment (McKay, Todaro, Neziroglu, & Yaryura-Tobias, 1996; McKay, Todaro, et al., 1997). It is essential to devote specific sessions to providing patients with psychoeducation regarding this issue, in addition to bringing up the concept in the midst of treatment. Providing patients with a specific plan and ERP techniques when they experience a setback helps to prevent a minor worsening of symptoms that may lead to relapse. It is also helpful to list common situations that typically trigger worsening of symptoms and to educate the patient to be careful and family members to keep an extra close eye on the child during those situations. Setbacks can occur during life changes or transitions, such as from middle school to high school, or in the case of loss or illness of a family member (especially in the case of HC). Other situations that can trigger a setback are social stressors, such as losing a best friend or being bullied.

In addition to psychoeducation, follow-up sessions with decreasing frequency should ideally be scheduled for 6 months to 1 year after active treatment, allowing a patient to be monitored and to maintain the connection with the therapist. After active treatment, sessions can be scheduled bimonthly, then monthly, and eventually every 6–8 weeks, until the patient and family are confident that the patient is symptom free, even during a variety of stressful life situations.

CONCLUSION

Obsessive–compulsive spectrum disorders demonstrate certain symptom dimensions such as obsessions, compulsions–avoidance behaviors, overvalued ideation, and shifting. In this chapter, we discussed these symptoms within the context of OCD, HC, and BDD. Differential diagnosis between these disorders and others, and among themselves, was presented. A case example of a child with OCD, HC, and BDD to varying degrees was depicted. Treatment suggestions were provided, along with step-by-step guidelines. Variables that affect treatment outcome were noted, and finally data demonstrating the development of anxiety hierarchies were provided.

REFERENCES

Abramowitz, J. S., Whiteside, S. P., & Deacon, B. J. (2005). The effectiveness of treatment for pediatric obsessive compulsive disorder: A meta-analysis. *Behavior Therapy, 36*, 55–63.

Achenbach, T. M. (1991). *Manual for the Child Behavior Checklist/4–18 and 1991 profile.* Burlington: University of Vermont, Department of Psychiatry.

Albertini, R. S., & Phillips, K. A. (2003). Thirty-three cases of body dysmorphic disorder in children and adolescents. In M. E. Hertzig & E. A. Farber (Eds.), *Annual progress in child psychiatry and child development: 2000–2001* (pp. 335–348). New York: Brunner-Routledge.

Amir, N., Freshman, M., & Foa, E. B. (2000). Family distress and involvement in relatives of obsessive compulsive disorder patients. *Journal of Anxiety Disorders, 14*, 501–519.

Barrett, P., Healy, B. L., & March, J. S. (2003). Behavioral avoidance test for childhood obsessive–compulsive disorder: A home-based observation. *American Journal of Psychotherapy, 57*(1), 80–101.

Barrett, P., Healy-Farrell, L., & March, J. S. (2004). Cognitive behavioral family treatment of childhood obsessive compulsive disorder: A controlled trial. *Journal of the American Academy of Child and Adolescent Psychiatry, 43*, 46–62.

Barrett, P., Shortt, A., & Healy, L. (2002). Do parent and child behaviours differentiate families whose children have obsessive compulsive disorder from other clinic and non-clinic families? *Journal of Child Psychology and Psychiatry, 43,* 597–607.

Benazon, N. R., Ager, J., & Rosenberg, D. R. (2002). Cognitive behavior therapy in treatment naive children and adolescents with obsessive compulsive disorder: An open trial. *Behaviour Research and Therapy, 40,* 529–540.

Calvocoressi, L., Lewis, B., Harris, M., & Trufan, S. J. (1995). Family accommodation in obsessive compulsive disorder. *American Journal of Psychiatry, 152,* 441–443.

Calvocoressi, L., Mazure, C. M., Kasl, S. V., Skolnick, J., Fisk, D., Vegso, S. J., et al. (1999). Family accommodation of obsessive compulsive symptoms: Instrument development and assessment of family behavior. *Journal of Nervous and Mental Disease, 187,* 636–642.

Carson, R. C., Butcher, J. N., & Mineka, S. (2000). *Abnormal psychology and modern life* (11th ed.). Boston: Allyn & Bacon.

Conners, C. K., Sitarenios, G., Parker, J. D. A., & Epstein, J. N. (1998). The Revised Conners Parent Rating Scale (CPRS-R): Factor structure, reliability, and criterion validity. *Journal of Abnormal Child Psychology, 26,* 257–268.

Cooper, M. (1996). Obsessive compulsive disorder: Effects on family members. *American Journal of Orthopsychiatry, 66,* 296–304.

Dollard, J., & Miller, E. (1950). *Personality and psychotherapy: An analysis in terms of learning, thinking, and culture.* New York: McGraw-Hill.

Fireman, B., Koran, M., Leventhal, J. L., & Jacobson, A. (2001). The prevalence of clinically recognized obsessive–compulsive disorder in a large health maintenance organization. *American Journal of Psychiatry, 158,* 1904–1910.

Fischer, D. J., Himle, J. A., & Hanna, G. L. (1998). Group behavioral therapy for adolescents with obsessive–compulsive disorder: Preliminary outcomes. *Research on Social Work Practice, 8,* 629–636.

Foa, E. B. (1979). Failure in treating obsessive–compulsives. *Behaviour Research and Therapy, 17,* 169–176.

Foa, E. B., & Kozak, M. J. (1995). DSM-IV field trial: Obsessive–compulsive disorder. *American Journal of Psychiatry, 152,* 90–96.

Franklin, M. E., & Foa, E. B. (2002). Cognitive behavioral treatments for obsessive–compulsive disorder. In P. E. Nathan & J. M. Gorman (Eds.), *A guide to treatments that work* (pp. 367–386). New York: Oxford University Press.

Fritz, G. K., Fritsch, S., & Hagino, O. (1991). Somatoform disorders in children and adolescents: A review of the past 10 years. *Journal of the American Academy of Child and Adolescent Psychiatry, 36*(10), 1329–1339.

Grunes, M. S., Neziroglu, F., & McKay, D. (2001). Family involvement in the behavioral treatment of obsessive–compulsive disorder: A preliminary investigation. *Behavior Therapy, 32,* 803–820.

Hertzig, M. E., & Farber, E. A. (2003). *Annual progress in child psychiatry and child development: 2000–2001.* New York: Brunner-Routledge.

Hibbs, E., Hamburger, S., & Lenane, M. (1991). Determinants of expressed emotion in families of disturbed and normal children. *Journal of Child Psychology and Psychiatry, and Allied Discipline, 32,* 757–770.

Hoehn-Saire, R., & McLeod, D. R. (1991). Clinical management of generalized anxiety disorder. In W. Coryell & G. Winokur (Eds.), *The clinical management of anxiety disorders* (pp. 79–100). New York: Oxford University Press.

Jaspers, K. (1913). *Psicopatologia general* [General psychopathology] (R. O. Saubidet, Trans.). Buenos Aires: Beta.

Kozak, M. J., & Foa, E. B. (1994). Obsessions, overvalued ideas, and delusions in obsessive–compulsive disorder. *Behaviour Research and Therapy, 32*, 343–353.

Lahey, B. B., Applegate, B., Waldman, I. D., Loft, J. D., Hankin, B. L., & Rick, J. (2004). The structure of child and adolescent psychopathology: Generating new hypotheses. *Journal of Abnormal Psychology, 113*(3), 358–385.

Leonard, H. L., Lenane, M. C., Swedo, S. E., Rettew, D. C., Gershon, E. S., & Rapoport, J. L. (1992). Tics and Tourette's disorder: A 2- to 7-year follow-up of 54 obsessive–compulsive children. *American Journal of Psychiatry, 149*, 1244–1251.

Lopatka, C., & Rachman, S. J. (1995). Perceived responsibility and compulsive checking: An experimental analysis. *Behaviour Research and Therapy, 33*, 673–684.

March, J. S., & Mulle, K. (1998). *OCD in children and adolescents: A cognitive-behavioral treatment manual.* New York: Guilford Press.

March, J. S., Mulle, K., & Herbel, B. (1994). Behavioral psychotherapy for children and adolescents with obsessive compulsive disorder: An open trial of a new protocol driven treatment package. *Journal of the American Academy of Child and Adolescent Psychiatry, 33*, 333–341.

Martin, J. L., & Thienemann, M. (2005). Group cognitive-behavior therapy with family involvement with middle school age children with obsessive compulsive disorder: A pilot study. *Child Psychiatry and Human Development, 36*, 113–127.

McKay, D., Neziroglu, F., & Yaryura-Tobias, J. A. (1997). Comparison of clinical characteristics in obsessive–compulsive disorder and body dysmorphic disorder. *Journal of Anxiety Disorders, 11*(4), 447–454.

McKay, D., Todaro, J. F., Neziroglu, F. A., & Yaryura-Tobias, J. A. (1996). Evaluation of a naturalistic maintenance program in the treatment of obsessive–compulsive disorder: A preliminary investigation. *Journal of Anxiety Disorders, 10*(3), 211–217.

McKay, D., Todaro, J., Neziroglu, F. A., Campisie, T., Moritz, K., & Yaryura-Tobias, J. A. (1997). Body dysmorphic disorder: Preliminary evaluation of treatment and maintenance using exposure with response prevention. *Behaviour Research and Therapy, 35*, 67–70.

Moritz, E. K. (1998). *Behavior therapy in game format for the treatment of childhood obsessive compulsive disorder.* Unpublished dissertation, Hofstra University, Hempstead, NY.

Mowrer, H. (1947). On the dual nature of learning: A reinterpretation of "conditioning" and "problem solving." *Harvard Educational Review, 17*, 102–148.

Muris, P., Dreesen, L., Bogels, S., Weckx, M., & van Melick, M. (2004). A questionnaire for screening a broad range of DSM-defined anxiety disorder symptoms in clinically referred children and adolescents. *Journal of Child Psychology and Psychiatry, 45*(4), 813–820.

Neziroglu, F., Henriksen, J., & Yaryura-Tobias, J. A. (2006). Psychotherapy of obsessive–compulsive disorder: Established facts and advances between 1995–2005. *Psychiatric Clinics of North America, 29*, 585–604.

Neziroglu, F., & Khemlani-Patel, S. (2005). Overlap of body dysmorphic disorder and hypochondriasis with OCD. In J. S. Abramowitz & A. C. Houts (Eds.), *Concepts and controversies in obsessive–compulsive disorder.* New York: Springer.

Neziroglu, F., McKay, D., & Yaryura-Tobias, J. A. (2000). Overlapping and distinctive features of hypochondriasis and obsessive–compulsive disorder. *Journal of Anxiety Disorders, 14*, 603–614.

Neziroglu, F., McKay, D., Yaryura-Tobias, J. A., Stevens, K. P., & Todaro, J. (1999). The Overvalued Ideas Scale: Development, reliability and validity in obsessive–compulsive disorder. *Behaviour Research and Therapy, 37*, 881–902.

Neziroglu, F., Peterson, I., Yaryura-Tobias, J. A., & Weisman (2007). Clinical characteristics of compulsive hoarding and obsessive–compulsive disorders. *Behaviour Research and Therapy.*

Neziroglu, F., Stevens, K. P., McKay, D., & Yaryura-Tobias, J. A. (2001). Predictive validity of the overvalued ideas scale: Outcome in obsessive–compulsive and body dysmorphic disorders. *Behaviour Research and Therapy, 39*, 745–756.

Noyes, R. J., Kathol, R. G., Fisher, M., Phillips, B. M., Suelzer, M. T., & Holt, C. S. (1993). The validity of DSM-III-R hypochondriasis. *Archives of General Psychiatry, 50*, 961–970.

Obsessive Compulsive Cognitions Working Group (OCCWG). (1997). Cognitive assessment of obsessive compulsive disorder. *Behaviour Research and Therapy, 35*, 667–681.

Obsessive Compulsive Cognitions Working Group (OCCWG). (2001). Development and initial validation of the Obsessive Beliefs Questionnaire and the Interpretation of Intrusions Inventory. *Behaviour Research and Therapy, 39*, 987–1006.

Ollendick, T. H. (1983). Reliability and validity of the revised Fear Survey Schedule for children (FSSC-R). *Behaviour Research and Therapy, 21*, 685–692.

Otto, M. W., Wilhelm, S., & Cohen, L. S. (2001). Prevalence of body dysmorphic disorder in a community sample of women. *American Journal of Psychiatry, 158*, 2061–2063.

Pediatric OCD Treatment Team. (POTS). (2004). Cognitive-behavior therapy, sertraline, and their combination for children and adolescents with obsessive–compulsive disorder: The pediatric OCD treatment team (POTS) randomized controlled trial. *Journal of the American Medical Association, 292*, 1969–1976.

Phillips, K. A. (2000). Body dysmorphic disorder: Diagnostic controversies and treatment challenges. *Bulletin of the Menninger Clinic, 64*(1), 18–36.

Phillips, K. A., & Castle, D. J. (2002). Body dysmorphic disorder. In D. J. Castle & K. A. Phillips (Eds.), *Disorders of body image* (pp. 101–120). Petersfield, UK: Wrightson Biomedical Publishing.

Phillips, K. A., & Diaz, S. F. (1997). Gender differences in body dysmorphic disorder. *Journal of Nervous and Mental Disease, 185*, 570–577.

Quay, H. C., & Peterson, D. R. (1993). *The Revised Behavior Problem Checklist: Manual.* Odessa, FL: Psychological Assessment Resources.

Rachman, S., & de Silva, P. (1978). Abnormal and normal obsessions. *Behaviour Research and Therapy, 16*, 233–248.

Robins, L. N., & Regier, D. A. (Eds.). (1991). *Psychiatric disorders in America: The Epidemiologic Catchment Area Study* (with a foreword by D. X. Freedman). New York: Free Press.

Salkovskis, P. M. (1985). Obsessional–compulsive problems: A cognitive-behavioural analysis. *Behaviour Research and Therapy, 23*, 571–583.

Salkovskis, P. M., Wroe, A. L., Gledhill, A., Morrison, N., Forrester, E., Richards, C., et al. (2000). Responsibility attitudes and interpretations are characteristic of obsessive compulsive disorder. *Behaviour Research and Therapy, 38*, 347–372.

Scahill, L., Riddle, M. A., McSwiggin-Hardin, M., Ort, S. I., King, R. A., Goodman, W. K., Cicchetti, D., et al. (1997). Children's Yale–Brown Obsessive–Compulsive

Scale: Reliability and validity. *Journal of the American Academy of Child and Adolescent Psychiatry, 36*(6), 844–852.

Shafran, R. (1997). The manipulation of responsibility in obsessive–compulsive disorder. *British Journal of Clinical Psychology, 36*, 397–407.

Silverman, W. K., & Albano, A. M. (1996). *Anxiety Disorder Interview Schedule for DSM-IV: Child and parent interview schedule.* San Antonio, TX: Psychological Corporation.

Siqueland, L., Rynn, M., & Diamond, G. S. (2005). Cognitive behavioral and attachment based family therapy for anxious adolescents: Phase I and II studies. *Journal of Anxiety Disorders, 19*, 361–381.

Spielberger, C. D. (1973). *Manual for the State–Trait Anxiety Inventory for Children.* Palo Alto, CA: Consulting Psychologists Press.

Steketee, G. (1993). Social support and treatment outcome in obsessive–compulsive disorder at 9 month follow-up. *Behavioral Psychotherapy, 21*, 81–95.

Steketee, G., & Van Noppen, B. (2003). Family approaches to treatment for obsessive compulsive disorder. *Revista Brasileira de Psiquiatria, 25*, 43–50.

Swedo, S. E., Leonard, H. L., & Garvey, M. (1998). Pediatric autoimmune neuropsychiatric disorders associated with streptococcal infections: Clinical description of the first 50 cases. *American Journal of Psychiatry, 155*, 264–271.

Taylor, S. (2002). Cognition in obsessive–compulsive disorder: An overview. In R. O. Frost & G. Steketee (Eds.), *Cognitive approaches to obsessions and compulsions: Theory, assessment, and treatment* (pp. 1–12). New York: Pergamon Press.

Valleni-Basile, L., Garrison, C., & Jackson, K. (1995). Family and psychosocial predictors of obsessive–compulsive disorder in a community sample of young adolescents. *Journal of Child and Family Studies, 4*, 193–206.

Wagner, A. P. (2003). Cognitive behavioral therapy for children and adolescents with obsessive–compulsive disorder. *Brief Treatment and Crisis Intervention, 3*, 291–306.

Wernicke, C. (1906). *Grundrisse der psychiatrie* [Foundations of psychiatry]. Leipzig: Verlag.

Williams, D. T., & Hirsch, G. (1988). The somatizing disorders: Somatoform disorders, factitious disorders and malingering. In C. J. Kestenbaum & D. T. Williams (Eds.), *Handbook of clinical assessment of children and adolescents* (Vol. 1, pp. 734–768). New York: New York University Press.

Wright, K. D., & Asmundson, G. J. G. (2003). Health anxiety in children: Development and psychometric properties of the Childhood Illness Attitude Scales. *Cognitive Behaviour Therapy, 32*(4), 194–202.

Yaryura-Tobias, J. A., Grunes, M. S., Walz, J., & Neziroglu, F. (2000). Parental obsessive–compulsive disorder as a prognostic factor in a year long fluvoxamine treatment in childhood and adolescent obsessive–compulsive disorder. *International Clinical Psychopharmacology, 15*(3), 163–168.

Yaruyra-Tobias, J. A., & Neziroglu, F. A. (1997a). *Obsessive–compulsive disorder spectrum: Pathogenesis, diagnosis, and treatment.* Washington, DC: American Psychiatric Association.

Yaruyra-Tobias, J. A., & Neziroglu, F. A. (1997b). *Biobehavioral treatment of obsessive–compulsive spectrum disorders.* New York: Norton.

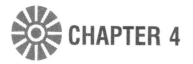 **CHAPTER 4**

Inattentiveness

Linda A. Reddy and James B. Hale

Inattention, although central to diagnosing attention-deficit/hyperactivity disorder, may result from a variety of neurocognitive and/or social–emotional conditions, and may overlap with both internalizing and externalizing disorders. In this chapter, the authors describe their cognitive hypothesis-testing model (CHT) to help explain the nature of inattention and its relationship to children's social–emotional, behavioral, and academic deficits. Through the cases of "Thomas" and "Lisa," the authors help us make sense of inattention both with and without executive function deficits. More importantly, through CHT and behavioral consultation, the authors demonstrate how individualized, empirically based interventions are designed and implemented for each case to address the child's unique social–emotional, behavioral and academic needs. Practitioners from mental health, school-based, and medically related fields, as well as other professionals who work with children, should find the chapter contents immensely useful.—A. R. E.

INTRODUCTION

Inattention is one of the most common referral problems for psychologists and pediatricians, with affected children likely to require intensive service delivery. This is not because inattention is a pervasive and distinct clinical disorder, but because it is found in children with a wide range of disorders and conditions (Hale, Fiorello, & Brown, 2005; Reddy & De Thomas, 2006). When evaluating and treating attention problems, it is imperative that practitioners consider how many childhood conditions have overlapping symptoms that are expressed differently within the context of the child's natural environment. Identifying the causes of inattention requires practitioners to engage in intensive investigation of both the neurocognitive and behavioral domains. Practitioners' efforts are realized and rewarded when accurate case conceptualizations lead to the design and implementation of empirically supported interventions for children.

Inattention is commonly associated with a constellation of symptoms that can lead to attention-deficit/hyperactivity disorder (ADHD), a clinical disorder that provides the conceptual impetus for this chapter's four objectives. First, we provide a discussion of ADHD-related symptoms found among common childhood disorders (i.e., learning disabilities, pervasive developmental disorders, auditory processing disorders, anxiety disorders, and mood disorders). Second, we present the historical antecedents and the biological, psychological, and psychosocial determinants of ADHD-related symptoms. Third, we review common cognitive–neuropsychological and social–emotional assessment approaches used with this population. Finally, we describe two cases studies that illustrate the link between assessment and treatment of children who experience significant inattention.

Symptom Dimensions and Relationship to Specific Disorders

ADHD encompasses a complex mix of neurocognitive deficits that include impairments in attention, hyperactivity, impulsivity, planning, organization, and evaluation skills across settings. ADHD comprises a heterogeneous group of deficits, often including comorbid conditions that complicates the assessment and intervention process. The comorbidity rate for this population varies across clinical samples (learning disabilities, anxiety disorders, etc.), gender, and age. For example, research indicates that the comorbidity of ADHD and specific learning disabilities (LD) range from 25 to 70% (Kellner, Houghton, & Douglas, 2003). The comorbidity rates of ADHD and depressive disorders range from 10.3 (Souza, Pinheiro, Denardin, Mattos, & Rohde, 2004) to approximately 33–50% (Pfiffner et al., 1999). Approximately one-third of youth with ADHD are diagnosed with anxiety disorders (e.g., Perrin & Last, 1996; Safren, Lanka, Otto, & Pollack, 2001; Souza et al., 2004) and in a sample with central auditory processing disorder, about 50% of youth met criteria for ADHD (Riccio, Hynd, Cohen, Hall, & Molt, 1994). As a result, ADHD-related symptoms of inattentiveness, hyperactivity, and impulsivity are often confused with other disorders and conditions, such as anxiety, depression, poor nutrition, and medical illness (Cushman & Johnson, 2001). Meta-analyses reveal that children diagnosed with ADHD and comorbid internalizing disorders may differ from those with ADHD and externalizing disorders (Angold, Costello, & Erkanli, 1999), but there are at least 38 different causes of inattention (Goodman & Poillion, 1992). Thus, an accurate diagnosis of ADHD requires an understanding of many disorders, and their neurocognitive functions and behavioral patterns (Reddy & De Thomas,

2006). The next section highlights this comorbidity by examining symptom dimensions of ADHD found in some common childhood disorders.

Specific Learning Disabilities

Estimating the prevalence rate of LD in school-age children is a difficult task. Research has reported rates as low as 1% and as high as 30% (Ingalls & Goldstein, 1999). This wide range in prevalence is likely due to the lack of consensus on what defines the construct of LD (Bradley & Danielson, 2004). For example, some studies define LD through teacher reports of school performance (DuPaul & Stoner, 2003), whereas others have used significant intelligence and achievement discrepancies, or simply low achievement scores (Fletcher, Denton, & Francis, 2005). Additionally, the failure to respond to empirically valid interventions has been advocated as a method for identifying LD (e.g., Reschly, 2004), but all these practices are limited given that they do not address specifically whether children have a deficit in the basic psychological processes that leads to unexpected learning failure, a critical component of the federal LD definition (Hale, Naglieri, Kaufman, & Kavale, 2006). As a result, LD should be conceived as a heterogeneous category, encompassing a wide array of specific cognitive and academic asset and deficit areas that are differentially affected by whether affected children have or do not have comorbid disorders.

Children with ADHD are often found to have one or more LD, and comorbidity rates are difficult to estimate. Although the comorbidity between ADHD and LD across studies is approximately 31% (DuPaul & Stoner, 2003), results of individual studies range from 7 (e.g., August & Holmes, 1984) to 92% (e.g., Silver, 1981). The majority of LD subtypes tend to be more common in the inattentive and combined types of ADHD, rather than the hyperactive–impulsive type (Tannock & Brown, 2000; Wilcutt & Pennington, 2000). One notable exception that has received much attention is nonverbal LD (NLD), sometimes referred to as right-hemisphere LD (RHLD; Hale & Rubenstein, 2006).

Children with NLD often exhibit deficits in visual, spatial, and motor skills, and implicit language (Hale & Fiorello, 2004; Rourke, 1995). They commonly have difficulties perceiving social cues, attending to visual stimuli, and shifting mental sets. Poor social judgment, procedural skills, and semantic memory also characterize these children (Ingalls & Goldstein, 1999). Because they lack awareness of self and environment (Hale & Fiorello, 2004), their clinical presentation is similar to that seen in children with ADHD, especially the inattentive type (Hale et al., 2005). However, NLD, and indeed, LD in general, are conceptualized as faulty processing skills (i.e., deficits in input), whereas ADHD is conceptualized as deficits in performance (i.e., output). Children with ADHD generally know what they are supposed to do and fail to do it consistently, because their inattentiveness, impulsivity, and hyperactivity interfere with their ability to sustain effort to complete assigned tasks

(Goldstein, 1999). The question of whether ADHD is a performance deficit affecting a child's availability for learning or actually a skills deficit due to executive dysfunction and poor academic skills remains a point of contention, with causes for learning problems in different ADHD subtypes.

As noted, LD broadly conceptualized as reading disorders (RD), mathematics disorders (MD), and written expression disorders. Children with these specific disorders often exhibit a number of deficits that are also associated with ADHD, particularly the inattentive and combined types. Both ADHD and RD are associated with deficits in naming speed (amount of time it takes to name various stimuli, such as colors, letters, numbers, objects, etc.), motor skills, and time perception (e.g., awareness of time of day or time passed since a specific event; Tannock & Brown, 2000). However, children with RD also exhibit problems in phonological awareness and verbal memory (Tannock & Brown, 2000), and automatic-processing skills, as measured by rapid letter identification tasks (e.g., timed naming responses to cards with random letters; August & Garfinkel, 1990; O'Connor & Jenkins, 1999). These children often have difficulties following verbal and/or written directions, and appear confused because of their lack of basic comprehension skills. Children with ADHD tend to have normal automatic processing skills but exhibit difficulties in sustained and effortful processing (e.g., rote memorization; August & Garfinkel, 1990; Muir-Broaddus, Rosenstein, Medina, & Soderberg, 2002) and executive control (e.g., planning, shifting mental set) of learning (Hale et al., 2006; Tannock & Brown, 2000; Cepeda, Cepeda, & Kramer, 2000). Additionally, children with ADHD tend to understand instructions but often react before processing them and/or fail to process them because of their inability to sustain attention, suggesting specifically that ADHD may be a disorder of *intention*, not attention (Denckla, 1996).

Difficulties in mathematics can result from a number of factors, such as limited opportunities to learn, poor instruction, and specific LD and/or ADHD. MD can occur because of procedural difficulties that affect computation, deficits in semantic memory that affect retrieval of number facts, visual–spatial deficits that result in number misalignment and misinterpretation, and/or not understanding basic operations (Geary, 1993; Hale, Fiorello, Bertin, & Sherman, 2003). Children with ADHD often experience limited math productivity (Tannock & Brown, 2000), completing fewer problems with more errors than children with MD (Benedetto-Nasho & Tannock, 1999).

Disorders of written expression include spelling errors and poor handwriting, but these problems are also common in children with ADHD, with approximately 65% experiencing this comorbidity (Mayes, Calhoun, & Crowell, 2000). For a diagnosis of written expression disorder, children must display difficulties in articulation and fluency in written communication (Tannock & Brown, 2000). One possible reason for this is the wide range of skills necessary for the production of developmentally appropriate written expression. It has been suggested that to effectively express ideas through writing, one must be able to collect and retrieve relevant information; organize the information, so that a plan for communication can be developed; translate those ideas into written words; and review and edit the product for optimal communication (Kellogg, 1994). Therefore, the executive functions required to plan, organize, monitor, evaluate, and revise the written language product (Hale & Fiorello, 2004) are common problems in children with ADHD (Hale et al., 2005).

Differential diagnosis of ADHD and LD can be challenging because of the overlapping symptomatology. A diagnosis of ADHD is likely when assessment data clearly indicate that a child has good cognitive functioning, but poor executive control of attention, impulsivity, and hyperactivity, which leads to academic underachievement and behavior problems. In contrast, an LD diagnosis is likely when data consistently identify specific academic problems in the absence of clinically elevated ADHD symptoms. Other factors may aid in the assessment process, such as early onset of disruptive behaviors (e.g., impulsivity, disinhibition, aggression), which are less common in children with LD. Children with ADHD display patterns of inattention and behavior problems that are pervasive across social contexts (e.g., school, home) and functional domains (e.g., silent reading, writing, participating in group sports, making and maintaining friends), but children with LD are more likely to have a specific academic area of weakness. Additionally, children with ADHD are likely to perform in the average range on standardized achievement tests (e.g., Woodcock–Johnson Tests of Achievement; Bradley-Johnson, Morgan, & Nutkins, 2004), whereas children with LD are likely to perform in the below average to low range in specific domain areas (DuPaul & Stoner, 2003).

Pervasive Developmental Disorders

As a diagnostic spectrum, the pervasive developmental disorders (PDD) are also quite heterogeneous in composition. Children with PDD, including autism and Asperger syndrome, have significant attention and executive problems that lead to academic and behavioral impairments (Liss et al., 2001). Although the intellectual and social deficits in these children are often seen as a the key to differential diagnosis of PDD, neither adequately differentiates between children with PDD and ADHD, because both groups may experience these types of impairments, and these comorbid diagnoses are seen frequently in clinical practice (e.g., Baron-Cohen, 1995; Goldstein & Schwebach, 2004), with as many as 65% of children with high-functioning autism/Asperger syndrome showing clinically significant attention problems (Holtmann, Bolte, & Poustka, 2005).

The nature of attention and executive problems may differ among PDD subtypes, with children with autism having internal distraction, and those with Asperger syndrome having external distraction (Hale & Fiorello, 2004), similar to children with ADHD and those with NLD/RHLD (Hale & Rubenstein, 2006). In fact, some children with NLD/RHLD experience poor attention to self (e.g., asomatognosia, anosodiaphoria) and to the environment (e.g., attentional neglect), which can result in a diagnosis of ADHD, especially the inattentive type (Hale et al., 2005), a point we discuss later in the chapter. As a result, some have argued that Asperger syndrome is a more severe form of NLD/RHLD, and that at least some of these children should not be included on the PDD spectrum as a result (Hale & Fiorello, 2004; Klin, Volkmar, Sparrow, Cicchetti, & Rourke, 1995), although this position is not shared by many who study PDD, who suggest that autism and Asperger syndrome differences are largely a matter of symptom severity (e.g., Miller & Ozonoff, 2000; Wing, 1998).

Auditory Processing Disorder

Central auditory processing disorder (CAPD), or auditory processing disorder (APD), is defined by the American Speech–Language–Hearing Association (1996) as an "inability to discriminate auditory patterns, localize sound, and understand speech with competing or degraded stimuli" (Katz & Tillery, 2004, p. 191). Prevalence rates of APD among school-age children range from 5 to 10%, with 45–75% of children with ADHD experiencing APD (Riccio et al., 1994; Tannock & Brown, 2000). However, these estimates may be confounded by the high prevalence of LD among children with ADHD (Gomez & Condon, 1999).

Common symptoms associated with ADHD and APD include inattentiveness, listening problems, distractibility, and difficulty following oral instructions (Chermak, Tucker, & Seikel, 2002; Katz & Tillery, 2004; Tannock & Brown, 2000). ADHD hyperactive–impulsive and combined types may be distinguished from APD because of the behavioral control problems experienced by those with ADHD. However, some assert that the ADHD inattentive type represents a cognitive rather than a behavioral disorder, with symptoms resembling those who display characteristics of APD (Chermak et al., 2002).

Despite some similarities between ADHD inattentive type and APD, differences in symptomatology do exist. As discussed, ADHD inattentive type is characterized by output rather than input problems. Thus, executive functions such as organization, planning, and purposeful, sustained attention are compromised. These children appear absentminded, careless, and forgetful. In contrast, APD, much like LD, is characterized by input problems. The inattentiveness exhibited in children with this disorder results from difficulties with selective and divided attention to auditory cues due to a dysfunction in the auditory cortex (e.g., lesions, structural abnormalities; Bellis, 1996; Chermak et al., 2002). Children with APD have difficulties following directions because of poor auditory processing skills as opposed to poor sustained attention. These children often have problems discriminating speech and need to have things repeated (Chermak et al., 2002; Meister, von Wedel, & Walger, 2004). Additionally, children with ADHD inattentive type display a pervasive pattern of inattentiveness across social contexts (e.g., homework, meals, class) and modalities (e.g., auditory, visual), whereas children with APD tend to display inattention during activities that require the use of auditory processing skills. However, children with ADHD are likely to have difficulty with frontal–basal ganglia–thalamic regulation of input processes (e.g., Hale et al., 2005), so differential diagnosis can be challenging.

Anxiety Disorders

Anxiety is believed to be the most common psychiatric problem in children and adolescents. An estimated 10% of children and adolescents meet criteria for at least one anxiety disorder (Breton et al., 1999) and roughly 33% have more than one anxiety disorder (Kashani & Orvaschel, 1990; Strauss & Last, 1993). Approximately 25% of children with ADHD meet criteria for one or more anxiety disorders (e.g., separation anxiety, generalized anxiety disorder, panic disorder; Biederman, Newcorn, & Sprich, 1991; Lee, 1999).

The relationship between ADHD and anxiety is controversial. Some researchers have found that anxiety is associated with ADHD inattentive symptoms but not with ADHD hyperactive–impulsive symptoms (e.g., fidgeting, talking excessively, interrupting; e.g., Angold et al., 1999; Lahey, Schaughency, Hynd, Carlson, & Nieves, 1987; Newcorn et al., 2001; Pliszka, 1992). Other researchers have hypothesized that the presence of anxiety can inhibit the display of externalizing behaviors (e.g., inability to sit still and/or wait for one's turn, impulsivity; Gray, 1987; Quay, 1997); still others have found that anxiety does not significantly suppress externalizing behaviors often found in ADHD populations (Abikoff et al., 2002). However, Abikoff and colleagues acknowledge that the type of comorbid anxiety disorder likely influences the clinical presentation of ADHD symptomatology.

The symptoms of anxiety disorders can resemble those found among children with ADHD. For example, children with generalized anxiety disorder (GAD) often manifest restlessness, irritability, and difficulty concentrating (APA, 2000), symptoms commonly seen in children with ADHD. However, restlessness and irritability exhibited by children with GAD are associated with excessive and uncontrollable worrying (APA, 2000) rather than the difficulties with behavioral inhibition and hyperactivity often seen in children with ADHD (Pliszka & Olvera, 1999). Children with anxiety disorders tend to be worrisome, fidgety, and distractible, and consequently have concentration and academic difficulties.

Approximately 30% of children with ADHD experience comorbid obsessive–compulsive disorder (OCD) symptoms (Geller, Biederman, Griffin, & Jones, 1996), which is not surprising considering they are both likely disorders of the cortical–subcortical circuits (e.g., Lichter & Cummings, 2001). Children who meet criteria for both disorders exhibit high levels of inattention, distractibility, and restlessness. Questions have been raised as to whether these children truly meet criteria for ADHD, or whether their ADHD-like symptoms result from the obsessional nature of OCD. Although research supports the coexistence of both diagnoses when this symptom profile is present (Geller et al., 2002, 2004), OCD is likely due to overactivity of the frontal–subcortical circuits that leads to *internal* inattention, whereas ADHD is due to underactivity of the same circuits, leading to *external* inattention (Hale & Fiorello, 2004; Hale et al., 2005). The repetitive behaviors often exhibited by children with OCD reduce distress experienced during the obsessional thought process and are not due to hyperactivity or impulsivity. As with GAD, obsessional thoughts frequently interfere with children's attention to academic and social tasks. Panic disorder (PD) and posttraumatic stress disorder (PTSD) are considered low-prevalence childhood disorders (e.g., Wittchen, Reed, & Kessler, 1998) that also manifest inattentive, disorganized, and agitated behaviors distinguishable from ADHD. Children with PD exhibit severe physiological signs (e.g., racing heart, shortness of breath) of anxiety that can be triggered by perceived and/or nonperceived threats in their environment. PTSD anxiety symptoms may result from prior trauma and/or perceived threats of injury and/or death (APA, 2000). Both PD and PTSD result in intrusive thoughts that can significantly interfere with children's attention and academic success.

The behavioral symptoms of anxiety disorders in general are more narrowly focused and accompanied by excessive worries and/or intrusive thoughts that significantly interfere with attention. In cases where the behavioral symptoms of ADHD and anxiety disorders are not easily differentiated, a clinician may obtain a differential diagnosis by assessing the presence and type of thoughts and worries that accompany the behavior (e.g., test anxiety, fear of speaking in a group, preoccupation with problems at home). Children with anxiety disorders tend to have less academic impairments than children with ADHD (Pliszka & Olvera, 1999). However, when children exhibit symptoms of both ADHD and anxiety disorder, the clinical picture may be more severe. These children tend to have academic and social problems, and to worry excessively about these problems (Tannock, 2000). In addition, pharmacological treatment may be different for these conditions based on whether the anxiety or ADHD symptoms predominate (e.g., Hale & Fiorello, 2004; Hale et al., 2005).

Mood Disorders

Mood disorders have become increasingly more common among school-age children (e.g., Beidel, 1991; Kessler, Avenevoli, & Merikangas, 2001). For example, dysthymic disorder has been found in approximately 3% of children (e.g., Kashani et al., 1987; Lewinsohn, Hops, Roberts, Seeley, & Andrews, 1993). The National Comorbidity Survey Replication (NCS-R; Kessler et al., 2005) recently reported that approximately 28% of their dysthymic disorder sample met criteria for ADHD, whereas approximately 5% of their ADHD sample were dysthymic. Dysthymia is characterized by a depressed or irritable mood persisting for at least 1 year, accompanied by at least two other depressive symptoms. Irritability, as well as other symptoms such as low self-esteem and poor concentration, are common in both dysthymia and ADHD (e.g., APA, 2000; Wasserstein, 2005).

Major depressive disorder (MDD) has been estimated to occur in approximately 2.5% of children (e.g., Ford, Goodman, & Meltzer, 2003; Hammen & Rudolph, 1996; Lewinsohn, Rhode, & Seeley, 1998), with rates increasing with age (e.g., Ford et al., 2003; Kashani & Orvaschel, 1988). For example, MDD has a lifetime prevalence of up to 20% by the end of high school (Ford et al., 2003; Lewinsohn et al., 1998). Attention and executive deficits are common in MDD (Mayberg, 2001); approximately 14% of children with ADHD also have MDD (Kessler et al., 2005). Depressive symptoms in MDD occur in greater numbers and with more severity than in dysthymic disorder, and persist for at least 2 weeks (APA, 2000). As noted, some depressive symptoms are similar to ADHD symptoms (e.g., irritability, low self-esteem, poor concentration). However, other depressive symptoms, such as fatigue and psychomotor retardation, are incompatible with ADHD symptoms and have been associated with milder forms of hyperactivity, impulsivity, and conduct problems (e.g., Perrin & Last, 1996; Pliszka, Carlson, & Swanson, 1999).

The presentation of symptoms in depressive disorders is often similar to that of ADHD. Both ADHD and depression can manifest in sleep disturbances, psychomotor agitation, irritability, and difficulty concentrating (APA, 2000). Feelings of worthlessness are reported as a common characteristic among depressed youth. Likewise, youth with ADHD provide similar reports, typically related to academic and social failure (Hechtman & Weiss, 1986). Differential diagnosis between depressive disorders and ADHD can be accomplished by assessment of symptoms of depression that are not often seen in children with ADHD. Examples of symptoms may include diminished interest in activities, changes in weight or diet, and recurrent thoughts about death, dying, and/or suicide (APA, 2000). Practitioners are also encouraged to assess whether the child's current social and academic functioning represents a negative change in comparison to previous functioning.

The prevalence and nature of early-onset bipolar disorder (BPD) among children and adolescents has received much attention. Some researchers have reported that BPD is nonexistent in child samples (Costello et al., 1996), whereas others have reported that up to 2% of children meet criteria for BPD (Verhulst, van der Ende, Ferdinand, & Kasius, 1997). The inconsistency in findings is partially due to a lack of consensus among scholars on what constitutes this disorder in children (e.g., Biederman et al., 2000; Pavuluri, Birmaher, & Naylor, 2005). Researchers have concluded that the criteria for BPD in the *Diagnostic and Statistical Manual of Mental Disorders*, fourth edition, text revision (DSM-IV-TR, APA, 2000), are developmentally inappropriate for children. For example, children with BPD do not usually display discrete episodes of depression and mania; rather, they display depressive and manic symptoms simultaneously or cycle between them several times a day (e.g., Findling et al., 2001; Kowatch et al., 2005). Both depressed and elevated moods in children may manifest as severe irritability, as well as classic depression and euphoria (e.g., Findling et al., 2001; Geller, Zimerman, & Williams, 2000).

Among children with BPD, the comorbidity of ADHD is approximately 80% (Shear, DelBello, Lee-Rosenberg, & Strakowski, 2002), whereas 22% of children with ADHD have BPD (Butler, Arredondo, & McCloskey, 1995). Similar to ADHD symptoms, BPD symptoms may include irritability, pressured speech, distractibility, and increased energy (Wozniak, 2005), with attention and executive deficits common in both disorders (Shear et al., 2002). To aid in differential diagnosis, Geller et al. (2003) outlined "cardinal symptoms" of BPD, such as elated mood, grandiosity (e.g., believe that one is a superhero or that one can fly), uncontrollable laughter for no reason, and decreased need for sleep (i.e., without fatigue).

Next, we outline historical antecedents, biological, psychological, and psychosocial factors associated with ADHD-related symptoms. Following this section, we review assessment approaches for this population.

Differential Diagnosis

Historical Antecedents

A number of child and family conditions and factors (e.g., health status, family history, and development) are important considerations for evaluating and treating children with ADHD-related symptoms. For example, several medical conditions have been linked to ADHD symptoms. Children with ADHD display higher rates of allergies, asthma, stomachaches, ear infections (Schnoll, Burshteyn, & Cea-Aravena, 2003), and sleep difficulties (Ball, Tiernan, Janusz, & Furr, 1997) than do controls. Hauser et al. (1993), using structured interviews, found that whereas 61% of children resistant to thyroid hormone were diagnosed with ADHD, only 13% of children without this condition were diagnosed with ADHD. Hearing and vision impairments, head injuries, lead toxicity, thyroid disorders, pediatric autoimmune neuropsychiatric disorders associated with streptococcal infections (PANDAS), and/or seizure disorders may manifest in clinical levels of inattention, impulsivity, insomnia, hyperactivity, anxiety, and/or depression (Schnoll et al., 2003). Research results on the role of prenatal and perinatal characteristics (e.g., toxemia, long labor, low birthweight) in the development of ADHD symptoms in children are mixed. Some researchers report high rates of ADHD symptoms among children with chronic exposure to lead (e.g., Needleman et al., 1979; Tuthill, 1996), whereas others report inconclusive findings (Schroeder & Gordon, 2002).

Family psychiatric history is related to ADHD-related symptoms in children. For example, first-degree relatives of children with ADHD are more susceptible to having ADHD symptoms than relatives of children without ADHD (e.g., Samudra & Cantwell, 1999; Schroeder & Gordon, 2002; Whalen &

Henker, 1998). Greater levels of anxiety, depression, and ADHD have been found in siblings of children with ADHD compared to siblings of controls (Samudra & Cantwell, 1999). There is some evidence that parents and relatives of children with ADHD have higher rates of LD, antisocial tendencies, and alcohol abuse than do those of controls (e.g., Edwards, Schulz, & Long, 1995; Johnston & Mash, 2001). Furthermore, Chi and Hinshaw (2002) found an association between the severity of ADHD symptoms and levels of maternal depression. Similarly, children tend to have a higher propensity for the onset of depressive symptoms when their mothers are depressed (e.g., Ollendick, Shortt, & Sander, 2004). Symptoms of anxiety are more likely to occur in both offspring of anxious parents and parents of children with anxiety than in controls (McClure, Brennan, Hammen, & Le Brocque, 2001).

The development of ADHD-related symptoms is reported across informants and settings (Schroeder & Gordon, 2002). From birth to 2 years of age, parents and child care workers report that children with ADHD display difficult temperaments. For example, infants and toddlers have been described as overactive and display intense emotions, negative moods, and poor physiological regulation. Among preschool-age children, overactivity, impulsivity, noncompliance, aggression, immaturity, and difficulty with peer group activities have been reported. Children ages 3–5 with ADHD tend to toilet train later than their non-ADHD peers and have higher rates of accidental poisoning and injury. As children with ADHD enter elementary school, they continue to have peer relation, restlessness, and attentional difficulties, as well as child–adult interaction problems.

At approximately age 9 years, the number of problematic behaviors that children with ADHD exhibit increase exponentially (Schroeder & Gordon, 2002). Academic problems, such as frequent mistakes and incomplete assignments, as well as poor social skills, limited self-control, and difficulty in developing athletic skills, are found. Parents of children ages 9–12 years with ADHD often describe their children as irresponsible and forgetful. These children frequently receive comorbid diagnoses such as LD, oppositional defiant disorder, conduct disorder, and mood and/or anxiety disorders.

In adolescents, attentional problems may manifest in poor academic performance, forgetfulness, and incomplete and/or inaccurate homework assignments (Schroeder & Gordon, 2002). Adolescents with ADHD may also exhibit noncompliant behavior in dealing with authority figures (e.g., teachers, parents, coaches) and behave more immaturely than their nondisabled peers. Drug use, impaired social functioning, depressive symptoms, diminished self-esteem, and car accidents are not uncommon among adolescents with ADHD (DuPaul & Stoner, 2003).

Biological Factors

Several biological factors, such as genetics, brain structure and chemical imbalance, and temperament, are linked to the development of ADHD-related symptoms. Genetics research, often conducted with twins and adopted youth, focuses on the degree to which symptoms develop because they are inherited from one's relatives. Evidence exists that ADHD symptoms such as inattentiveness and hyperactivity can be accounted for by genetics (Levy & Hay, 2001). High heritability estimates of ADHD suggest a strong genetic influence. However, the influence of genetics associated with this population varies by informant (e.g., parents, teachers) and diagnostic criteria used (Goodman & Stevenson, 1989). Additionally, research has suggested that the development of a disorder (e.g., ADHD) may be attributed to a general genetic vulnerability for inattention and hyperactivity rather than to a specific disorder (Eley & Stevenson, 1999).

Brain structure and chemical imbalances have been linked to the development of ADHD-related symptoms. Among youth with ADHD, research indicates that frontal lobes (e.g., Castellanos et al., 2002; Filipek, 1999), basal ganglia (e.g., Semrud-Clikeman et al., 2000; Hynd et al., 1993), anterior cingulate (e.g., Rubia, Smith, Brammer, Toone, & Taylor, 2005; Shultz et al., 2004) and corpus callosum (e.g., Giedd et al., 1994; Semrud-Clikeman et al., 1994) can impact symptom expression. Low levels of dopamine and norepinephrine are linked to ADHD symptoms (Whalen & Henker, 1998), which accounts for the beneficial effects of central nervous system stimulants in treating the disorder (Hale & Fiorello, 2004; Hale et al., 1998; Hoeppner et al., 1997). However, children with depression experience low levels of serotonin, dopamine, norepinephrine, and the monoamines (Wagner & Ambrosini, 2001), which lead to attention and executive function deficits (Mayberg, 2001). As a result, differential diagnosis requires not only examination of the behavioral manifestations of these disorders but also assessment of the attention and executive function deficits associated with the various cortical–subcortical circuits (Hale et al., 2005).

Temperament may play a significant role in the development of children's adaptive and maladaptive functioning. Difficulty with emotional regulation, irritability, negative emotionality, and risk-taking behavior are common temperamental characteristics of ADHD children (Schroeder & Gordon, 2002). Research has shown that 3- to 5-year-old boys who score in the clinical range on the Total Behavior Problems subscale of the Child Behavior Checklist (CBCL; Achenbach, 1991) are more likely to have difficult temperaments (e.g., high motor activity, distractibility, reactivity, inattention, and irregular patterns of sleeping and eating) than boys who score in the nonclinical range (Jansen, Fitzgerald, Ham, & Zucker, 1995). However, the relationship between children's temperament and subsequent problematic behaviors may be influenced by levels of parental psychopathology (e.g., Mun, Fitzgerald, von Eye, Puttler, & Zucker, 2001).

Temperamental characteristics may also influence children's academic achievement and classroom behavior. For example, increased rates of fidgeting, energy, and distractibility, and decreased rates of persistence (especially on difficult tasks) in first-graders have been linked to low scores on measures of academic achievement in fifth-graders (Martin, Olejnik, & Gaddis, 1994). Similar results have been found between temperament and reading and math achievement scores among adolescents (Guerin, Gottfried, Oliver, & Thomas, 1994). Temperament factors, such as level of activity, distractibility, and persistence, may also influence teachers' and peers' responses to children with ADHD, which may impact their academic self-concept and academic performance (Martin, 1988).

Differentiating between children with ADHD and those with difficult temperaments may be challenging due to the overlapping characteristics found in each. Keogh (2003) suggested that children who exhibit hyperactivity, inattentiveness, and/or impulsivity across settings may warrant a diagnosis of ADHD, whereas children with difficult temperaments often have behavioral problems that are more situation-specific (e.g., morning routine, homework). Temperament factors, such as persistence, adaptability, and task orientation, may influence the development of learning difficulties and/or LD (Keogh, 1994). Teglasi, Cohn, and Meshbesher (2004) stated that temperamental characteristics have a direct relationship with "disrupted learning and development of self or others, dysfunctional relationships with families, peers, or teachers, (and) distressing emotions" (p. 15). Thus, children who display intense patterns of emotional outbursts in class are likely to develop learning and/or interpersonal relationships problems.

Psychological Factors

Psychological factors, such as parental stress, role dissatisfaction, perceived control, and expectancies, may influence the display of ADHD-related symptoms.

Parents of children with ADHD report higher levels of psychological distress than the parents of children without ADHD (Murphy & Barkley, 1996). In comparison to parents of controls, parents of children with ADHD (i.e., combined and/or inattentive subtypes) were more dissatisfied with their roles as parents (Podolski & Nigg, 2001). However, dissatisfaction in parenting roles may differ between mothers and fathers of children with ADHD. For example, mothers' dissatisfaction was associated with their children's inattention and oppositional behaviors, whereas fathers' dissatisfaction was associated with their children's aggressive and oppositional behaviors. Hyperactivity did not contribute to role distress or dissatisfaction for mothers and fathers.

Parents' perceived control of their children's behavior has been found to be related to parental stress and symptom severity among ADHD children (Harrison & Sofronoff, 2002). For example, research has suggested that the severity of children's behavioral problems and mothers' perceived control over their children's behavior are predictors of maternal stress. Harrison and Sofronoff hypothesized that mothers who report high levels of stress related to caring for their children may experience learned helplessness, a belief that they cannot control or modify their children's behavior.

Parental expectancies differ between parents of youth with and without ADHD. For example, Sonuga-Barke and Goldfoot (1995) found that mothers of children with ADHD in general have lower expectations of their own children (e.g., developmental milestones, academics) than mothers of controls, when children's cognitive functioning (IQ scores) was controlled. Findings were similar among other clinical populations. For example, mothers of anxious children, with respect to their children's future performance, report fewer positive expectations and more negative expectations than do mothers of controls (Kortlander, Kendall, & Chansky, 1994). Mothers of anxious children also misjudge their children's coping skills, expecting them to be more distressed and less able to calm themselves during stressful situations, than do mothers of controls (Kortlander, Kendall, & Panichelli-Mindel, 1997).

Psychosocial Factors

Factors related to the family environment, parent and child attachment, peer relations, and academic performance may influence the presentation of ADHD-related symptoms. Families of children with ADHD are more likely to exhibit lower levels of family cohesion and higher levels of parental disagreement than do families of controls (Samudra & Cantwell, 1999). The quality of mothers' caregiving has been shown to predict distractibility in 3½-year-olds and hyperactivity in 6- to 8-year-olds (Carlson, Jacobvitz, & Sroufe, 1995). For example, mothers' use of inappropriate control strategies with children (e.g., harsh comments without explanation and physical restraints), as well as a lack of affection and approval of their children, is associated with ADHD symptoms (Johnston, Murray, Hinshaw, Pelham, & Hoza, 2002). Similarly, Ollendick et al. (2004) reported finding higher levels of control and emotional overinvolvement, and lower levels of acceptance and psychological independence among parents of anxious children than among those of controls.

Attachment theory has been used to explain how early parent–child relationships may serve as protective or risk factors for mental illness. Some research has indicated that attachment issues among children with ADHD are linked to stress related to mothers' pregnancy and children's first year of life (Stiefel, 1997). Examples of factors that negatively impact child–parent attachment are insecurity about parenting, lack of significant other/familial support, mothers' negative views of fathers' behavior, significant life stressors (e.g., death of a close relative), and pregnancy/birth complications. According to this line of research, a demand–dissatisfaction cycle and insecure attachment patterns develop in the parent and child interaction and may lead to ADHD symptoms. As one example, Stiefel (1997) suggests that children who are unsure of whether to approach or avoid their mothers might have difficulty concentrating and paying attention.

Attachment theorists have also proposed that ADHD symptoms are linked to poor attachment between mothers and their children, because the disrupted attachment pattern, in part, leads to impairments in children's self-regulation and interpersonal functioning (Clarke, Ungerer, Chahoud, Johnson, & Stiefel, 2002). Clarke et al. found significantly lower scores on measures of attachment and parent–child relationship and higher rates of aggressive coping skills (e.g., hitting or kicking others or objects out of frustration) among children with ADHD than among controls. Because research supports attachment theory and its role in the development of ADHD-like symptoms, some assert that parent–child interactions, and the context of these interactions (e.g., homework, meals), should be the primary focus of treatment rather than the use of medication and child-focused behavioral techniques (Labauve, 2003).

The peer relations of children with ADHD are often dissimilar to those of nondisabled peers. For example, children with ADHD are invited less frequently to participate in games and activities than are controls (Pelham & Milich, 1984). Children with ADHD tend to have interpersonal deficits (i.e., problems with the "give-and-take" in social situations), higher levels of interpersonal intensity, problems with social information processing and friendship development, and more aggressive and noisier play (Whalen & Henker, 1998). Youth with ADHD combined type and those with the predominantly inattentive type may display discrepant social difficulties (Maedgen & Carlson, 2000). For example, children with the combined type tend to have aggressive social interactions and difficulties inhibiting their emotions and behaviors, whereas children with the inattentive type tend to approach social situations passively and exhibit a general lack of social knowledge.

Children diagnosed with ADHD and LD tend to be at greater risk for social deficits (Kellner et al., 2003). However, comorbid LD may impact children with ADHD combined type differently than children with ADHD inattentive type. For example, Kellner et al. (2003) found that children with ADHD combined type and LD reported "significantly more interpersonal difficulties [and] social interaction anxiety and significantly lower levels of social self-concept (i.e., specific feelings of peer isolation and peer hostility) and social self confidence" in comparison to children with ADHD inattentive type and controls (p. 130). Although differences in social skills were not found between children with ADHD combined type only and ADHD combined type and LD, children with ADHD inattentive type and controls reported lower levels of social anxiety and higher levels of social self-concept and self-confidence than children with ADHD inattentive type and LD.

Children with ADHD often struggle academically from the onset of their education. For example, young children with ADHD perform more poorly (i.e., one standard deviation lower) on tests of cognitive functioning and preacademic competencies (e.g., basic math concepts, prereading abilities, and fine-motor coordination skills) than their nondisabled peers (DuPaul, McGoey, Eckert, & VanBrakle, 2001). Unfortunately, these discrepancies do not vanish as children become adolescents. Adolescents without ADHD symptoms are more likely than adolescents with ADHD to complete high school (Barkley, Fischer, Edelbrock, & Smallish, 1990).

Keogh's (1971) pioneer work outlined that ADHD-related symptoms impact learning in two distinct ways. First, increased hyperactivity influences children with ADHD to pay less attention to their teachers; thus, they may acquire less academic information than their peers. Second, children with ADHD may exhibit poorer performance on academic tasks, because they impulsively record their answers. Difficulties with inattention and disorganization may also manifest as carelessness, resulting in incorrect answers to class work and homework and disorganized desks/work areas (DuPaul & Stoner, 2003). These children may focus on activities other than those presented by their classroom teachers and subsequently do not complete in-class assignments (Goldstein, 1999). However, some children with ADHD are observed watching their teachers' instruction and are able to answer questions and perform well academically. These inconsistencies in observed behavior may result in teachers' describing children with ADHD as being "noncompliant" as opposed to having a true deficit. Thus, a comprehensive assessment is warranted to ascertain the behavioral and neurocognitive function of behaviors observed in the home and school.

In the next section, we present some of the common cognitive–neuropsychological and social–emotional assessment approaches used with this population. This review is intended to offer practitioners an appreciation of the range of measures used with youth with ADHD. It is not intended to be an exhaustive list.

ASSESSMENT APPROACHES

Prior to a comprehensive evaluation, a pretesting assessment (i.e., intake) is recommended to determine whether a set of tests and/or full evaluation is appropriate for a child. Pretesting can take different forms, such as a parent interview that includes developmental, social, and educational history; review of school records (i.e., report cards, behavior data, current academic assignments); classroom-based observations/data; teacher consultation; and the completion of parent and teacher behavior rating scales. Parents' and children's responses (i.e., verbal and nonverbal) during pretesting also provide important information on parents' and children's social, emotional, and behavioral functioning, and overall comfort with testing. Feedback from other professionals (e.g., physicians, social workers, and school personnel), family members, and coaches can also be helpful. The importance of the pretesting phase in the overall evaluation process is highlighted in the forthcoming case studies.

Like all evaluations, a comprehensive ADHD evaluation rests on the type of referral provided, the referring agent or agency, and the unique child, family, and school system factors. We recommend that practitioners adopt an idiographic assessment approach that includes multiple methods, informants, and contexts to assess a child's cognitive, learning, speech–language, sensory, social–emotional, cultural–linguistic, and adaptive–maladaptive functioning. It is also recommended that practitioners assess the clinical nuances of comorbid externalizing and internalizing disorders; learning characteristics and/or disabilities; previous assessment and/or treatment experiences; parent and teacher observations/feedback; personality; and children's parent, teacher, and peer interactions.

Cognitive–Neuropsychological Assessment

A number of cognitive–neuropsychological assessment instruments exist that can assist practitioners in the assessment of ADHD-related symptoms. Probably the most popularly used intelligence instrument is the Wechsler Intelligence Scale for Children—Fourth Edition (Wechsler, 2003). The WISC-IV more closely adheres to a neuropsychological model of cognitive functioning that includes a psychometrically strong four-factor model (i.e., Verbal Comprehensive; Perceptual Reasoning, formerly Perceptual Organization; Working Memory, former Freedom from Distractibility; and Processing Speed indices). The WISC-IV possesses considerable evidence of reliability and validity, including concurrent validity with the WISC-III (Wechsler, 2003). In the technical manual, large practical (i.e., effect sizes) group differences were reported between children with ADHD and LD and controls on Full Scale IQ, Processing Speed, and Working Memory indices, whereas moderate effect sizes were reported between children with ADHD and controls on the Processing Speed index (Wechsler, 2003). Independent research on the clinical utility of the WISC-IV for children with ADHD is limited, but these scales may be used to differentiate childhood disorders, including ADHD (Mayes & Calhoun, 2004). The application of the WISC-IV with ADHD and ADHD-related disorders is illustrated in the case studies.

Based on Cattell–Horn–Carroll theory of cognitive abilities, the Woodcock–Johnson Tests of Cognitive Abilities (WJ-III-COG) is a comprehensive cognitive assessment battery that comprises 20 tests, classified into three categories: Verbal Ability, Thinking Ability, and Cognitive Efficiency (Woodcock, McGrew, & Mather, 2001). The WJ-III-COG also includes five clinical clusters that measure aspects of executive functioning (i.e., Phonemic Awareness, Working Memory, Broad Attention, Cognitive Fluency, and Executive Processes). The WJ-III-COG possesses good reliability and validity indices (Woodcock et al., 2001). Studies on the clinical utility of the WJ-III-COG for children with ADHD have been mixed. For example, Ford, Keith, Floyd, Fields, and Schrank (2003) reported that the two most significant test predictors of ADHD group members were Auditory Working Memory and Planning, whereas Reddy, Dumont, and Bray (2005) reported for the same group Auditory Attention and Rapid Picture Naming.

Based on CHC G*f*-G*c* theory, the Differential Abilities Scales (DAS; Elliott, 1990a) includes 17 cognitive subtests designed to produce a composite General Conceptual Ability (GCA) score. The subtests produce Verbal, Nonverbal, and Spatial Clusters that correspond to the verbal, fluid, and visualization factors in the G*f*-G*c* model. The DAS includes three Diagnostic subtests (i.e., Recall of Digits, Recall of Objects, and Speed of Information Processing). The DAS school-age version is reported to have good reliability and validity (see Elliott, 1990a, 1990b). The DAS Sequential and Quantitative Reasoning and the Recall of Digits subtests correctly classify ADHD only and controls 72.5% of the time (Gibney, McIntosh, Dean, & Dunham, 2002). With a comorbid ADHD sample, Reddy, Braunstein, and Dumont (2005) reported that the four Diagnostic subtests accurately classified 67% of the sample, and the Recall of Digits subtest was the most significant predictor for ADHD status.

Based on Luria's model of neuropsychological processing, the Cognitive Assessment System (CAS; Naglieri & Das, 1997) includes a full scale score, four clusters referred to as the PASS model (i.e., planning, attention, simultaneous processing, and successive processing), and 12 subtests. Reliability and validity indices are good, and most subscales show good technical characteristics (Naglieri & Das, 1997). Children with ADHD exhibit lower CAS Planning scores than anxiety–depressed and control samples, whereas no group differences were found on the WISC-III (Naglieri, Goldstein, & Iseman, 2003). In a sample of 119 children (i.e., 48 with ADHD, 23 with RD, and 48 with regular education), the ADHD group had lower Planning and Simultaneous scores than the regular education group, whereas the RD group had lower Successive scores than the regular education group (Naglieri, Salter, & Edwards, 2004). Although cross-battery analyses have suggested that the Planning and Attention factors should be combined and not interpreted separately (Keith, Kranzler, & Flanagan, 2001), the CAS offers the first treatment validity studies of any cognitive measure (e.g., PASS Remedial Program [PREP]; Das, Carlson, Davidson, & Longe, 1997).

The NEPSY is designed to assess neuropsychological development in children between the ages of 3 and 12 (Korman, Kirk, & Kemp, 1998). It comprises 14 subtests that assess five core domains: Attention/Executive Functions, Language, Sensorimotor Functions, Visuospatial Processing, and Memory and Learning. The NEPSY includes a Core Assessment that provides an overview of a child's neuropsychological status, an Expanded or Selective Assessment that provides an analysis of specific cognitive disorders, and a Full Assessment for a comprehensive neuropsychological evaluation. The NEPSY includes good reliability, and concurrent and criterion-related validity (Korman et al., 1998). As reported by the authors, children with ADHD yield lower Attention/Executive Function core domain scores and perform more poorly on the Tower, Auditory Attention and Response Set, Statue, and Knock and Tap subtests compared to matched controls. Children with ADHD also demonstrate impaired performance on all language subtests (except

Speeded Naming) and the Sensorimotor Functions core domain. Also, children with ADHD exhibit decreased List Learning, Sentence Repetition, and Narrative Memory within the Memory and Learning domain. A sample of children at risk for ADHD (age 4½ to 6½ years) had lower Tower and Statue scores than did controls (Perner, Kain, & Barchfeld, 2002). Independent research on the NEPSY with ADHD-related disorders is limited. The NEPSY does offer a flexible assessment tool that taps basic and complex cognitive processes for this population.

The Delis–Kaplan Executive Function System (D-KEFS; Delis, Kaplan, & Kramer, 2001), an efficient and flexible approach for assessing children's executive functions, comprises nine subtests that measure flexibility of thinking, inhibition, attention, language, perception, and abstract thought: Trail Making, Verbal Fluency, Design Fluency, Color–Word Interference, Sorting, 20 Questions, Word Context, Tower, and Proverb. These subtest can be individually or group-administered to children and adults ages 8–89 years. The D-KEFS allows practitioners to "pick and choose" tests to evaluate clinical hypotheses on executive functioning by comparing and contrasting a child's performance on multiple tests and testing conditions. The authors outline extensive information on the test's technical characteristics and interpretation strategies (Delis et al., 2001), but research on children with ADHD is missing. However, numerous studies have demonstrated the utility of tests similar to D-KEFS in the diagnosis of ADHD, such as the Trail Making Test, art B, Stroop Color–Word Test, Wisconsin Card Sorting Test, and Controlled Oral Word Association Test (e.g., Hale & Fiorello, 2004; Hale et al., 1998, 2005; Hoeppner et al., 1997). Unlike these measures, which often have limited child samples, the D-KEFS provides the first set of executive function tests co-normed on a large national sample.

The Brief Rating Inventory of Executive Function (BRIEF; Gioia, Isquith, Guy, & Kenworthy, 2000) is the first scale for parents and teachers that assess children's executive function behaviors. The BRIEF comprises eight clinical subscales (i.e., Inhibit, Shift, Emotional Control, Initiate, Working Memory, Plan/Organize, Organization of Materials, and Monitor) and two validity subscales (i.e., Inconsistency, Negativity). The clinical subscales comprise a Global Executive Composite and two indices, Behavioral Regulation and Metacognition. The BRIEF has strong psychometric properties (Gioia et al., 2000). As reported by the authors, the Working Memory and Inhibit subscales accurately discriminate between ADHD subtypes from controls. Parents rate children with ADHD as having significantly more problems than controls on all of the BRIEF scales. The Behavioral Regulation Index differentiated between children with ADHD inattentive type and ADHD combined type (Pratt, Campbell-La Voie, Isquith, Gioia, & Guy, 2000). Similarly, teachers rated children with ADHD as having significantly more problems than controls on the BRIEF scales. The Inhibit, Shift, Emotional Control, and Monitor subscales differentiated between children with ADHD inattentive and ADHD from combined type, with children with the ADHD combined type scoring higher on all scales.

The use of continuous performance tests (e.g., Test of Variables of Attention [TOVA, Greenberg, 1988–1999]; Conners Continuous Performance Test–II [CPT-II, Conners & MHS Staff, 2000]) have become increasingly popular among practitioners. Much research has been conducted on the use of continuous performance tests (CPTs) with children with ADHD and ADHD-related disorders (Riccio & Reynolds, 2003). Overall, CPTs tend to yield high positive predictive power (i.e., a child's poor performance strongly confirm the presence of ADHD-related symptoms) and poor negative predictive power (i.e., a child's passing performance yields inconclusive results). Like other measures, CPT results are complicated by the high rate of comorbidity in this population and differential patterns of performance among ADHD subtypes (e.g., Hale et al., 2005).

Next, we present some of the common social, emotional, and behavioral assessments used with this population. It is important that practitioners recognize the relationship between cognition, achievement, and social–emotional functioning. The assessment of emotional and behavioral functioning in children with ADHD requires an understanding of the interplay of biological, cognitive, and environmental factors in brain development.

Social–Emotional Assessment

Behavior Rating Scales

Popular among practitioners, behavior rating scales (BRS) are efficient and effective tool to assess social, emotional, and behavioral functioning in children with ADHD across informants (i.e., parent, teacher) and settings (i.e., home, school; Pelham, Fabiano, & Massetti, 2005). Many excellent BRS exist. Next, we provide a description of some of the well-known BRS.

The Achenbach System of Empirically Based Assessment (ASEBA; Achenbach & Rescorla, 2001) evaluates the adaptive and maladaptive functioning of children ages 1½ to 18 years. The ASEBA includes parent (CBCL), teacher (Teacher Report Form [TRF]), and child (Youth Report Form [YRF]) forms. The CBCL and TRF include preschool (1½ to 5 years) and school-age forms (6–18 years) that assess teachers' and parents' perceptions of children's externalizing and internalizing behaviors. The CBCL includes a total scale, two composite scales (i.e., Externalizing and Internalizing), eight clinical subscales (i.e., Anxious/Depressed, Withdrawn/Depressed, Somatic Complaints, Social Problems, Thought Problems, Attention Problems, Rule-Breaking Behavior, and Aggressive Behavior), and three competence scales (i.e., Activities, Social, and School). Like the CBCL, the TRF includes the same composite and clinical scales, as well as four competence subscales (i.e., Working Hard, Behaving, Learning, and Happy). The CBCL and TRF are well researched and have extensive reliability and validity information across a broad range of child clinical populations, including children with ADHD (e.g., Achenbach & Rescorla, 2001; Doyle, Ostrander, Skare, Crosby, & August, 1997; Eiraldi, Power, Karustis, & Goldstein, 2000).

The Conners' Parent and Teacher Rating Scales—Revised (CPRS-R and CTRS-R, respectively; Conners, 1997a) is one of the most widely used BRS for children with ADHD. The CPRS-R and CTRS-R assess childhood psycho-pathology for children ages 3–17 years. The CPRS-R has seven primary factors (i.e., Oppositional, Inattention, Hyperactivity, Anxious–Shy, Perfectionism, Social Problems, and Psychosomatic). The CTRS-R has six primary factors (i.e., Oppositionality, Inattention, Hyperactivity–Impulsivity, Anxious–Shy, Perfectionism, and Social Problems). The CPRS-R and CTRS-R have excellent reliability, concurrent, and criterion-related validity with children with ADHD (Conners, 1997a). For example, the CPRS-R scales correctly identify ADHD from nonreferred children 92.3% of the time (Conners, Sitarenios, Parker, & Epstein, 1998a), and the CTRS-R scales correctly discriminate between ADHD and nonreferred children 78.1% of the time (Conners, Sitarenios, Parker, & Epstein, 1998b). However, they do not discriminate well between childhood disorders with attention problems, including differentiation of ADHD subtypes (Hale, How, DeWitt, & Coury, 2001).

The Behavior Assessment System for Children–2 (BASC-2; Reynolds & Kamphaus, 2004) evaluates the adaptive and maladaptive behaviors of children and adults ages 2–25 years. The BASC-2 includes a Teacher Rating Scale (TRS), a Parent Rating Scale (PRS), and a Self-Report of Personality (SRP, discussed in the personality inventory section). The PRS and TRS have Preschool (2–5 years), Child (6–12 years), and Adolescent (12–21 years) forms that assess parents' and teachers' perceptions of children's adaptive and problem behaviors. The PRS includes four composite subscales (i.e., Adaptive Skills, Behavioral Symptoms Skills, Externalizing Problems, and Internalizing Problems); 14 primary subscales (i.e., Adaptability, Activities of Daily Living, Aggression, Anxiety, Attention Problems, Atypicality, Conduct Problems [child and adolescent form only], Depression, Functional Communication, Hyperactivity, Leadership [child and adolescent only], Social Skills, Somatization, and Withdrawal); and seven content subscales (i.e., Anger Control, Bullying, Developmental Social Disorders, Emotional Self-Control, Executive Functioning, Negative Emotionality, and Resiliency). The TRS includes all of the composites and primary subscales in the PRS, as well as a composite subscale on school problems and two subscales on learning problems and study skills. BASC-2 has good reliability and concurrent validity (i.e., ASEBA, BRIEF, CPRS-R, CTRS-R) and criterion-related validity with nonclinical and clinical groups (e.g., ADHD, LD, depressive disorders; Reynolds & Kamphaus, 2004). The BASC (Reynolds & Kamphaus, 1992) accurately differentiates between children with and without ADHD (e.g., Manning, 2001; Pizzitola, Riccio, & Siekierski, 2005). However, research on the BASC-2 with ADHD children has yet to be conducted.

The Social Skills Rating System (SSRS; Gresham & Elliot, 1990) assesses children's social behaviors and includes Parent (PF), Teacher (TF), and Student (SF) forms. The SSRS-PF and SSRS-TF have Preschool, Elementary, and Secondary forms, and the SSRS-SF has forms for grades 3–6 and 7–12. The SSRS-PF and SSRS-TF assess parents' and teachers' perceptions of children's social skills and behavioral difficulties. Both the PF and TF include Social Skills and Problem Behaviors Scales, and the TF also includes an Academic Competence Scale (i.e., Elementary and Secondary Forms only). The Social Skills Scale includes five subscales (i.e., Cooperation, Assertion, Responsibility, Empathy, and Self-Control), and the Problem Behaviors Scale includes three subscales (i.e., Externalizing Problems, Internalizing Problems, and Hyperactivity). The Academic Competence Scale includes nine items that assess concerns about student academic functioning. The SSRS has good reliability, concurrent validity (e.g., TRF), and criterion-related validity with clinical and nonreferred children (Gresham & Elliot, 1990). The SSRS differentiates between African American preschoolers at low and high risk for ADHD (Bain & Pelletier, 1999). Limited independent research has been conducted with ADHD-related populations.

Personality Inventories

Personality inventories provide valuable information on the social–emotional functioning of children with ADHD. Many excellent child and adolescent personality inventories exist, such as the Minnesota Multiphasic Personality Inventory—Adolescents (MMPI-A, Butcher, 1992), the Millon Adolescent Personality Inventory (Millon, Green, & Meagher, 1982), the Personality Inventory for Children–II (Lachar & Gruber, 2001), the Personality Inventory for Youth (PIY, Lachar & Gruber, 1995), and the Student Behavior Survey (SBS, Lachar, Wingenfeld, Kline, & Gruber, 2000).

A new child self-report measure of personality, the Self-Report of Personality (SRP) of the BASC-2 (Reynolds & Kamphaus, 2004), has Child (8–11 years), Adolescent (12–21 years), and College (18–25 years) levels that assess perceptions of personality. The child and adolescent levels have the same composite (i.e., Emotional Symptoms Index, Inattention/Hyperactivity, Internalizing Problems, Personal Adjustment, School Problems) and primary subscales (i.e., Anxiety, Attention Problems, Attitude to School, Attitude to Teacher, Atypicality, Interpersonal Relations, Locus of Control, Relations with Parents, School Adjustment, Self-Esteem, Self-Reliance, Sensation Seeking, Sense of Inadequacy, Social Stress, Somatization). The SRP also has content subscales (i.e., Anger Control, Ego Strength), available only for the adolescent level. The SRP is reported to have good reliability, concurrent validity (ASEBA-YRF [Achenbach & Rescorla, 2001]; Conners–Wells Adolescent Self-Report Scale [Conners, 1997b]; Children's Depression Inventory [CDI; Kovacs, 2003]; Revised Children's Manifest Anxiety Scale [RCMAS; Reynolds & Richmond, 2000]), and criterion-related validity with clinical groups (e.g., ADHD, depressive disorders, LD, and mental retardation; Reynolds & Kamphaus, 2004).

Next, we present two case studies that illustrate the use of some common cognitive–neurocognitive and social–emotional measures for children with inattention. The case of "Thomas" describes a boy who displays inattention but does not have executive functioning deficits. The case of "Lisa" describes a girl who displays both inattention and executive functioning deficits. Treatment plans are detailed for each.

CASE FORMULATION: CONCEPTUAL MODEL OF ASSESSMENT AND TREATMENT

The cases of "Thomas" and "Lisa" were formulated by using a cognitive hypothesis-testing (CHT) model and behavioral consultation approach. The CHT model provides a step-by-step method for identifying and serving children with attention and other problems, as highlighted in Figure 4.1. However, as a model of practice, emphasis is placed on helping a majority of children before they ever need a CHT evaluation. Whether conceived as a systematic prereferral service, intervention assistance team, or a response-to-intervention approach, practitioners must *intervene to assess* children in a problem-solving consultation before they are referred for testing (Hale & Fiorello, 2004). If a majority of children respond to interventions implemented with integrity, then fewer children will need formal CHT evaluations, and if they are needed, this intervention data may be essential in helping to develop referral questions and hypotheses about children's strengths and needs. This is the only way that comprehensive CHT evaluations are feasible in practice: Reducing referrals means more time to conduct both interventions and more comprehensive evaluations.

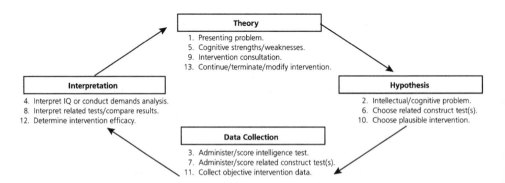

FIGURE 4.1. The cognitive hypothesis-testing (CHT) model. From Hale and Fiorello (2004). Copyright 2004 by The Guilford Press. Reprinted by permission.

Despite our best efforts, some children will not respond to standard or problem solving interventions, and may require formal CHT evaluations. As depicted in Figure 4.1, the first CHT step is to develop a *theory* based on the referral question, history, and previous interventions. Next, a cognitive–neuropsychological *hypothesis* is developed, in part to explain the attentional, academic, or behavioral deficit areas. Based on this information, the clinician then chooses, administers, and scores an intellectual–cognitive assessment measure in the *data collection/analysis* step. The nomothetic and idiographic *data interpretation* step follows, based on both psychometric and neuropsychological knowledge (Hale & Fiorello, 2004), which leads to the *theory* about the child's cognitive strengths and weaknesses. The clinician then examines the theory by choosing additional measures (*hypothesis*) to confirm or refute the intellectual test data (*data collection/analysis*), examining results in light of the record review/history, systematic observations, behavior ratings, and parent–teacher interviews to gain a thorough understanding of the child (*data interpretation*).

Although this initial evaluation provides a good picture of the child's strengths and needs, this is where CHT *begins*, not ends. This information is then used in collaborative problem-solving meetings (i.e., behavioral consultation) with teachers and/or parents to develop a *theory* about an intervention that might address the child's needs, which is the next *hypothesis*. The intervention is undertaken with a single-subject design and ongoing progress monitoring in the *data collection/analysis* step, and is systematically evaluated during the *data interpretation* stage to determine intervention efficacy. If the intervention is effective, then it is terminated, but practitioners can revise or recycle the intervention until beneficial results are achieved. In this way, the CHT model is self-correcting, providing a method to link assessment and other data to effective interventions for individual children.

Case Presentation: Thomas

This case highlights how multiple strategies, including comprehensive cognitive and neuropsychological assessment, may be necessary as part of a larger problem-solving model for children with attention problems. As noted throughout the chapter, children with attention problems typically present with many other difficulties, including academic, behavioral, and social–emotional concerns, and these problems may be caused by multiple factors, both individually and environmentally determined. Although comprehensive evaluation may not be the first step in addressing attention concerns, it may be necessary when initial attempts at ameliorating the problems are unsuccessful. The case of "Thomas" begins with relevant background information that describes the problem. After initial attempts at addressing his attention, learning, and social–emotional needs were equivocal at best, the clinician used CHT. These results confirmed that Thomas had attention problems, but due to a cause (spatial inattention) other than the one initially posited (ADHD).

As a result, Thomas received individualized interventions designed to meet his needs, both academic and behavioral. The clinician's results using ongoing progress monitoring to evaluate the efficacy of these interventions suggest that Thomas has been making progress toward overcoming his inattention, progress that had been limited by traditional strategies for children with ADHD.

Background

At the time of referral, Thomas was a 10 year, 10-month-old boy, who was first seen by a pediatrician when he was 9 years old. The pediatrician used a typical evaluation for children with attention problems, including physical examination, standardized parent and teacher rating scales, and DSM-IV-TR criteria, and arrived at ADHD and developmental coordination disorder (DCD) diagnoses and a treatment plan during Thomas's first visit. The diagnoses were largely based on a parent report that Thomas had difficulty with following directions, paying attention for long periods, and completing his work in a timely fashion (if at all). He was not impulsive or hyperactive, which could be a sign that his attention problems were different than those found in children with "true" ADHD (Hale et al., 2005). Consistent with his DCD diagnosis, Thomas had very poor handwriting, and difficulty with fine-motor coordination, which may in part explain his reluctance and difficulty with writing and math computation. However, his mother noted that his written language also did not appear to make sense at times, and Thomas also had considerable difficulty with math word problems. Fortunately, he had above average reading skills. He read clearly, without hesitation, and his answers to comprehension questions, especially factual information and detail-oriented questions, were typically "right on target." His parents and teacher both noted that Thomas was a "nice kid," describing him as "cooperative" and "not a behavior problem." However, Thomas struggled with social relationships, because he was often anxious, quiet, and withdrawn. Both his parents and teacher reported that Thomas was frequently inattentive, but he vacillated between being actively engaged and "in his own world" at times.

Following ADHD and DCD diagnoses, the pediatrician provided Thomas with a trial of stimulant medication and an order for the school to provide occupational therapy (OT). The school team developed an Americans with Disabilities Act (ADA)/Section 504 plan that included math fact drill and repetition, and OT for the "fine-motor problems." The teacher thought Thomas's attention improved during the first few days of the intervention, but as seen in Figure 4.2, the 10 mg dose of Ritalin (methylphenidate [MPH]) was not effective according to teacher's Conners ratings, and neither was the higher dose of 20 mg. The use of a systematic math intervention with flashcards to develop math fact automaticity improved Thomas's acquisition of math facts, but he continued to have problems with math computation, math word problems, and written language. Because his response to these interventions was limited, Thomas was referred for a CHT evaluation in preparation for more targeted interventions designed to meet his needs.

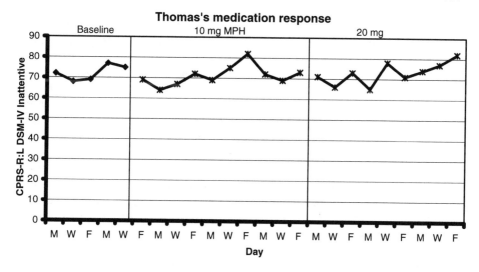

FIGURE 4.2. Thomas's response to medication treatment.

Assessment

A teacher interview, classroom observation, and examination of permanent products revealed that Thomas had good reading decoding skills, a good fund of information, and compliance with instruction, but he had some difficulty with transitions and was frequently off-task and stared blankly on occasion. Although Thomas's developmental history suggested delayed initial language acquisition and fine- and gross-motor difficulties, his language had improved dramatically when he was 2, and he could be quite verbose when discussing trains or animals. He knew facts and details that astonished his parents and teachers, and at one point was considered for placement in a gifted program. However, when Thomas approached other children, he was mostly ignored, and peers some times made fun of him. The teacher reported that he had no real friends in the classroom. Thomas was compliant with direct teacher requests, but he had difficulty following multistep directions and was frequently distracted or disorganized, especially in unstructured or ambiguous situations. Thomas's work pace was slow and methodical, and if he completed tasks, then he was often the last one in the class to finish.

During the evaluation, Thomas was quiet, reserved, and fidgety. His responses were often limited in content, but he became surprisingly talkative when he talked about his favorite mammals, and he even tried to humor the examiner with several "knock-knock" jokes. Despite his apparent linguistic skills, Thomas's responses were at time tangential and often unrelated to the questions posed of him. Throughout the evaluation, Thomas had minimal eye contact, flat affect, and a stilted prosody, with his voice sounding strangely mechanical. Thomas reported having many friends ("Everybody likes me, I have so many friends") and no difficulty with academic subjects ("I'm the best at everything"), but he did note his dislike of gym and recess, saying it was "stupid" and "boring." He also said he hated tests and that they made him feel "sick."

Thomas's teacher and parent behavior ratings (CBCL, CPRS-R:L [Long Form], TRF, CTRS-R:L) suggested difficulty with internalizing symptoms such as anxiety, withdrawal, dysphoria, and poor self-esteem, and significant attention problems. Although his parents and teachers rated Thomas as fidgety and overactive at times, they did not endorse other hyperactivity items or rate him as impulsive. Upon further questioning and observation, Thomas's overactivity seemed to be related to performance or social anxiety. He also had significant social problems (i.e., peer rejection, preferred younger friends, poor social discourse) and some thought problems (i.e., repetitive speech, peculiar interests, preservative behaviors), but few externalizing oppositional or conduct problem behaviors.

The CHT model was then used to examine Thomas's cognitive and neuropsychological functioning. As can be seen in Table 4.1, Thomas's performance on the WISC-IV was in the average range, and although there were no significant factor score differences, there were many subtest differences within factors, which suggests the Full Scale IQ and factor scores may not be an accurate representation of his overall functioning (e.g., Fiorello, Hale, McGrath, Ryan, & Quinn, 2001). On the Verbal Comprehension index, Thomas had good categorical or convergent thought on Similarities subtest (also supported by Picture Concepts results), and although his language was somewhat tangential and pedantic on the Vocabulary subtest, he showed a good knowledge base on Vocabulary and Information subtests, suggesting adequate verbal concept formation and crystallized abilities. However, his social knowledge, judgment, and commonsense problem-solving skills were relatively impaired on the Comprehension subtest, one of the strongest Wechsler predictors of

TABLE 4.1. WISC-IV Intellectual Assessment Results for Thomas

Measure/subtest	SS/ss	Measure/subtest	SS/ss
	Global scores		
Verbal Comprehension	96	Perceptual Reasoning	92
Working Memory	102	Processing Speed	94
	Subtest scores		
Similarities	10	Block Design	8
Vocabulary	12	Picture Concepts	13
Comprehension	6	Matrix Reasoning	5
(Information	11)	(Picture Completion	4)
Digit Span	11	Coding	7
Letter–Number Sequencing	10	Symbol Search	11

Note. Global scores are reported in SS; subtest scores are reported in ss: SS, Standard Score, $M = 100$, $SD = 15$; ss, scaled score, $M = 10$, $SD = 3$. From Hale, Nagleri, Kaufman, and Kavale (2006). Copyright (2006) by John Wiley & Sons. Reprinted by permission.

psychopathology (Hale, Rosenberg, Hoeppner, & Gaither, 1997). His Working Memory index was strong, and he showed little difference between Digits Forward (scaled score [ss] = 11) and Digits Backward (ss = 9), which would be inconsistent with executive dysfunction and ADHD (Hale, Hoeppner, & Fiorello, 2001). Although his Block Design score was in the average range, Thomas's two configuration errors and his complaint that he did not have enough blocks to complete the task were associated with right-hemisphere spatial problems (Hale & Fiorello, 2004). Together with his Picture Completion and Matrices performance, these results suggest difficulty with global–spatial–holistic or simultaneous processing, nonverbal problem solving, and fluid reasoning, but it should also be noted that attention deficits are more likely to impact these Perceptual Reasoning than Verbal Comprehension subtest measures (e.g., Denckla, 1996), so these findings may be related to ADHD. Thomas's Processing Speed varied, with adequate Symbol Search but was quite low Coding, possibly because of the increased graphomotor requirements on this task.

In CHT, the intellectual measure is used as a screening tool, then additional measures are used to examine clinical hypotheses, because subtest or profile analysis is of questionable value without corroborating evidence (Hale & Fiorello, 2004). Based on his diagnosis and other data (but not necessarily his WISC-IV findings), it was important to evaluate further Thomas's attention, working memory, and executive function as one possible cause for his difficulties. It was also important to examine his visual–spatial–holistic and novel problem-solving skills to see whether he had what is often considered an NLD. Although Thomas's language skills appeared adequate, one of the characteristics of NLD is difficulty with implicit, ambiguous, or contextual language (Bryan & Hale, 2001), which may account for part of Thomas's difficulty on the Comprehension subtest, so this, too, needed to be evaluated.

The results presented in Table 4.2 suggest that Thomas's "fine-motor" problem is really secondary to visual–spatial–simultaneous processing deficits. The area of the brain responsible for these skills is also associated with poor self-awareness and inattention to the environment, sometimes referred to as "neglect" (Hale & Fiorello, 2004). Although attention problems are typical with this condition, Thomas is not as likely to benefit from medication treatment as those children with "true" ADHD that affects attention and executive function (Hale et al., 2005). His novel problem-solving or fluid-reasoning skills were inconsistent, likely because the WJ-III Analysis and Synthesis subtest can be solved using a trial-and-error approach. Thomas had considerable difficulty with the Comprehensive Assessment of Spoken Language (CASL) Supralinguistic subtests, and his Memory for Faces was impaired, suggesting that a more proper diagnosis may be a "nonverbal" learning disorder or Asperger syndrome (Klin et al., 1995). Instead of focusing the intervention on what initially appeared to be executive and motor problems, results had provided a better understanding of Thomas's true difficulties, leading to more targeted interventions as a result.

TABLE 4.2. Cognitive Hypothesis-Testing Results for Thomas

Measure/subtest	SS	Measure/subtest	SS
Woodcock Johnson–III		Developmental Test of VMI	
Concept formation	80	Visual	76
Analysis and synthesis	92	Motor	100
		Visual–motor integration	86
Cognitive Assessment System			
Figure memory	75	NEPSY	
Planned connections	90	Arrows	75
Expressive attention	100	Memory for faces	80
		Visual–Motor precision	95
Continuous Performance Test–II		Finger tapping	95
Omissions	98	Tower	100
Commissions	111		
Reaction time	94	Test of Memory and Learning (ss)	
Detectability	87	Memory for location	70
Perseverations	91		
Reaction time block change	104	Hale Cancellation Task	
Reaction time ISI change	102	Correct	92
Comprehensive Assessment of Spoken Language (SS)			
Nonliteral language	70		
Inference	80		
Pragmatic judgment	75		

Note. VMI, Visual–Motor Integration. All scores are reported as standard scores (SS), with higher scores equal to better performance. The Conners Continuous Performance Test (CPT-II) was changed from T to z to SS, with reversed scoring, so higher scores again equal better performance. From Hale, Naglieri, Kaufman, and Kavale (2006). Copyright 2006 by John Wiley & Sons. Reprinted by permission.

Treatment

Behavioral consultation, a collaborative problem-solving approach, was implemented with Thomas's parents and teacher (Bergen & Kratochwill, 1990). Behavioral consultation includes four stages—problem identification, problem analysis, plan implementation, and plan evaluation—and has had a rich history of outcome effectiveness (Reddy, Barboza-Whitehead, Files, & Rubel, 2000). In the case of Thomas, six sessions were implemented.

SESSION 1

During Session 1, problem identification and problem analysis were conducted. The consultant reviewed Thomas's CHT and behavior data with his parents and teacher. Based on the data, four treatment goals were collaboratively identified: (1) increase Thomas's self-awareness and attention to the environment (using apparently intact executive skills), (2) improve spatial processing for feedback to the apparently intact motor system, (3) foster attention through self-monitoring of on-task performance, and (4) better comprehend language prosody and vocal–facial affect (i.e., improve relationships and social skills). It was agreed that the consultant, parent, and teacher would meet to design interventions for each goal.

SESSIONS 2 AND 3

During Sessions 2 and 3, problem analysis and plan implementation were conducted. Targeted interventions were designed specifically to improve Thomas's four behavioral goals. A brief description of each intervention implemented is presented.

Because Thomas's executive skills seemed to be intact, self-monitoring and charting were designed and implemented to improve his attention and increase his self-awareness using a 1- (*Unfocused/off-task*) to 3-point (*Highly focused/on-task*) Likert scale that he completed after the teacher randomly tapped his desk five times per class period (total possible = 15 points). For the spatial–holistic processing problems, Thomas's teacher recommended use of graph paper to improve letter shape, formation, and spacing. After Thomas completed his writing sample, he was encouraged by his teacher to compare his letter writing and word spacing for 10 words to a "best writing" template he created with teacher instruction. He received 1 point for each word with the letters written correctly and 1 point for each correct word spacing (total possible = 19).

Finally, to improve his relationships and social skills, Thomas was taught to discriminate among facial expressions and tape recordings of vocal affect. Outside the classroom, Thomas had to rate 10 pictures and audiotaped voices on a 3-point Likert scale (–1, *Negative affect*; 0, *Neutral affect*; 1, *Positive affect*), and indicate whether they were the same or different. Thomas received 1 point for judging valence (2 points total per trial) and 1 point for judging the congruence of facial and vocal affect (3 points possible per trial). Thomas was rewarded with computer game time (i.e., 1 minute per point) during free time at school. Given that this intervention occurred only one time per week for 30 minutes per session for 8 weeks, a pre- to postevaluation approach was used, with the SSRS (Gresham & Elliott, 1990) scores used to evaluate intervention effectiveness.

SESSIONS 4 AND 5

During Sessions 4 and 5 (plan evaluation), the consultant, parents, and teacher evaluated each intervention. Thomas's parents and teacher reviewed the data and concluded that the self-charting program improved his on-task performance in Language Arts class (see Figure 4.3). However, his parents and teacher noted that his progress was not quite as good in math class. His

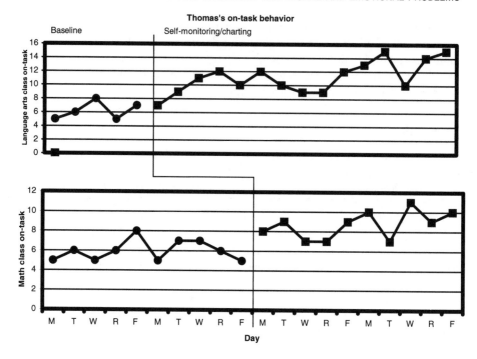

FIGURE 4.3. Thomas's response to self-monitoring intervention.

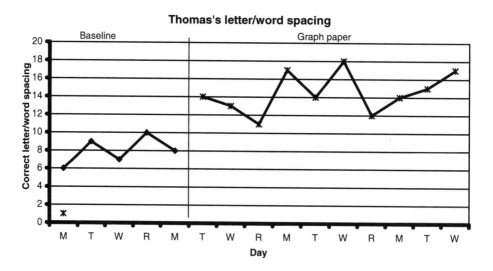

FIGURE 4.4. Thomas's response to handwriting intervention.

teacher speculated that Thomas still found this academic area difficult. Results suggested that the math intervention described earlier was not sufficient to remediate Thomas's difficulty in this area.

For his second treatment goal, Thomas's letter and word spacing improved. His parents and teacher noted that he reached the goal of 90% correct on several occasions (see Figure 4.4).

After social skills instruction, Thomas's Total Social Skills went from the lower end (SS = 73; 2nd percentile) to the upper end (standard score [SS] = 82; 12th percentile) of the below average range according to teacher report. His parents and teacher concluded that Thomas's social skills were improving and that the intervention should continue.

SESSION 6

Approximately 1 month after plan evaluation (i.e., booster session), Thomas's consultant, parents, and teacher met to review his progress.

TEACHER: I am very pleased with Thomas's progress.

MOTHER: I am happy too, but would like to improve his math skills. Do you have any suggestions on what I can do to help him here?

TEACHER: Yes, I have a math workbook you can use with him. I would suggest doing these exercises at home, three times a week, for about 20 to 30 minutes and provide him a reward immediately following the assignment. This will reinforce the skills he has learned this year. Kids tend to lose some academic skills over the summer, so doing this will help keep him on track for the fall.

CONSULTANT: I would also suggest that you continue to use graph paper for writing and encourage him to evaluate his writing of letters and space between words.

MOTHER: Thank you for all of your help.

CONSULTANT: It was a pleasure to work with you two.

Because of the collaborative nature of behavioral consultation, Thomas's parents and teacher were encouraged to contribute equally to the identification of treatment goals, design, implementation, and evaluation of interventions used. Thus, high parent and teacher treatment acceptability and treatment adherence led to favorable initial outcomes (Springer & Reddy, 2004). Likewise, treatment resistance was low for all involved. A booster session was conducted with Thomas's parents and teacher to monitor and sustain outcomes and to troubleshoot any potential obstacles that might hinder treatment implementation in the future. Outcome data were evaluated continuously for each intervention throughout plan implementation.

Case Presentation: Lisa

Background

"Lisa," a 6 year, 10-month-old girl, was struggling in all her academic sub-jects in first grade and was at risk for retention when she was referred for eval-uation. Although her pediatrician was concerned about her attention and achievement problems, Lisa had never obtained a formal evaluation by the physician or the school. She was described as a friendly, outgoing child who loved adult attention. Although Lisa was eager to please, this did not always translate into appropriate behavior in the classroom, because her name was frequently written on the board for rule violations. Lisa's mother had received many calls home about Lisa's inappropriate behavior, and despite frequent parental discussions and removal of privileges, nothing seemed to work. The mother had read some information on "ADHD" but did not want her child on medication, because she had heard "lots of bad things" about stimulants. Lisa reported having good peer relationships, but both the parent and teacher reported limited social skills and frequent conflicts with peers. When asked about these conflicts, Lisa said, "I don't know. I'm nice to them; sometimes they just mess with me, and we fight."

Assessment

A teacher interview, classroom observation, and examination of permanent products revealed that Lisa had attentional difficulties during whole-group in-struction and when completing her work. According to the teacher, Lisa strug-gled in most academic areas but seemed quite "capable" at times. When the teacher worked individually with Lisa, she did "quite well," but these advances were short-lived when whole-class instruction occurred. Writing was particularly difficult for Lisa. Seldom writing more than a few sentences, Lisa would often make comments such as "I don't know what to say." In addition, her grammar was poor, her word choice was inaccurate at times, and her handwriting was often illegible. When asked specifically about problem behaviors, the teacher reported that Lisa was often inattentive, easily dis-tracted, frequently fidgety, and typically off-task unless redirected. Lisa talked frequently with teachers and peers, blurted out answers without raising her hand, and often began assignments before directions were given. She fre-quently asked for repeated directions or teacher comments, which caused the teacher to be concerned about her hearing or auditory processing. However, her grasp of sound–symbol relationships seemed to be quite good. Her school desk and room at home were frequently in disarray. Lisa was highly resistant to organizing and/or cleaning them when instructed to do so. Not surpris-ingly, homework was a real challenge. Lisa not only had difficulty completing the typical homework assignments but also she often had to finish in-class assignments at home, because she did not complete them during allotted seatwork time. Lisa had frequent confrontations with her parents during homework sessions and often took several hours to complete the assignments. In addition, she often "forgot" to write down the assignments correctly, or if she did write down and complete them, she "forgot" to turn them in. Prior to the comprehensive evaluation, Lisa's desk had been moved to the front of the room next to the teacher, but this seemed to help very little. In an attempt to foster homework completion, the teacher regularly sent home notes to Lisa's parents regarding homework completion. Despite this effort, Lisa's behavior pattern with homework continued, with some progress noted.

During the evaluation, Lisa was friendly and talkative. Having a full range of affect, Lisa's eye contact was good, her prosody was typical, and her facial expressions were often animated. She was often fidgety, impulsive, and stood up or left her seat without permission. Although she seemed motivated to perform tasks, her interest was often limited, as was her frustration tolerance, and Lisa required regular encouragement to complete more difficult items. With frequent breaks, she was able to comply with task demands. Although Lisa was talkative, her verbal responses were often disorganized, and she had word-finding difficulties. Her graphomotor skills were poor.

Lisa's teacher and parent behavior ratings suggested difficulty with attention, impulse control, and hyperactivity, but few internalizing problems. She also had significant social problems and rule-breaking, and aggressive behavior, but few internalizing anxious, depressive, or withdrawal behaviors. Although Lisa had some somatic complaints, the teacher and parent thought this was in response to her academic difficulties, because Lisa often complained about these things in the morning before school, and attempted to stay home because she was "sick."

The CHT model (Hale & Fiorello, 2004) was then used to examine Lisa's cognitive and neuropsychological functioning. As seen in Table 4.3, Lisa's WISC-IV performance was mostly in the average range, but her Processing Speed score was low average, and there were several subtest differences within factors, suggesting that the Full Scale IQ and factor scores might not be an accurate representation of her overall functioning (e.g., Fiorello et al., 2001). On the Verbal Comprehension scale, Lisa's receptive and expressive language appeared to be adequate, but her sentences were poorly formed, and her word choice was inaccurate at times. Although her Information score was in the low average range, it should be noted that her errors were interspersed throughout the subtest, which was also the case on the Matrix Reasoning subtest. Although her Working Memory score was adequate, largely because of her good performance on Digits Forward (ss = 13), she struggled with the Digits Backward (ss = 8), Letter–Number Sequencing, and Arithmetic subtests, which is consistent with a deficit in working memory and/or other executive functions (Hale, Hoeppner, & Fiorello, 2001). Lisa also struggled with speed and graphomotor skills on the Coding subtest, and her Symbol Search performance was notable for quick, inaccurate responding.

The results of the WISC-IV cognitive screening suggested further evaluation of Lisa's attention, working memory, and executive function as one possi-

TABLE 4.3. WISC-IV Intellectual Assessment Results for Lisa

Measure/subtest	SS/ss	Measure/subtest	SS/ss
	Global scores		
Verbal Comprehension	98	Perceptual Reasoning	96
Working Memory	91	Processing Speed	83
	Subtest scores		
Similarities	9	Block Design	9
Vocabulary	9	Picture Concepts	11
Comprehension	11	Matrix Reasoning	8
Information	7	Picture Completion	9
Digit Span	11	Coding	6
Letter–Number Sequencing	6	Symbol Search	8
Arithmetic	5		

Note. Global scores are reported in SS; subtest scores are reported in ss. SS, standard score, $M = 100$, $SD = 15$; ss, scaled score, $M = 10$, $SD = 3$. From Hale, Naglieri, Kaufman, and Kavale (2006). Copyright 2006 by John Wiley & Sons. Reprinted by permission.

ble cause for her difficulties. It was also important to examine her visual–spatial–motor coordination skills to determine whether the graphomotor deficits reported and observed during testing were the result of visual–spatial, motor, or visual–motor integration deficits. Although Lisa's language skills appeared to be adequate, she seemed to have some difficulty with language formulation and word retrieval. This might suggest an expressive language deficit, the history, observations, but the data suggested that these difficulties could be secondary to attention and executive problems, not a typical expressive language deficit. Although these causes of expressive language problems are highly related, it is important in CHT to try to limit the number of additional measures, if at all possible, because too much testing can lead to significant "problems" based on chance alone (Hale & Fiorello, 2004). As a result, the clinician decided that only expressive language tests sensitive to word retrieval issues would be used during CHT, and that additional language evaluation could be undertaken if those results suggested further language testing was warranted.

The results presented in Table 4.4 suggest that Lisa shows many of the signs of attention and executive problems characteristic of children with ADHD (Hale et al., 2005). Although there were some inconsistencies, her performance suggested difficulty with sustained attention, planning, organization, self-monitoring, mental flexibility, set shifting, and working memory. Consistent with the hemispheric encoding–retrieval asymmetry model (Tulving & Markowitsch, 1997) and how this relates to brain structures that regulate attention and executive function (Lichter & Cummings, 2001), Lisa seems to have considerable difficulty with verbal and design fluency. She struggles with word retrieval in free recall or unstructured situations, and

TABLE 4.4. Cognitive Hypothesis-Testing Results for Lisa

Measure/subtest	SS/ss	Measure/subtest	SS/ss
Wisconsin Card Sort Test		Developmental Test of VMI	
Total errors	86	Visual	93
Perseverative responses	87	Motor	84
Perseverative errors	84	Visual–motor integration	83
Nonperseverative errors	91		
Categories completed[a]	3(> 16th%ile)	NEPSY Sensorimotor	
Failure to maintain set[a]	4(2nd-5th%ile)	Finger tapping	95
Trials to first category[a]	23(> 16th%ile)	Visuomotor precision	80
WJ-III Tests of Cognitive Abilities		Boston Naming Test	
Numbers reversed	85	Free recall + semantic cue	81
Auditory working memory	91	Recall with phonemic cue	101
NEPSY Attention/Executive		Controlled Oral Word Association Test	
Tower	85	Letters	84
Auditory Attention and Response Set	80	Animals	105
Visual attention	90	WISC-PI	
Design fluency	80	Information multiple choice	95
		Written arithmetic	100

Note. VMI, Visual–Motor Integration; WISC-PI, Wechsler Intelligence Scale for Childen—Process Instrument; WJ-III, Woodcock–Johnson–III.
[a] Raw scores reported. All other scores are reported as standard scores (SS), with higher scores equal to better performance. From Hale, Naglieri, Kaufman, and Kavale (2006). Copyright 2006 by John Wiley & Sons. Reprinted by permission.

when memory is structured for her, she does well. This suggests that her memories are adequate; it is the executive search for memory (i.e., working memory) that is impaired, which is typical in children with ADHD (Hale & Fiorello, 2004). Unlike Thomas, Lisa's graphomotor problems seem to be related specifically to motor skills, or visual–motor integration rather than visual–spatial processing problems. Taken together, these findings are consistent with ADHD combined type, in which "brain manager" executive deficits in planning, organizing, strategizing, inhibiting, monitoring, evaluating, and changing behavior interfere with both academic and behavioral competence (Hale & Fiorello, 2004). This type of attention problem is really an *intention* problem (Denckla, 1996) or one of attention *control*, the hallmark of "true" ADHD (Hale et al., 2005).

Treatment

In a behavioral consultation with Lisa's parents and teacher, the consultant designed and evaluated targeted interventions for Lisa at school. A total of eight sessions were implemented.

SESSION 1

During Session 1, problem identification was conducted with Lisa's consultant, mother, and teacher. The CHT and behavioral data were reviewed. Lisa's deficits were explained in terms of her "brain manager" being "partly asleep." The consultant explained that ADHD was due to *underactive* "brain manager" areas, and that stimulant medication "wakes the brain manager so that it can control the rest of the brain." Lisa's mother agreed that maybe it was time to reconsider her thinking on a trial of stimulant medication. The consultant, Lisa's mother, and the teacher also agreed that targeted behavioral interventions were also needed to meet Lisa's needs. However, the implementation of behavioral interventions would be done after the medication trial.

SESSION 2

During Session 2, problem analysis was conducted. On her own, Lisa's mother read some literature on the use and effectiveness of stimulant treatment and consulted with her pediatrician. The consultant, Lisa's mother, and her teacher discussed the pros and cons of medication and possible side effects.

The consultant offered Lisa's mother an option of participating in a double-blind placebo controlled trial of MPH to see whether the medication would help Lisa's "brain boss" overcome her attention, impulse control, and overactivity problems. It was agreed that Lisa's pediatrician would prescribe the medication and assist the consultant and Lisa's mother in monitoring the use of medication and evaluating its effectiveness.

SESSION 3

During Session 3, plan implementation was conducted. It was agreed that four conditions would be implemented: the 4 weeks of baseline assessment, 3 blinded weeks of placebo, 1 week of low-dose MPH (i.e., 5 mg), and 1 week of high-dose MPH (i.e., 10 mg). During each condition, neuropsychological testing of Attention, Working Memory, and Executive Function were completed (see Table 4.4). These data were summarized and rank-ordered across conditions to assess Lisa's cognitive response to the medication (see Table 4.5). Behavioral response was determined by the consultant, using weekly parent and teacher ratings, and systematic classroom observations of five behaviors, using momentary time sampling for 5 school days (see Table 4.6). These data were rank-ordered across conditions for evaluating behavioral response. The mean cognitive and behavioral ranks (lower ranks indicate better performance and behavior) were then graphically displayed to aid in determining clinical response (see Figure 4.5). In addition, both the cognitive and behavioral ranks were subjected to nonparametric randomization tests for ranks using

TABLE 4.5. Medication Trial Results for Lisa

Cognitive variables[a1]	Baseline	Placebo	5 mg MPH	10 mg MPH
			Blinded conditions	
Go–No Go correct	17(4)	21(3)	27(1)	26(2)
SRTM word storage	41(3.5)	41(3.5)	53(1)	48(2)
SRTM consistent retrieval	24(3)	21(4)	43(1)	36(2)
Stroop Color–Word correct	14(4)	17(1)	15(3)	16(2)
Stroop Color–Word errors	4(3)	4(3)	2(1)	4(3)
TOMAL Digits Backward	10(4)	12(3)	20(1)	14(2)
Hale Cancellation correct	13(4)	18(3)	26(1.5)	26(1.5)
Hale Cancellation time	172(2)	199(4)	163(1)	191(3)
Trail Making Test B errors	6(4)	3(3)	1(1)	2(2)
Trail Making Test B time	534(4)	56(2)	44(1)	60(3)
CPT-II omissions	65(4)	62(3)	55(1)	60(2)
CPT-II commissions	60(3)	64(4)	43(2)	34(1)
CPT-II reaction time[b2]	41(3)	47(1)	54(2)	63(4)
CPT-II block change	57(3)	61(4)	44(2)	41(1)
CPT-II interstimulus intervals change	57(3)	69(4)	51(2)	42(1)
Mean cognitive rank	3.43	3.03	1.43	2.10

Note. Lower ranks indicate better performance and behavior. SRTM, Selective Reminding Test of Memory; TOMAL, Test of Memory and Learning; CPT-II, Conners Continuous Performance Test—Second Edition.

[a] All cognitive scores are raw scores except CPT-II T-scores.

[b] Low scores indicate impulsivity, and high scores suggest slow response time, so ranks are determined by deviation from the standardization mean (50).

the NPStat computer program to determine statistical medication response. This objective protocol not only helps to determine whether the child benefits from medication treatment but also explores both cognitive and behavioral medication responses, which are not always consistent (e.g., Hale et al., 1997, 1998, 2005, 2006).

SESSION 4

During Session 4 (problem evaluation), the effectiveness of the medication trial was examined by the consultant, Lisa's mother, and the pediatrician, based on its impact on Lisa's cognitive and behavioral responsiveness. The results of the double-blind, placebo controlled medication trial of 5 mg and 10 mg of MPH are displayed in Table 4.5, and the mean ranks are graphically displayed in Figure 4.3. The results of the neuropsychological measures revealed that Lisa did respond cognitively to the medication (Friedman Fr = 22.08, p < .001), with both the 5 mg (Wilcoxon signed-rank T = 9.50, p = .002) and 10 mg (Wilcoxon signed-rank T = 20.50, p = .048) conditions different from the placebo condition, but not each other (Wilcoxon signed-

TABLE 4.6. Medication Trial and Behavioral Intervention Results for Lisa

Behavioral variables[a]	Baseline	Placebo	Blinded conditions		
			5 mg MPH	10 mg MPH	Behavior therapy
Parent ratings					
CPRS-R:L oppositional	60(3.5)	52(1)	56(2)	60(3.5)	56
CPRS-R:L cognitive problems	89(4)	81(2)	72(1)	87(3)	74
CPRS-R:L hyperactivity index	87(4)	84(3)	80(2)	70(1)	64
CPRS-R:L DSM-IV inattentive	90(4)	80(2)	74(1)	84(3)	73
CPRS-R:L DSM-IV hyperactivity–impulsivity	83(2)	90(4)	89(3)	75(1)	67
HSQ-R mean score	7.4(3.5)	7.5(3.5)	7.4(2)	6.9(1)	—
Side Effects Rating Scale	0	3	0	21	—
Teacher ratings					
CTRS-R:L oppositional	65(3.5)	58(1)	63(2)	65(3.5)	62
CTRS-R:L cognitive problems	89(3.5)	81(2)	76(1)	89(3.5)	75
CTRS-R:L hyperactivity index	77(4)	74(3)	71(2)	70(1)	64
CTRS-R:L DSM-IV inattentive	82(4)	72(2)	66(1)	74(3)	64
CTRS-R:L DSM-IV hyperactivity–impulsivity	73(2)	80(4)	79(3)	65(1)	63
SSQ-R mean score	6.5(4)	6.0(2)	6.3(3)	4.6(1)	—
APRS learning ability	18(2.5)	18(2.5)	16(4)	22(1)	—
APRS impulse control	15(3)	15(3)	15(3)	18(1)	—
APRS academic performance	22(2)	21(3)	18(4)	28(1)	—
APRS social problems	10(4)	12(3)	13(2)	17(1)	—
Side Effects Rating Scale	7	11	12	18	—
Classroom observations					
RAT off-task	28(2)	35(4)	10(1)	33(3)	—
RAT fidgeting	33(3)	38(4)	28(2)	15(1)	—
RAT plays with objects	20(3)	25(4)	5(1)	10(2)	—
RAT vocalizes	13(3.5)	10(2)	13(3.5)	3(1)	—
RAT out of seat	3(2)	5(3)	10(4)	0(1)	—
Mean behavior rank	3.19	2.76	2.26	1.79	

Note. Lower ranks indicate performance and behavior. CPRS-R:L = Conners Parent Rating Scale—Revised: Long Form; HSQ-R, Home Situations Questionnaire—Revised; CTRS-R:L, Conners Teacher Rating Scale—Revised: Long Form; SSQ-R, School Situations Questionnaire—Revised; APRS, Academic Performance Rating Scale; RAT, Restricted Academic Task.
[a] All behavior rating scores are raw scores except CPRS-R:L and CTRS-R:L T-scores.

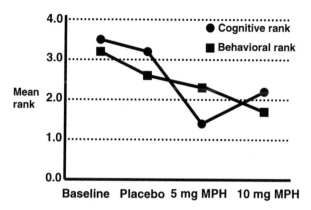

FIGURE 4.5. Lisa's mean cognitive and behavioral ranks for medication conditions.

rank $T = 22.00$, $p = .052$). The lowest rank (best performance) was obtained during the 5 mg condition, in which working memory and executive control seemed best. However, several measures were comparable across active drug conditions, and impulse control seemed to be qualitatively better during the high-dose condition. For the behavioral ranks, a similar pattern was obtained (Friedman $Fr = 14.01$, $p = .001$), but this time the lowest rank was obtained for the high-dose condition, which was different than the placebo condition (Wilcoxon signed-rank $T = 52.00$, $p = .026$), but the low-dose condition was not different from placebo (Wilcoxon signed-rank $T = 69.50$, $p = .181$). This common response pattern (e.g., Hale et al. 1997, 1998, 2005, 2006), with the lower dose best for cognition and the higher dose best for behavior, makes medication titration difficult. Does one choose the best dose for cognition or the best dose for behavior? As a result of these findings, the consultant, pediatrician, and mother decided to try Lisa on the 5 mg MPH dose in an attempt to maximize executive functions, with behavior interventions designed to target Lisa's impulsive responding and work compliance.

SESSION 5

Behavioral consultation was used to design, implement, and evaluate Lisa's behavioral interventions at school. Lisa continued to take 5 mg of MPH. Lisa's mother, teacher, and consultant participated in the problem-solving process. During Session 5, problem identification was conducted and two school-based behavioral goals were identified for Lisa: *follow directions* and *complete assigned work*. Given Lisa's disability, it was agreed that Lisa's goal, follow directions, would include "with two reminders" as an accommodation to assist her with goal-directed behavior.

SESSIONS 6 AND 7

During Sessions 6 and 7, problem analysis and plan implementation were conducted. After much discussion, it was decided that a positive behavior system at home and school would enhance Lisa's impulsive responding, because she seeks out and responds well to adult attention and praise. A daily good behavior chart was created that outlined Lisa's school day in approximately 40-minute time periods (see Figure 4.6). It was agreed that Lisa would be given positive verbal feedback and written feedback (i.e., showing that she earned a point) for working toward her two behavioral goals at the end of each time period. Lisa's teacher agreed to provide verbal and written feedback throughout Lisa's day. The consultant suggested that feedback be given briefly (i.e., 3–5 seconds) and focus on what Lisa earned rather than what she did not earn. Examples of structured verbal statements included "Lisa (*pause*), good job following directions" and "Lisa (*pause*), good job completing your work." When Lisa did not earn a point, an example of a structured verbal statement might include "Lisa (*pause*), you did not earn a point this time, but I know

Date: _____

Lisa's Good Behavior Chart

Class	Follow Directions (w/ 2 reminders)	Complete Assigned Work
8:20–8:30 A.M.		
8:30–9:15 A.M.		
9:20–10:05 A.M.		
10:10–10:55 A.M.		
11:00–11:45 A.M. A.M. Reward (6 out of 10 points)		
11:45–12:35 P.M. Lunch/Recess		
12:40–1:25 P.M.		
12:30–2:15 P.M.		
2:20–3:05 P.M. P.M. Reward (4 out of 6 points)		

Home Reward Earned   **YES**

(Must earn 6 out of 10 points in the A.M. *and* 4 out of 6 points in the P.M. for home reward.)

FIGURE 4.6. Lisa's good behavior chart.

you can in the next time period." It was also discussed that the teacher would decide whether Lisa earned a point (i.e., place a check on the chart) or did not earn a point (i.e., left blank, no zeros would be used) before approaching Lisa to avoid her arguing and/or negotiating about points. It was agreed that Lisa would *not* be given verbal threats when she was not following her goals, such as "Lisa, if you do not get started on your work soon you will loss your point." Points are earned and not taken away.

It was also discussed that Lisa would benefit from nonverbal reminders (prompts). Thus, it was decided that her two behavioral goals (follow directions, complete assigned work) would be taped on her desk (one on the left corner and the other on the right corner of Lisa's desk). When needed, her teacher would point to Lisa's behavioral goal on her desk to prompt her nonverbally toward the goal.

Using the good behavior chart, the consultant created a home–school-based reward system. Lisa's progress at school would be reviewed by her mother and rewarded at home. Initially, it was agreed that Lisa would need to earn 6 out of 10 points (60% criteria) in the morning (prior to lunch and recess) *and* 4 out of 6 points (approximately 60% criteria) in the afternoon to earn a daily home reward. If Lisa earned her morning or afternoon point goals, her teacher would give her additional praise and a special sticker. A discussion of the choice of home rewards then followed.

MOTHER: I am not sure what to give her for a home reward. She already gets a lot.

CONSULTANT: Typically the most powerful reward for children is parent time. I would not use rewards that required special trips to Toy "R" Us or fast-food restaurants because of the expense and chance you may not be able to follow through on giving the reward on a daily basis. Let's think of things you can reasonably give her on a daily basis in the house.

TEACHER: How about a special treat or dessert? Does your family eat dessert often?

MOTHER: Yes, we have vanilla ice cream. Her favorite ice cream is chocolate chip mint.

TEACHER: That could work as one of the rewards.

CONSULTANT: How about 15 minutes of time with you or your husband?

MOTHER: We spend a lot of time together.

CONSULTANT: What I am thinking of is time that is child-centered with her, that is, her choice of the activity in the house for 15 minutes. Lisa identifies the activity and you go along with it.

MOTHER: OK, we could do that each day. Lisa also loves getting back rubs.

The following home rewards were identified: (1) 15 minutes of special time with her mother or father, (2) a 10-minute back rub, and (3) a special dessert (i.e., chocolate chip mint ice cream) or an extra snack. After 2–3 weeks of successful goal attainment, the criterion for home rewards would be slowly increased.

Despite cognitive improvements from the medication, the teacher indicated that Lisa has difficulties sustaining her attention on tasks and at times disrupted the class. Further discussion revealed that Lisa at times became overwhelmed, stressed, and got out of her seat during the day. Therefore, it was decided that Lisa would benefit from one or two brief structured breaks (i.e., 10 minutes) during the school day. It was agreed that she could take a 10-minute break (to use the class computer) between 10 and 11 A.M. and, if needed, between 2 and 3 P.M.. Lisa would not be permitted to take a break during an exam or in the middle of a class assignment.

Because Lisa sometimes forgot to write her homework assignments completely, a homework log was developed (see Figure 4.7). Lisa was required to write her homework assignments down for each class period or write "no homework" when homework was not assigned. For each class period, her teacher would review and initial Lisa's homework log. In addition, a "get ready checklist" was created to improve Lisa's planning and organization skills for the school morning routine and at the end of the day (Figure 4.8). Her teacher would encourage her to check off each step she completed in the

Date: _____

Class	Teacher's Initials	Write Down Assignments and Due Dates or "No Homework"
1.		
2.		
3.		
4.		
5.		
6.		
7.		
8.		

FIGURE 4.7. Lisa's homework log.

Get Ready in the A.M.	Check when Completed
1. Hang up my coat	
2. Unpack backpack	
3. Put lunch box in my cubby	
4. Put my homework in the basket	
5. Take out my pencils	
Get Ready at 3:13 P.M.	
1. Get backpack from my cubby	
2. Put my homework log in backpack	
3. Place folders in backpack	
4. Put on my coat	
5. Put lunchbox in my backpack	

FIGURE 4.8. Lisa's get ready checklist.

morning and afternoon. Home and school daily collaboration is vital for out-come effectiveness with this population (Reddy, Springer, Hall, Benisz, Braunstein, Hauch, et al., 2005). A copy of Lisa's daily good behavior chart was sent home each day, so her mother could review and reinforce Lisa's progress toward her goals. As mentioned, Lisa earned one home-based reward for meeting her morning *and* afternoon reward criteria.

SESSION 8

During Session 8 (problem evaluation), each behavioral intervention was eval-uated. The effectiveness of the behavioral intervention plan was assessed through a pre- to postassessment approach (problem evaluation). A 1 week baseline (i.e., pretest) of Lisa's following directions and completion of in-class work was accomplished by a momentary time sample approach. After the behavioral intervention plan was in place for 4 weeks, a postassessment was conducted. Results revealed 40% improvement in direction following and 35% improvement in completion of assigned work since baseline. At baseline, Lisa's percentage of direction following was 45% and completion of in-class assigned work was 60%. In addition, the Conners Parent and Teacher Rating Scales were readministered after 4 weeks of implementation. As shown on Table 4.6, results revealed that the behavior intervention plan resulted in improvements in impulsivity and hyperactivity at home and at school.

Consultation with Lisa's pediatrician, mother, and teacher on the effec-tiveness of the medication trial was informative and valuable in helping Lisa's cognitive processing and learning. The school-based behavioral interventions provided further additive benefits in improving Lisa's goal-directed behavior, and planning and organizational skills. Lisa's mother and her teacher developed a positive working partnership that was rewarding and resulted in high treatment acceptability and adherence.

CONCLUSIONS

This chapter highlights the multidimensional nature of inattention reported in school-age children and adolescents. As shown in the case studies, the manifestation of inattention may result from several neurocognitive disabilities and/or social–emotional conditions, and can easily be misinterpreted as ADHD. Comprehensive evaluations that embrace a CHT approach can serve as a valuable tool for identifying possible sources of inattention and aid in the design of empirically based behavioral interventions for a child's unique needs. Through behavioral consultation and ongoing progress monitoring, targeted interventions can meet the needs of all children with inattention.

REFERENCES

Abikoff, H. B., Jensen, P. S., Arnold, L. L. E., Hoza, B., Hechtman, L., Pollack, S., et al. (2002). Observed classroom behavior of children with ADHD: Relationship to gender and comorbidity. *Journal of Abnormal Child Psychology, 30*, 349–359.

Achenbach, T. M. (1991). *Manual of the Achenbach System of Empirically Based Assessment—Child Behavior Checklist, Teacher Report Form, and Youth Report.* Burlington: University of Vermont, Research Center for Children, Youth, and Families.

Achenbach, T. M., & Rescorla, L. A. (2001). *Manual of the Achenbach System of Empirically Based Assessment—Child Behavior Checklist, Teacher Report Form, and Youth Report.* Burlington: University of Vermont, Research Center for Children, Youth, and Families.

American Psychiatric Association (APA). (2000). *Diagnostic and statistical manual of mental disorders* (4th ed., text rev.). Washington, DC: Author.

American Speech–Language–Hearing Association Task Force on Central Auditory Processing Consensus Development. (1996). Central auditory processing: Current status of research and implications for clinical practice. *American Journal of Audiology, 5*, 41–54.

Angold, A., Costello, E. J., & Erkanli, A. (1999). Comorbidity. *Journal of Child Psychology and Psychiatry, and Allied Disciplines, 40*, 57–87.

August, G. J., & Garfinkel, B. D. (1990). Comorbidity of ADHD and reading disability among clinic-referred children. *Journal of Abnormal Child Psychology, 18*, 29–45.

August, G. J., & Holmes, C. S. (1984). Behavior and academic achievement in hyperactive subgroups and learning-disabled boys. A six-year follow-up. *American Journal of Diseases of Children, 138*, 1025–1029.

Ball, D., Tiernan, M., Janusz, J., & Furr, A. (1997). Sleep patterns among children with attention deficit hyperactivity disorder: A reexamination of parent perceptions. *Journal of Pediatric Psychology, 22*, 389–398.

Bain, S. K., & Pelletier, K. A. (1999). Social and behavior differences among a predominately African American preschool sample. *Psychology in the Schools, 36*(3), 249–259.

Barkley, R. A., Fischer, M., Edelbrock, C. S., & Smallish, L. (1990). The adolescent outcome of hyperactive children diagnosed by research criteria: I. An 8-year prospective follow-up study. *Journal of the American Academy of Child and Adolescent Psychiatry, 29,* 546–557.

Baron-Cohen, S. (1995). *Mindblindfulness: An essay on autism and theory of the mind.* Cambridge, MA: MIT Press.

Beidel, D. C. (1991). Social phobia and overanxious disorder in school-age children. *Journal of the American Academy of Child and Adolescent Psychiatry, 30,* 545–552.

Bellis, T. J. (1996). *Assessment and management of central auditory processing disorders in the educational setting.* San Diego: Singular Publishing Group.

Benedetto-Nasho, E., & Tannock, R. (1999). Math computation, error patterns and stimulant effects in children with attention deficit hyperactivity disorder. *Journal of Attention Disorders, 3,* 121–134.

Bergen, J. R., & Kratochwill, T. R. (1990). *Behavioral consultation and therapy.* New York: Plenum Press.

Biederman, J., Mick, E., Faraone, S. V., Spencer, T., Wilens, T. E., & Wozniak, J. (2000). Pediatric mania: A developmental subtype of bipolar disorder? *Biological Psychiatry, 48,* 458–456.

Biederman, J., Newcorn, J., & Sprich, S. (1991). Comorbidity of attention deficit hyperactivity disorder with conduct, depressive, anxiety, and other disorders. *American Journal of Psychiatry, 148,* 564–577.

Bradley, R., & Danielson, L. (2004). The Office of Special Education Program's LD Initiative: A context for inquiry and consensus. *Learning Disability Quarterly, 27,* 186–188.

Bradley-Johnson, S., Morgan, S. K., & Nutkins, C. (2004). The Woodcock–Johnson Tests of Achievement. *Journal of Psychoeducational Assessment, 22,* 261–274.

Breton, J.-J., Bergeron, L., Valla, J.-P., Berthiaume, C., Gaudet, N., Lambert, J., et al. (1999). Quebec Child Mental Health Survey: Prevalence of DSM-III-R mental health disorders. *Journal of Child Psychology and Psychiatry, and Allied Disciplines, 40,* 375–384.

Bryan, K. L., & Hale, J. B. (2001). Differential effects of left and right hemisphere cerebral vascular accidents on language competency. *Journal of the International Neuropsychological Society, 7,* 655–664.

Butcher, J. N. (1992). *Essential of MMPI-2 and MMPI-A interpretation.* Minneapolis: University of Minnesota Press.

Butler, S. F., Arredondo, D. E., & McCloskey, V. (1995). Affective comorbidity in children and adolescents with attention deficit hyperactivity disorder. *Annals of Clinical Psychiatry, 7,* 51–55.

Carlson, E. A., Jacobvitz, D., & Sroufe, L. A. (1995). A developmental investigation of inattentiveness and hyperactivity. *Child Development, 66,* 37–54.

Castellanos, F. X., Lee, P. P., Sharp, W., Jeffries, N. O., Greenstein, D. K., Clasen, L. S., et al. (2002). Developmental trajectories of brain volume abnormalities in children with attention-deficit/hyperactivity disorder. *Journal of the American Medical Association, 288,* 1740–1748.

Cepeda, N. J., Cepeda, M. L., & Kramer, A. F. (2000). Task switching and attention deficit hyperactivity disorder. *Journal of Abnormal Child Psychology, 28,* 213–226.

Chermak, G. D., Tucker, E., & Seikel, J. A. (2002). Behavioral characteristics of auditory processing disorder and attention-deficit hyperactivity disorder: Predominately inattentive type. *Journal of the American Academy of Audiology, 13,* 332–338.

Chi, T. C., & Hinshaw, S. P. (2002). Mother–child relationships of children with ADHD: The role of maternal depressive symptoms and depression-related distortions. *Journal of Abnormal Child Psychology, 30*(4), 387–400.

Clarke, L., Ungerer, J., Chahoud, K., Johnson, S., & Stiefel, I. (2002). Attention deficit hyperactivity disorder is associated with attachment insecurity. *Clinical Child Psychology and Psychiatry, 7*(2), 179–198.

Conners, C. K., Sitarenios, G., Parker, J. D. A., & Epstein, J. N. (1998a). The revised Conners Parent Rating Scale (CPRS-R): Factor structure, reliability, and criterion validity. *Journal of Abnormal Child Psychology, 26*(4), 257–268.

Conners, C. K., Sitarenios, G., Parker, J. D. A., & Epstein, J. N. (1998b). The revised Conners Teacher Rating Scale (CTRS-R): Factor structure, reliability, and criterion validity. *Journal of Abnormal Child Psychology, 26*(4), 279–291.

Conners, K. (1997a). *Conners Parent and Teacher Rating Scale—Revised.* North Tonawanda, NY: Multi-Health Systems.

Conners, K. (1997b). *Conners Adolescent Self-Report Scale.* North Tonawanda, NY: Multi-Health Systems.

Conners, K., & MHS Staff. (2000). *Conners Continuous Performance Test–II User's Manual.* Toronto: Multi-Health Systems.

Costello, E. J., Angold, A., Burns, B. J., Stangl, D. K., Tweed, D. L., Erkanli, A., & Worthman, C. M. (1996). The Great Smoky Mountains Study of youth: Goals, design, methods, and the prevalence of DSM-III-R disorders. *Archives of General Psychiatry, 53,* 1129–1136.

Cushman, T. P., & Johnson, T. B. (2001). Understanding "inattention" in children and adolescents. *Ethical Human Sciences and Services, 3,* 107–125.

Das, J. P., Carlson, J., Davidson, M. B., & Longe, K. (1997). *PREP: PAS Remedial Program.* Seattle, WA: Hogrefe.

Delis, D. C., Kaplan, E., & Kramer, J. H. (2001). *Delis–Kaplan Executive Function System.* San Antonio, TX: Psychological Corporation.

Denckla, M. B. (1996). Biological correlates of learning and attention: What is relevant to learning disability and attention-deficit/hyperactivity disorder. *Journal of Developmental and Behavioral Pediatrics, 17,* 114–119.

Doyle, A., Ostrander, R., Skare, S., Crosby, R. D., & August, G. J. (1997). Convergent and criterion-related validity of the Behavior Assessment System for Children—Parent Rating Scale. *Journal of Clinical Child Psychology, 26*(3), 276–284.

DuPaul, G. J., McGoey, K. E., Eckert, T. L., & VanBrakle, J. (2001). Preschool children with attention-deficit/hyperactivity disorder: Impairments in behavioral, social, and school functioning. *Journal of the American Academy of Child and Adolescent Psychiatry, 40,* 508–515.

DuPaul, G. J., & Stoner, G. (2003). *ADHD in the schools: Assessment and intervention strategies* (2nd ed.). New York: Guilford Press.

Edwards, M. C., Schulz, E. G., & Long, N. (1995). The role of the family in the assessment of attention deficit hyperactivity disorder. *Clinical Psychology Review, 15*(5), 375–394.

Eiraldi, R. B., Power, T. J., Karustis, J. L., & Goldstein, S. G. (2000). Assessing ADHD and comorbid disorders in children: The child behavior checklist and the devereux scales of mental disorders. *Journal of Clinical Child Psychology, 29*(1), 3–16.

Eley, T. C., & Stevenson, J. (1999). Exploring the covariation between anxiety and depression symptoms: A genetic analysis of the effects of age and sex. *Journal of Child Psychology and Psychiatry, 40*, 1273–1282.

Elliott, C. D. (1990a). *Differential Ability Scales: Administration and scoring manual.* San Antonio, TX: Psychological Corporation.

Elliott, C. D. (1990b). *Differential Ability Scales: Introductory and technical handbook.* San Antonio, TX: Psychological Corporation.

Filipek, P. A. (1999). Neuroimaging in the developmental disorders: The state of the science. *Journal of Child Psychology and Psychiatry, 40*, 113–128.

Findling, R. L., Gracious, B. L., McNamara, N. K., Youngstrom, E. A., Demeter, C. A., Branicky, L. A., et al. (2001). Rapid, continuous cycling and psychiatric comorbidity in pediatric bipolar I disorder. *Bipolar Disorders, 3*, 202–210.

Fiorello, C. A., Hale, J. B., McGrath, M., Ryan, K., & Quinn, S. (2001). IQ interpretation for children with flat and variable test profiles. *Learning and Individual Differences, 13*, 115–125.

Fletcher, J. M., Denton, C., & Francis, D. J. (2005). Validity of alternative approaches for the identification of learning disabilities: Operationalizing unexpected underachievement. *Journal of Learning Disabilities, 38*, 545–552.

Ford, L. Keith, T. Z., Floyd, R., Fields, C., & Schrank, F. J. (2003). WJ III and children with ADHD. In F. Schrank & D. Flanagan D. (Eds.), *The Woodcock–Johnson III: Clinical use and interpretation.* San Diego: Academic Press.

Ford, T., Goodman, R., & Meltzer, H. (2003). The British Child and Adolescent Mental Health Survey 1999: The Prevalence of DSM-IV disorders. *Journal of the American Academy of Child and Adolescent Psychiatry, 42*, 1203–1211.

Geary, D. C. (1993). Mathematical disabilities: Cognitive, neuropsychological, and genetic components. *Psychological Bulletin, 114*, 345–362.

Geller, B., Craney, J. L., Bolhofner, K., DelBello, M. P., Axelson, D., Luby, J., et al. (2003). Phenomenology and longitudinal course of children with a prepubertal and early adolescent bipolar disorder phenotype. In B. Geller & M. P. DelBello (Eds.), *Bipolar disorder in childhood and early adolescence* (pp. 25–50). New York: Guilford Press.

Geller, B., Zimerman, B., & Williams, M. (2000). Diagnostic characteristics of 93 cases of a prepubertal and early adolescent bipolar disorder phenotype by gender, puberty and comorbid attention deficit hyperactivity disorder. *Journal of Child and Adolescent Psychopharmacology, 10*, 157–164.

Geller, D. A., Biederman, J., Faraone, S. V., Cradock, K., Hagermoser, L., Zaman, N., et al. (2002). Attention-deficit/hyperactivity disorder in children and adolescents with obsessive–compulsive disorder: Fact or artifact? *Journal of the American Academy of Child and Adolescent Psychiatry, 41*, 52–58.

Geller, D. A., Biederman, J., Faraone, S. V., Spencer, T., Doyle, R., Mullin, B., et al. (2004). Re-examining comorbidity of obsessive compulsive and attention-deficit hyperactivity disorder using an empirically derived taxonomy. *European Child and Adolescent Psychiatry, 13*, 83–91.

Geller, D. A., Biederman, J., Griffin, S., & Jones, J. (1996). Comorbidity of juvenile obsessive–compulsive disorder with disruptive behavior disorders. *Journal of the American Academy of Child and Adolescent Psychiatry, 35*, 1637–1646.

Gibney, L. A., McIntosh, D. E., Dean, R. S., & Dunham, M. (2002). Diagnosing attention disorders with measures of neurocognitive functioning. *International Journal of Neuroscience, 112,* 539–564.

Giedd, J. N., Castellanos, F. X., Casey, B. J., Kozuch, P., King, A. C., Hamburger, S. D., et al. (1994). Quantitative morphology of the corpus callosum in attention deficit hyperactivity disorder. *American Journal of Psychiatry, 151,* 665–669.

Gioia, G. A., Isquith, P. K., Guy, S. C., & Kenworthy, L. (2000). *Brief Rating Inventory of Executive Function: Professional manual.* Lutz, FL: Psychological Assessment Resources.

Goldstein, S. (1999). Attention-deficit/hyperactivity disorder. In S. Goldstein & C. R. Reynolds (Eds.), *Handbook of neurodevelopmental and genetic disorders in children* (pp. 154–184). New York: Guilford Press.

Goldstein, S., & Schwebach, A. J. (2004). The comorbidity of pervasive developmental disorder and attention deficit hyperactivity disorder: Results from a retrospective chart review. *Journal of Autism and Developmental Disorders, 34,* 329–339.

Gomez, R., & Condon, M. (1999). Central auditory processing ability in children with ADHD with and without learning disabilities. *Journal of Learning Disabilities, 32,* 150–158.

Goodman, G., & Poillion, M. J. (1992). ADD: Acronym for any dysfunction or difficulty. *Journal of Special Education, 26,* 37–56.

Goodman, R., & Stevenson, J. (1989). A twin study of hyperactivity: II. The aetiological role of genes, family relationships and perinatal adversity. *Journal of Child Psychology and Psychiatry, and Allied Disciplines, 30,* 691–709.

Gray, J. A. (1987). Perspectives on anxiety and impulsivity: A commentary. *Journal of Research in Personality, 21,* 493–509.

Greenberg, L. M. (1988–1999). *The Test of Variables of Attention (TOVA).* Los Alamitos, CA: Universal Attention Disorders.

Gresham, F. M., & Elliott, S. N. (1990). *Social Skills Rating System.* Circle Pines, MN: American Guidance Service.

Guerin, D. W., Gottfried, A. W., Oliver, P. H., & Thomas, C. W. (1994). Temperament and school functioning during early adolescence. *Journal of Early Adolescence, 14,* 200–225.

Hale, J. B., & Fiorello, C. A. (2004). *School neuropsychology: A practitioner's handbook.* New York: Guilford Press.

Hale, J. B., Fiorello, C. A., Bertin, M., & Sherman, R. (2003). Predicting math achievement through neuropsychological interpretation of WISC-III variance components. *Journal of Psychoeducational Assessment, 21,* 358–380.

Hale, J. B., Fiorello, C. A., & Brown, L. (2005). Determining medication treatment effects using teacher ratings and classroom observations of children with ADHD: Does neuropsychological impairment matter? *Educational and Child Psychology, 22,* 39–61.

Hale, J. B., Hoeppner, J. B., DeWitt, M., Ritocco, D., Coury, D. L., & Trommer, B. L. (1998). Evaluating medication response in ADHD: Cognitive, behavioral, and single subject methodology. *Journal of Learning Disabilities, 31,* 595–607.

Hale, J. B., Hoeppner, J. B., & Fiorello, C. A. (2001). Analyzing Digit Span components for assessment of attention problems. *Journal of Psychoeducational Assessment, 20,* 128–143.

Hale, J. B., How, S. K., DeWitt, M. B., & Coury, D. L. (2001). Discriminant validity of the Conners scales for ADHD subtypes. *Current Psychology, 20,* 231–249.

Hale, J. B., Naglieri, J. A., Kaufman, A. S., & Kavale, K. A. (2006). Implementation of

IDEA: Integrating response to intervention and cognitive assessment methods. *Psychology in the Schools, 43,* 753–770.

Hale, J. B., Rosenberg, D., Hoeppner, J. B., & Gaither, R. (1997, April). *Cognitive predictors of behavior disorders in children with learning disabilities.* Paper presentation at the annual convention of the National Association of School Psychologists, Anaheim, CA.

Hale, J. B., & Rubenstein, J. (2006, March). *Reconceptualizing nonverbal learning disabilities for academic and behavioral intervention efficacy.* Workshop presented to the West Chester Association of School Psychologists, West Chester, PA.

Hammen, C., & Rudolph, K. D. (1996). Childhood depression. In E. J. Mash & R. A. Barkley (Eds.), *Child psychopathology* (pp. 153–195). New York: Guilford Press.

Harrison, C., & Sofronoff, K. (2002). ADHD and parental psychological distress: Role of demographics, child behavioral characteristics, and parental cognitions. *Journal of the American Academy of Child and Adolescent Psychiatry, 41*(6), 703–711.

Hauser, P., Zametkin, A. J., Martinez, P., Vitiello, B., Matochik, J. A., Mixson, A. J., et al. (1993). Attention deficit hyperactivity disorder in people with generalized resistance to thyroid hormone. *New England Journal of Medicine, 328,* 997–1001.

Hechtman, L., & Weiss, G. (1986). Controlled prospective fifteen year follow-up of hyperactive as adults: Non-medical drug and alcohol use and anti-social behaviour. *Canadian Journal of Psychiatry, 31,* 557–567.

Hoeppner, J. B., Hale, J. B., Bradley, A., Byrns, M., Coury, D. L., & Trommer, B. L. (1997). A clinical protocol for determining methylphenidate dosage levels in ADHD. *Journal of Attention Disorders, 2,* 19–30.

Holtmann, M., Bolte, S., & Poustka, F. (2005). ADHD, Asperger syndrome, and high functioning autism. *Journal of the American Academy of Child and Adolescent Psychiatry, 44,* 1101.

Hynd, G. W., Hern, K. L., Novey, E. S., Eliopulos, D., Marshall, R., Gonzalez, J. J., et al. (1993). Attention deficit-hyperactivity disorder and asymmetry of the caudate nucleus. *Journal of Child Neurology, 8,* 339–347.

Ingalls, S., & Goldstein, S. (1999). Learning disabilities. In S. Goldstein & C. R. Reynolds (Eds.), *Handbook of neurodevelopmental and genetic disorders in children* (pp. 101–153). New York: Guilford Press.

Jansen, R. E., Fitzgerald, H. E., Ham, H. P., & Zucker, R. A. (1995). Difficult temperament and problem behaviors in three- to five-year-old sons of alcoholics. *Alcoholism, Clinical and Experimental Research, 19,* 501–509.

Johnston, C., & Mash, E. J. (2001). Families of children with ADHD: Review and recommendations for future research. *Clinical Child and Family Psychology Review, 4*(3), 183–207.

Johnston, C., Murray, C., Hinshaw, S. P., Pelham, W. E., & Hoza, B. (2002). Responsiveness in interactions of mothers and sons with ADHD: Relations to maternal and child characteristics. *Journal of Abnormal Child Psychology, 30*(1), 77–88.

Kashani, J. H., Carlson, G. A., Beck, N. C., Hoeper, E. W., Corcoran, C. M., McAllister, J. A., et al. (1987). Depression, depressive symptoms, and depressed mood among a community sample of adolescents. *American Journal of Psychiatry, 144,* 931–934.

Kashani, J. H., & Orvaschel, H. (1988). Anxiety disorders in mid-adolescence: A community sample. *American Journal of Psychiatry, 145,* 960–964.

Kashani, J. H., & Orvaschel, H. (1990). A community study of anxiety in children and adolescents. *American Journal of Psychiatry, 147,* 313–318.

Katz, J., & Tillery, K. (2004). Central auditory processing. In L. Verhoeven & H. van Balkom (Eds.), *Classification of developmental language disorders: Theoretical issues and clinical implications* (pp. 191–208). Mahwah, NJ: Erlbaum.

Keith, T. Z., Kranzler, J. H., & Flanagan, D. P. (2001). What does the Cognitive Assessment System (CAS) measure?: Joint confirmatory factor analysis of the CAS and Woodcock–Johnson Tests of Cognitive Ability (3rd edition). *School Psychology Review, 30,* 89–119.

Kellner, R., Houghton, S., & Douglas, G. (2003). Peer-related personal experiences of children with attention-deficit/hyperactivity disorder with and without comorbid learning disabilities. *International Journal of Disability, Development and Education, 50*(2), 119–136.

Kellogg, R. T. (1994). *The psychology of writing.* New York: Oxford University Press.

Keogh, B. A. (1971). Hyperactivity and learning disorders: Review and speculation. *Exceptional Children, 38,* 101–109.

Keogh, B. K. (1994). Temperament and teachers' views of teachability. In W. B. Carey & S. C. McDevitt (Eds.), *Prevention and early intervention: Individual differences as risk factors for the mental health of children* (pp. 246–256). New York: Brunner/Mazel.

Kessler, R. C., Adler, L. A., Barkley, R., Biederman, J., Conners, C. K., Faraone, S. V., et al. (2005). Patterns and predictors of attention-deficit/hyperactivity disorder persistence into adulthood: Results from the National Comorbidity Survey Replication. *Biological Psychiatry, 57,* 1442–1451.

Kessler, R. C., Avenevoli, S., & Merikangas, K. R. (2001). Mood disorders in children and adolescents: An epidemiological perspective. *Biological Psychiatry, 49,* 1002–1014.

Klin, A., Volkmar, F. R., Sparrow, S. S., Cicchetti, D. V., & Rourke, B. P. (1995). Validity and neuropsychological characterization of Asperger syndrome: Convergence with nonverbal learning disabilities syndrome. *Journal of Child Psychology and Psychiatry, 36,* 1127–1140.

Korman, M., Kirk, U., & Kemp, S. (1998). *NEPSY: A developmental neuropsychological assessment manual.* San Antonio, TX: Harcourt Assessment.

Kortlander, E., Kendall, P. C., & Chansky, T. (1994, November). *Parental expectations and attributions associated with childhood anxiety disorders.* Paper presented at the annual convention of the Association of the Advancement of Behavior Therapy, San Diego, CA.

Kovacs, M. (2003). *Children's Depression Inventory.* North Tonawanda, NY: Multi-Health Systems.

Kowatch, R. A., Fristad, M., Birmaher, B., Wagner, K. D., Findling, R. L., & Hellander, M., & the Child Psychiatric Workgroup on Bipolar Disorder. (2005). Treatment guidelines for children and adolescents with bipolar disorder. *Journal of the American Academy of Child and Adolescent Psychiatry, 44,* 213–235.

Labauve, B. J. (2003). Systemic treatment of attention deficit hyperactivity disorder. *Journal of Systemic Therapies, 22*(2), 45–55.

Lachar, D., & Gruber, C. P. (1995). *Personality Inventory for Youth (PIY).* Los Angeles: Western Psychological Services.

Lachar, D., & Gruber, C. P. (2001). *Personality Inventory for Children (PIC-2)* (2nd ed.). Los Angeles: Western Psychological Services.

Lachar, D., Wingenfeld, S. A., Kline, R. B., & Gruber, C. P. (2000). *Student Behavior Survey manual.* Los Angeles: Western Psychological Services.

Lahey, B. B., Schaughency, E. A., Hynd, G. W., Carlson, C. L., & Nieves, N. (1987).

Attention deficit disorder with and without hyperactivity: Comparison of behavioral characteristics of clinic-referred children. *Journal of the American Academy of Child and Adolescent Psychiatry, 26,* 718–723.

Lee, V. (1999). ADHD: The buzz letters of the 90's. *The School Psychologist: A Publication of the New York Association of School Psychologists, 17,* 8–10.

Levy, F., & Hay, D. A. (Eds.). (2001). *Attention, genes, and ADHD.* Philadelphia: Taylor & Francis.

Lewinsohn, P. M., Hops, H., Roberts, R. E., Seeley, J. R., & Andrews, J. A. (1993). Adolescent psychopathology: I. Prevalence and incidence of depression and other DSM-III-R disorders in high school students. *Journal of Abnormal Psychology, 102,* 133–144.

Lewinsohn, P. M., Rohde, P., & Seeley, J. R. (1998). Major depressive disorder in older adolescents: Prevalence, risk factors, and clinical implications. *Clinical Psychology Review, 18,* 765–794.

Lichter, D. G., & Cummings, J. L. (2001). *Frontal–subcortical circuits in psychiatric and neurological disorders.* New York: Guilford Press.

Liss, M., Fein, D., Allen, D., Dunn, M., Feinstein, C., Morris, R., et al. (2001). Executive functioning in children with high functioning autism. *Journal of Child Psychology and Psychiatry, 42,* 261–270.

Maedgen, J. W., & Carlson, C. L. (2000). Social functioning and emotional regulation in the attention deficit hyperactivity disorder subtypes. *Journal of Clinical Child Psychology, 29*(1), 30–42.

Manning, S. C. (2001). Identifying ADHD subtypes using the Parent and Teacher Rating Scales of the Behavior Assessment Scale for Children. *Journal of Attention Disorders, 5*(1), 41–51.

Martin, R. P. (1988). *The Temperament Assessment Battery for Children.* Brandon, VT: Clinical Psychology Publishing.

Martin, R. P., Olejnik, S., & Gaddis, L. (1994). Is temperament an important contributor to schooling outcomes in elementary school?: Modeling effects of temperament and scholastic ability on academic achievement. In W. B. Carey & S. C. McDevitt (Eds.), *Prevention and early intervention: Individual differences as risk factors for the mental health of children* (pp. 59–68). New York: Brunner/Mazel.

Mayberg, H. (2001). Depression and frontal-subcortical circuits: Focus on prefrontal–limbic interactions. In D. G. Lichter & J. L. Cummings (Eds.), *Frontal–subcortical circuits in psychiatric and neurological disorders* (pp. 177–206). New York: Guilford Press.

Mayes, S. D., & Calhoun, S. L. (2004). Similarities and differences in Wechsler Intelligence Scale for Children—Third Edition (WISC-III) profiles: Support for subtest analysis of clinical referrals. *Clinical Neuropsychologist, 18,* 559–572.

Mayes, S. D., Calhoun, S. L., & Crowell, E. W. (2000). Learning disabilities and ADHD: Overlapping spectrum disorders. *Journal of Learning Disabilities, 33,* 417–424.

McClure, E. B., Brennan, P. A., Hammen, C., & Le Brocque, R. M. (2001). Parental anxiety disorders, child anxiety disorders, and the perceived parent–child relationship in an Australian high-risk sample. *Journal of Abnormal Child Psychology, 9,* 1–10.

Meister, H., von Wedel, H., & Walger, M. (2004). Psychometric evaluation of children with suspected auditory processing disorders (APDs) using a parent-answered survey. *International Journal of Audiology, 43,* 431–437.

Miller, J. N., & Ozonoff, S. (2000). The external validity of Asperger disorder: Lack of evidence from the domain of neuropsychology. *Journal of Abnormal Psychology*, *109*, 227–238.

Millon, T., Green, C. J., & Meagher, R. B. (1982). *Millon Adolescent Personality Inventory*. Minneapolis, MN: National Computer Systems.

Muir-Broaddus, J. E., Rosenstein, L. D., Medina, D. E., & Soderberg, C. (2002). Neuropsychological test performance of children with ADHD relative to test norms and parent behavioral ratings. *Archives of Clinical Neuropsychology*, *17*, 671–689.

Mun, E. Y., Fitzgerald, H. E., von Eye, A., Puttler, L. I., & Zucker, R. A. (2001). Temperament characteristics as predictors of externalizing and internalizing child behavior problems in the contexts of high and low parental psychopathology. *Infant Mental Health Journal*, *22*, 393–415.

Murphy, K. R., & Barkley, R. A. (1996). Parents of children with attention-deficit/hyperactivity disorder: Psychological and attentional impairment. *American Journal of Orthopsychiatry*, *66*(1), 93–102.

Naglieri, J. A., & Das, J. P. (1997). *Das–Naglieri Cognitive Assessment System administration and scoring manual*. Itasca, IL: Riverside.

Naglieri, J. A., Goldstein, S., & Iseman, J. (2003). Performance of children with attention deficit hyperactivity disorder and anxiety/depression on the WISC-III and Cognitive Assessment System (CAS). *Journal of Psychoeducational Assessment*, *21*(1), 32–42.

Naglieri, J. A., Salter, C., & Edwards, G. (2004). Assessment of children with attention and reading difficulties using the PASS theory and Cognitive Assessment System. *Journal of Psychoeducational Assessment*, *22*(2), 93–105.

Needleman, H. L., Gunnoe, C., Leviton, A., Reed, R., Peresie, H., Maher, C., et al. (1979). Deficits in psychologic and classroom performance of children with elevated dentine levels. *New England Journal of Medicine*, *300*, 689–695.

Newcorn, J. H., Halperin, J. M., Jensen, P. S., Abikoff, H. B., Arnold, E., Cantwell, D. P., et al. (2001). Symptom profiles in children with ADHD: Effects of comorbidity and gender. *Journal of the American Academy of Child and Adolescent Psychiatry*, *40*, 137–146.

O'Connor, R. E., & Jenkins, J. R. (1999). Prediction of reading disabilities in kindergarten and first grade. *Scientific Studies of Reading*, *3*, 159–197.

Ollendick, T. H., Shortt, A. L., & Sander, J. B. (2004). Internalizing disorders of childhood and adolescence. In J. E. Maddux (Ed.), *Psychopathology: Foundations for contemporary understanding* (pp. 353–376). Mahwah, NJ: Erlbaum.

Pavuluri, M. N., Birmaher, B., & Naylor, M. W. (2005). Pediatric bipolar disorder: A review of the past 10 years. *Journal of the American Academy of Child and Adolescent Psychiatry*, *44*, 846–871.

Pelham, W. E., Fabiano, G. A., & Massetti, G. M. (2005). Evidenced-based assessment of attention deficit hyperactivity disorder in children and adolescents. *Journal of Clinical Child and Adolescent Psychology*, *34*(3), 449–476.

Pelham, W. E., & Milich, R. (1984). Peer relations of children with hyperactivity/attention deficit disorder. *Journal of Learning Disabilities*, *17*, 560–568.

Perner, J., Kain, W., & Barchfeld, P. (2002). Executive control and higher-order theory of mind in children at risk of ADHD. *Infant and Child Development*, *11*, 141–158.

Perrin, S., & Last, C. G. (1996). Relationship between ADHD and anxiety in boys:

Results from a family study. *Journal of the American Academy of Child and Adolescent Psychiatry, 35*(8), 988–996.

Pfiffner, L. J., McBurnett, K., Lahey, B. B., Loeber, R., Green, S., Frick, P. J., et al. (1999). Association of parental psychopathology to the comorbid disorders of boys with attention-deficit hyperactivity disorder. *Journal of Consulting and Clinical Psychology, 67,* 881–893.

Pizzitola, J. K., Riccio, C. A., & Siekierski, B. M. (2005). Assessment of ADHD using the BASC and BRIEF. *Applied Neuropsychology, 12*(2), 83–93.

Pliszka, S. R. (1992). Comorbidity of attention-deficit hyperactivity disorder and overanxious disorder. *Journal of the American Academy of Child and Adolescent Psychiatry, 31,* 197–203.

Pliszka, S. R., Carlson, C. L., & Swanson, J. M. (1999). *ADHD with comorbid disorders: Clinical assessment and management.* New York: Guilford Press.

Pliszka, S. R., & Olvera, R. L. (1999). Anxiety disorders. In S. Goldstein & C. R. Reynolds (Eds.), *Handbook of neurodevelopmental and genetic disorders in children* (pp. 216–246). New York: Guilford Press.

Podolski, C., & Nigg, J. T. (2001). Parent stress and coping in relation to child ADHD severity and associated child disruptive behavior problems. *Journal of Clinical Child Psychology, 30*(4), 503–513.

Pratt, B., Campbell-La Voie, F., Isquith, P. K., Gioia, G., & Guy, S. (2000). *Behavior Rating Inventory of Executive Function parent ratings in children with ADHD.* Unpublished raw data, New York.

Quay, H. C. (1997). Inhibition and attention deficit hyperactivity disorder. *Journal of Abnormal Child Psychology, 25,* 7–13.

Reddy L. A., Barboza-Whitehead, S., Files, T., & Rubel, R. (2000). Clinical focus of consultation outcome research with children and adolescents. *Special Services in the Schools, 16*(1/2), 1–22.

Reddy, L. A., Braunstein, D. J., & Dumont, R. (in press). Use of the Differential Ability Scale for children with attention-deficit/hyperactivity disorder. *School Psychology Quarterly.*

Reddy, L. A., & De Thomas, C. (2006). Assessment of attention-deficit/hyperactivity disorder with children. In S. R. Smith & L. Handler (Eds.), *The Clinical Assessment of Children and Adolescents: A Practitioner's Guide.* Mahwah, NJ: Erlbaum.

Reddy, L. A., Dumont, R., & Bray, N. (2005). *Use of the Woodcock–Johnson Tests of Cognitive Abilities for children with attention-deficit/hyperactivity disorder.* Presented at the American Psychological Association Conference in Washington, DC.

Reddy, L. A., Springer, C., Hall, T. M., Benisz, E., Braunstein, D., Hauch, Y., et al. (2005). Childhood ADHD Multimodal Program: An empirically-supported intervention for young children with ADHD. In L. Reddy, T. Hall, & C. Schaefer (Eds.), *Empirically-based play interventions for children* (pp. 145–168). Washington, DC: American Psychological Association Press.

Reschly, D. J. (2004). Commentary: Paradigm shift, outcomes criteria, and behavioral interventions: Foundations for the future of school psychology. *School Psychology Review, 33,* 408–416.

Reynolds, C. R., & Kamphaus, R. W. (1992). *Behavior Assessment System for Children–2 (BASC-2).* Circle Pines, MN: American Guidance Services.

Reynolds, C. R., & Kamphaus, R. W. (2004). *Behavior Assessment System for Children–2 (BASC-2).* Circle Pines, MN: American Guidance Services.

Reynolds, C. R., & Richmond, B. D. (2000). *Revised Children's Manifest Anxiety Scale*. Los Angeles: Western Psychological Services.

Riccio, C. A., Hynd, G. W., Cohen, M. J., Hall, J., & Molt, L. (1994). Comorbidity of central auditory processing disorder and attention-deficit hyperactivity disorder. *Journal of the American Academy of Child and Adolescent Psychiatry, 33*(6), 849–857.

Riccio, C. A., & Reynolds, C. R. (2003). The assessment of attention via continuous performance tests. In C. R. Reynolds & R. W. Kamphaus (Eds.), *Handbook of psychological and educational assessment of children: Personality, behavior, and context* (2nd ed., pp. 291–319). New York: Guilford Press.

Rourke, B. P. (1995). *Syndrome of nonverbal learning disabilities: Neurodevelopmental manifestations*. New York: Guilford Press.

Rubia, K., Smith, A. B., Brammer, M. J., Toone, B., & Taylor, E. (2005). Abnormal brain activation during inhibition and error detection in medication-naive adolescents with ADHD. *American Journal of Psychiatry, 162*, 1067–1076.

Safren, S. A., Lanka, G. D., Otto, M. W., & Pollack, M. H. (2001). Prevalence of childhood ADHD among patients with generalized anxiety disorder and a comparison condition, social phobia. *Depression and Anxiety, 13*, 190–191.

Samudra, K., & Cantwell, D. P. (1999). Risk factors for attention-deficit/hyperactivity disorder. In H. C. Quay & A. E. Hogan (Eds.), *Handbook of disruptive behavior disorders* (pp. 199–220). New York: Kluwer Academic/Plenum Press.

Schnoll, R., Burshteyn, D., & Cea-Aravena, J. (2003). Nutrition in the treatment of attention-deficit hyperactivity disorder: A neglected but important aspect. *Applied Psychophysiology and Biofeedback, 28*(1), 63–75.

Schroeder, C. S., & Gordon, B. N. (Eds.). (2002). *Assessment and treatment of childhood problems: A clinician's guide* (2nd ed., pp. 262–416). New York: Guilford Press.

Schultz, K. P., Fan, J., Tang, C. Y., Newcorn, J. H., Buchsbaum, M. S., Cheung, A. M., et al. (2004). Response inhibition in adolescents diagnosed with attention deficit hyperactivity disorder during childhood: An event-related fMRI study. *American Journal of Psychiatry, 161*, 1650–1657.

Semrud-Clikeman, M., Filipek, P. A., Biederman, J., Steingard, R., Kennedy, D., Renshaw, P., et al. (1994). Attention deficit hyperactivity disorder: Magnetic resonance imaging morphometric analysis of the corpus callosum. *Journal of the American Academy of Child and Adolescent Psychiatry, 33*, 875–881.

Semrud-Clikeman, M., Steingard, R. J., Filipek, P., Biederman, J., Bekken, K., & Renshaw, P. (2000). Using MRI to examine brain–behavior relationships in males with attention deficit disorder with hyperactivity. *Journal of the American Academy of Child and Adolescent Psychiatry, 39*, 477–484.

Shear, P. K., DelBello, M. P., Rosenberg, H., & Strakowski, S. M. (2002). Parental reports of executive dysfunction in adolescents with bipolar disorder. *Child Neuropsychology, 8*, 285–295.

Silver, L. B. (1981). The relationship between learning disabilities, hyperactivity, distractibility, and behavioral problems: A clinical analysis. *Journal of the American Academy of Child Psychiatry, 20*, 385–397.

Sonuga-Barke, E. J., & Goldfoot, M. T. (1995). The effect of child hyperactivity on mothers' expectations for development. *Child Care and Health Development, 21*, 17–29.

Souza, I., Pinheiro, M. A., Denardin, D., Mattos, P., & Rohde, L. A. (2004). Attention-deficit/hyperactivity disorder and comorbidity in Brazil: Comparisons between two referred samples. *European Child and Adolescent Psychiatry, 13*(4), 243–248.

Springer, C., & Reddy, L. A. (2005). Measuring adherence in behavior therapy: Opportunities for research and practice. *Behavior Therapist, 27*(4), 1–9.

Stiefel, I. (1997). Can disturbance in attachment contribute to attention deficit hyperactivity disorder?: A case discussion. *Clinical Child Psychology and Psychiatry, 2*(1), 45–64.

Strauss, C. C., & Last, C. G. (1993). Social and simple phobias in children. *Journal of Anxiety Disorders, 7*, 141–152.

Tannock, R. (2000). Attention-deficit/hyperactivity disorder with anxiety disorders. In T. E. Brown (Ed.), *Attention-deficit disorders and comorbidities in children, adolescents, and adults* (pp. 125–170). Washington, DC: American Psychiatric Publishing.

Tannock, R., & Brown, T. E. (2000). Attention-deficit disorders with learning disorders in children and adolescents. In T. E. Brown (Ed.), *Attention-deficit disorders and comorbidities in children, adolescents, and adults* (pp. 231–295). Washington, DC: American Psychiatric Publishing.

Teglasi, H., Cohn, A., & Meshbesher, N. (2004). Temperament and learning disability. *Learning Disability Quarterly, 27*, 9–20.

Tulving, E., & Markowitsch, H. J. (1997). Memory beyond the hippocampus. *Current Opinion in Neurobiology, 7*, 209–216.

Tuthill, R. W. (1996). Hair lead levels related to children's classroom attention deficit behavior. *Archives of Environmental Health, 51*, 214–220.

Verhulst, F. C., van der Ende, J., Ferdinand, R. F., & Kasius, M. C. (1997). The prevalence of DSM-III-R diagnoses in a national sample of Dutch adolescents. *Archives of General Psychiatry, 54*, 329–336.

Wagner, K. D., & Ambrosini, P. J. (2001). Childhood depression: Pharmacological therapy/treatment (pharmacology of childhood depression). *Journal of Clinical Child Psychology, 30*, 88–97.

Wasserstein, J. (2005). Diagnostic issues for adolescents and adults with ADHD. *Journal of Clinical Psychology, 61*, 535–547.

Wechsler, D. (2003). *Manual for the Wechsler Intelligence Scale for Children—Fourth Edition.* San Antonio, TX: Psychological Corporation.

Whalen, C. K., & Henker, B. (1998). Attention-deficit/hyperactivity disorders. In T. H. Ollendick & M. Hersen (Eds.), *Handbook of child psychopathology* (pp. 181–211). New York: Plenum Press.

Wilcutt, E. G., & Pennington, B. F. (2000). Comorbidity of reading disability and attention-deficit/hyperactivity disorder: Differences by gender and subtype. *Journal of Learning Disabilities, 33*, 179–191.

Wing, L. (1998). The history of Asperger syndrome. In E. Schopler, G. B. Mesibov, & L. J. Kunce (Eds.), *Asperger syndrome or high functioning autism?: Current issues in autism* (pp. 11–28). New York: Plenum Press.

Wittchen, H., Reed, V., & Kessler, R. C. (1998). The relationship of agoraphobia and panic in a community sample of adolescents and young adults. *Archives of General Psychiatry, 55*, 1017–1024.

Woodcock, R. W., McGrew, K. S., & Mather, N. (2001). *Woodcock–Johnson III Tests of Cognitive Abilities.* Itasca, IL: Riverside.

Wozniak, J. (2005). Recognizing and managing bipolar disorder in children. *Journal of Clinical Psychiatry, 66*(Suppl. 1), 18–23.

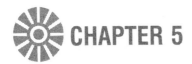

CHAPTER 5

Negative Affect

Kimberly D. Becker and Bruce F. Chorpita

Given that anxiety and depression share so many features, it is not surprising that youth are frequently at risk for both. Negative affect (NA), an individual's experience with negative mood states (e.g., sadness, fear, guilt, anger), accounts for much of the symptom overlap among anxiety, depressive, and adjustment disorders. Unlike diagnostic criteria for anxiety and depression, however, targeting NA allows for a broader examination of the cognitive, behavioral, and physical characteristics underlying emotional disturbances in youth. Presently, efficacious interventions target either anxiety or depressive disorders, but not both. In this chapter, the authors describe their distillation and matching model (Chorpita, Daleiden, & Weisz, 2005a) that draws from the most promising "practice elements" for treating anxiety and depressive disorders in youth. Through the case of "Erin," an adolescent with a diffuse mix of anxiety, depressive, anger, and avoidance behaviors, the authors reveal in remarkable detail how integrated clinical formulations addressing broad-based NA maximize positive treatment outcomes.—A. R. E.

INTRODUCTION

Anxiety and depression are among the most prevalent and highly related psychiatric disorders in youth (Costello, Mustillo, Erkanli, Keeler, & Angold, 2003). Theoretical and empirical advances over the last two decades have changed the way researchers and clinicians conceptualize and target the symptoms of anxiety and depression. Although once thought of as distinct disorders, anxiety and depression are now recognized as having both shared and unique characteristics. This chapter presents information regarding the symptomatology, etiology, assessment, and treatment of anxiety and depression syndromes (symptom clusters) under the rubric of the term "negative affect" (NA). NA, which is discussed in more detail later, essentially represents an individual's experience of negative mood states such as sadness, fear, guilt, and anger, which are distinguished from emotions subsumed by the construct of "positive affect" (PA), including joy, enthusiasm, and energy (Tellegen, 1985).

Nature of Symptom Dimensions

As indicated in *Diagnostic and Statistical Manual of Mental Disorders*, fourth edition, text revised (DSM-IV-TR; American Psychiatric Association [APA], 2000) diagnostic criteria, anxiety generally entails persistent and excessive fear of a particular situation or object, resulting in marked distress upon encountering, or complete avoidance of, the feared stimulus. However, the diversity of diagnoses (e.g., obsessive–compulsive disorder [OCD], posttraumatic stress disorder [PTSD], generalized anxiety disorder [GAD], social phobia, panic disorder) subsumed under the umbrella of anxiety disorders is evidence that anxiety may be manifested in many ways (Albano, Chorpita, & Barlow, 2003). The similarities among the more common depressive disorders, namely, major depressive disorder (MDD) and dysthymic disorder, are more readily recognizable as involving feelings of sadness or irritability (in the case of youth).

The conceptualization of the symptom dimensions rather than the diagnostic criteria of anxiety and depression in the broader context of NA allows for more general consideration of their many emotional, behavioral, cognitive, and physical manifestations. Emotional disturbances may take the form of fear, irritability, hostility, nervousness, sadness, distress, shame, guilt, anhedonia, and hopelessness (Joiner & Lonigan, 2000; Lonigan, Hooe, David, & Kistner, 1999). Behavioral indicators of NA include social withdrawal (Nilzon & Palmerus, 1998), behavioral avoidance (Barlow, 2002), and suicide attempts (Fennig et al., 2005). Cognitive components of NA may involve internal attributions and cognitive errors (e.g., overgeneralization and catastrophic thinking; Cole & Turner, 1993), as well as perceptions of diminished control (Chorpita, 2001). Physiological indicators of NA comprise somatic complaints such as headaches, stomachaches, and sleep difficulties, as well as tension, poor concentration, restlessness (Egger, Costello, Erkanli, & Angold, 1999), and "hypercortisolemia," a term referring to a dysregulated physiological response to stress (e.g., Dienstbier, 1989; Gunnar, 2001). The preceding is not even an exhaustive list of the pathological manifestations of NA, yet it suggests that the great variety of symptom dimensions challenges one's ability to comprehend these problems without some organizing conceptual framework.

Fortunately, a theoretical framework has emerged and developed over the past 20 years to organize these constructs. Originally proposed to articulate the relationship between anxiety and depression, Clark and Watson's (1991) tripartite model specified three subtypes of symptoms: (1) a general distress factor of NA reflecting symptomatology associated with both anxiety and depression, (2) a factor of (low) PA representing symptoms specific to depression, and (3) a factor of physiological hyperarousal (PH) uniquely associated with anxiety.

Empirical evidence provided strong support for the model (e.g., Watson, Clark, et al., 1995; Watson, Weber, et al., 1995). Specifically, within adult and child samples alike, it appears that NA is positively associated with both anxiety and depression, and PA is uniquely and negatively correlated with depression only (Brown, Chorpita, & Barlow, 1998; Chorpita, 2002; Lonigan, Phillips, & Hooe, 2003). Subsequent research on the relation of these constructs to specific dimensions of anxiety and depression (e.g., social anxiety, panic, depressed mood), however, demonstrated some inconsistencies in the model (e.g., Brown et al., 1998). In contrast to the original model, PH does not appear to be common to all anxiety syndromes; rather, when controlling for NA, PH appears uniquely associated with panic disorder in particular (Brown et al., 1998; Chorpita, 2002).

In light of this evidence, it became apparent that the original tripartite model did not entirely account for the heterogeneity of symptoms across specific anxiety disorders. Mineka, Watson, and Clark (1998) articulated a revised model that specified PH as being unique to panic disorder rather than to the entire class of anxiety disorders. Furthermore, Mineka et al. postulated the existence of specific factors, as yet unidentified, for the remaining anxiety disorders, a concept that has been elaborated more recently by Barlow (2002).

In addition to outlining these revisions to the model, Mineka and colleagues (1998) indicated that the proportions of both common and unique components of anxiety and depression differ substantially across syndromes. The implication of their hypothesis is that although each syndrome stems from NA, each has its own set of specific key features and dimensions. Some syndromes, such as generalized anxiety and depression, for example, are quite closely related to NA and are characterized by more pervasive distress than are anxiety syndromes that reflect more circumscribed fears, such as social or specific phobias. Although each anxiety syndrome appears to be related to NA, the strength of the association and the specific manifestation (e.g., worry, shyness, panic, sadness) of NA differs across the syndromes. Along the same lines, although there exist common cognitive, behavioral, and physiological symptoms among anxiety and depressive syndromes, there also exist differences. For example, cognitive biases in the form of automatic thoughts regarding personal failure or loss are more closely related to depression, whereas concerns such as threat or uncertainty more aptly describe the cognitive biases related to anxiety (Schniering & Rapee, 2004). As noted, physiological arousal reliably characterizes panic disorder, whereas somatic complaints that do not reflect sympathetic nervous system arousal (e.g., nausea) often occur with depression (Kasius, Ferdinand, van den Berg, & Verhulst, 1997) and other forms of anxiety, particularly separation anxiety disorder and GAD (Bell-Dolan & Brazeal, 1993; Kearney, 2001).

Prevalence

Symptoms of NA—hence, anxiety and depression—are normal experiences that reflect basic human emotions with specific purposes. For example, anxiety functions to alert an individual to novel or threatening stimuli (Thwaites & Freeston, 2005), thereby enabling the person to respond, and sadness serves to elicit assistance and support (Campos, Campos, & Barrett, 1989). What differentiates normal from maladaptive experiences of NA has to do with uncontrollable, chronic, and pervasive symptoms that cause significant distress and interference in the youth's functioning on a daily basis (Barlow, 2002). As an example, separation anxiety may be considered developmentally and situationally appropriate at certain times (e.g., for a young child who cries when his mother leaves him with a new babysitter), but these same symptoms in other contexts (e.g., an adolescent who consistently fabricates somatic complaints to avoid leaving his mother to go to school) may reflect psychopathology.

Subclinical symptoms of anxiety in the form of fears and worries are present in approximately 20% to as many as 70% of children and adolescents (Bell-Dolan, Last, & Strauss, 1990; Muris, Merckelbach, Gadet, & Moulaert, 2000). Similarly, depressed mood has been reported in between 10 and 40% of nonreferred youth (Achenbach, 1991a), and depressed mood appears to be a robust indicator of future referral for depression (Achenbach, 1991b). Fewer youth, however, exhibit symptomatology that warrants a clinical diagnosis. Nevertheless, anxiety and depressive disorders are among the most prevalent psychiatric disorders diagnosed in youth.

Benefits of a Dimensional Conceptualization

The benefits of utilizing a dimensional approach to conceptualizing the pathological manifestations of NA are multifold (e.g., Brown & Barlow, 2005). By focusing on symptom clusters, the dimensional approach allows for consideration of symptoms in the normative context. As such, a dimensional approach examines the pattern, severity, and degree of interference of a child's difficulties within the developmental context of the child's life, as well as the extent to which a child's manifestation of a particular dimension is extreme relative to age and gender norms. Such a conceptualization fosters the view of a child as a dynamic being, thereby encouraging the incorporation of evaluation and treatment strategies from a variety of perspectives, including developmental psychopathology and functional behavioral assessment. Furthermore, from a dimensional point of view, one need not understand entirely new concepts of human emotion and behavior, in that pathological manifestations are simply extremes of normal human experience (cf. Barlow, 1988).

A dimensional perspective also allows for consideration of symptoms as part of a response class, such that they co-occur and may represent manifestations of the same underlying difficulty. Such an approach allows for the application of treatment strategies that will bring about the most change with the greatest potential to generalize to other symptoms. Finally, a dimensional approach overcomes one of the obstacles that face taxonomic diagnoses, namely, the implicit etiological distinctions that underlie categories, by capitalizing on the commonalities and relationships among symptoms when one seeks to design interventions for children. As a result, one can develop a clearer understanding of the hierarchical relations among symptom dimensions than is offered by traditional categorical approaches, and that understanding allows improved predictions about things such as developmental course or comorbidity (e.g., Chorpita, 2002).

Relationship to Specific Disorders

As noted earlier, NA reflects the general distress factor shared by anxiety and depression syndromes that can be mapped onto DSM-IV-TR (APA, 2000) anxiety disorders (GAD, OCD, separation anxiety disorder [SAD], social phobia, specific phobia, panic disorder, and PTSD) and depressive disorders (MDD and dysthymic disorder), as well as adjustment disorders with depressed mood or anxiety.

As alluded to earlier, research has outlined in some detail the relation among the constructs of NA, other constructs in the tripartite model, and dimensions of DSM-IV-TR (APA, 2000) disorders (Brown et al., 1998; Chorpita, 2001; Chorpita, Albano, & Barlow, 1998; Chorpita, Plummer, & Moffitt, 2000; Joiner, Catanzaro, & Laurent, 1996; Lonigan et al., 1999). Figure 5.1 shows the basic relations identified in children among dimensions outlined in DSM-IV-TR and the constructs of NA, PA, and PH. This general model has been confirmed in four studies of children and adolescents in both clinical and nonclinical samples, and suggests that NA serves as a risk factor for all of the anxiety syndromes, whereas PH is related only to particular dimensions (Brown et al., 1998).

The dimensional conceptualization of NA naturally brings up diagnostic issues when considered in light of the taxonomic structure of DSM-IV-TR (APA, 2000). The first issue concerns the ubiquity of NA in normal emotional experiences. NA is a common part of emotion; worry, sadness, shyness, and other manifestations all have their place in normal child development. Clinicians may find themselves challenged to distinguish between the bad feelings that all youths experience now and again and feelings that reflect psychopathology. As is discussed later, assessment of the degree to which such feelings are uncontrollable, chronic, pervasive, distressing, and interfering is an important step in differentiating between normal and maladaptive experiences of NA. At the same time, recognizing subclinical symptoms of anxiety and depressive disorders can provide avenues for early intervention.

The mere presence of distressing feelings that impair a child's functioning does not provide sufficient basis for a diagnosis. The second diagnostic issue, therefore, concerns the appropriateness of such feelings given a child's circumstances. Whereas feelings of anxiety or depression may be considered excessive in some contexts, these same feelings may be entirely appropriate in truly

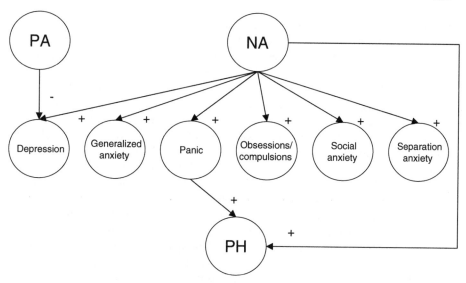

FIGURE 5.1. Relations between dimensions of the tripartite model of emotion and dimensions of anxiety disorders and depression. NA, negative affect; PA, positive affect; PH, physiological hyperarousal; "–" indicates negative association; "+" indicates positive association.

fear-provoking or depressing environments, such as abusive homes, and violent schools and neighborhoods (Barlow, 1988). Although youth in such situations may still require intervention, one should be careful not to pathologize the emotional responding of individuals who justifiably and naturally experience NA under such conditions.

Prevalence

Just as is true of the related symptom dimensions reviewed earlier, anxiety disorders and depression are common in youth, with prevalence estimates in epidemiological samples between 12 and 20% for anxiety (Gurley, Cohen, Pine, & Brook, 1996; Shaffer, Fisher, Dulcan, & Davies, 1996), and 15 and 25% for depression (Kessler, Avenevoli, & Merikangas, 2001; Lewinsohn, Rohde, Seeley, & Hops, 1991). Prevalence estimates vary somewhat depending on the diagnostic instrument utilized, with diagnostic interviews generally providing lower prevalence estimates than self-report symptom scales (Kessler & Walters, 1998).

Onset/Course

Anxiety disorders in general tend to develop earlier than depressive disorders (Avenevoli, Stolar, Li, Dierker, & Merikangas, 2001), with certain anxiety disorders, particularly SAD, developing earlier than others (Last, Hersen,

Kazdin, Finkelstein, & Strauss, 1987; Spence, Rapee, McDonald, & Ingram, 2001). Although certain disorders, such as SAD and phobias, may resolve over time without active treatment (Gullone, King, & Ollendick, 2001; Kearney, Sims, Pursell, & Tillotson, 2003), some anxiety disorders, such as OCD, tend to exhibit a more chronic course (Thomsen & Mikkelsen, 1995). Other anxiety disorders, such as GAD and social phobia, may also increase the risk for the development of comorbid disorders (Kessler et al., 1994). In general, however, the early onset of any anxiety disorder appears to increase risk for the development of comorbid disorders (Goodwin, Fergusson, & Horwood, 2004), to predict the chronicity of the disorder into adolescence and adulthood (Last, Hansen, & Franco, 1997), and to impair psychosocial functioning over time (Woodward & Fergusson, 2001).

Although depression was once considered a disorder afflicting only adults, its influence in children has become increasingly apparent. Research suggests that MDD has a stable course, especially in early onset and comorbid cases (Birmaher et al., 1996). The average duration of MDD is 7–9 months (Birmaher et al., 1996). Approximately 90% of major depressive episodes remit within 2 years (Cicchetti & Toth, 1998), although it appears that approximately 50% of depressed youth experience recurrent episodes into adulthood (Lewinsohn, Rohde, Seeley, Klein, & Gotlib, 2000).

By definition, dysthymic disorder (DD) requires fewer symptoms but lasts significantly longer than MDD, with an average length of 4 years (Cicchetti & Toth, 1998). Children often experience DD prior to depression (Goodman, Schwab-Stone, Lahey, Shaffer, & Jensen, 2000), with depressive episodes occurring approximately 2–3 years after the initial onset of DD (Cicchetti & Toth, 1998). Moreover, the early emergence of DD puts children at greater risk for subsequent mood disorders than does the appearance of MDD (Kovacs, Akiskal, Gatsonis, & Parrone, 1994). It appears, however, that children with comorbid diagnoses of DD and MDD ("double depression") may experience greater impairment in functioning than youth diagnosed with either MDD or DD alone (Goodman et al., 2000).

Comorbidity

Due to the shared influence of NA in both types of disorders, the considerable comorbidity among depressive and anxiety disorders in children is not surprising (e.g., Brady & Kendall, 1992). Research suggests that 30–75% of depressed youth have a diagnosable anxiety disorder (Kessler et al., 2001; Kovacs, Gatsonis, Paulauskas, & Richards, 1989), and that approximately the same proportion of anxious youth exhibit comorbid depression (Lewinsohn, Zinbarg, Seeley, Lewinsohn, & Sack, 1997; Strauss, Last, Hersen, & Kazdin, 1988).

Comorbidity estimates with other Axis I disorders are also high. For example, Last, Strauss, and Francis (1987) found that 80% of children with a principal diagnosis of an anxiety disorder had at least one additional Axis I disorder. Estimates of comorbidity with other Axis I disorders for youth with depression are between 40 and 70%, and between 20 and 50% of youth have two or more comorbid diagnoses (Cicchetti & Toth, 1998). In addition to following the occurrence of anxiety, depression also frequently follows the appearance of externalizing disorders (Biederman, Faraone, Mick, & Lelon, 1995; Kessler et al., 2001; Williamson, Birmaher, Axelson, Ryan, & Dahl, 2004). Research indicates that the type of primary disorder may be less important than the number of earlier disorders in predicting the onset of depression (Kessler & Walters, 1998).

How might NA account for the high comorbidity among anxiety and depressive disorders on the one hand, and other Axis I disorders on the other? When NA is considered from a dimensional perspective, it becomes apparent that disorders outside the mood and anxiety disorder classes also reflect varied proportions of NA (Mineka et al., 1998). Indeed, research indicates that NA is associated with conduct (McBurnett et al., 2005), eating (Leon, Fulkerson, Perry, Keel, & Klump, 1999), and substance use disorders (Pardini, Lochman, & Wells, 2004), as well as schizophrenia (Blanchard, Mueser, & Bellack, 1998). Although most research suggests that NA represents a risk for the development of anxiety and depressive disorders, the directionality of the relation between NA and the other Axis I disorders is less well understood.

Overall, research indicates that comorbidity has a number of long-term implications relative to prognosis. Specifically, comorbidity enhances the risk for chronic and recurrent psychopathology, functional impairment, delayed help-seeking behaviors, and possibly poor treatment outcome (Brent et al., 1998; Fombonne, Wostear, Cooper, Harrington, & Rutter, 2001a, 2001b), although the research is equivocal on this last point (Flannery-Schroeder, Suveg, Safford, Kendall, & Webb, 2004; Rapee, 2003). In the context of anxiety and depression, comorbidity may be interpreted as a marker for the degree of NA, which carries the risks noted earlier; that is, individuals with a greater number of anxiety and/or depressive diagnoses usually have a higher degree of NA, thus increasing the likelihood of risk for continued or chronic internalizing disorders.

Differential Diagnosis

The shared features of anxiety and depression at the symptom, syndrome, and disorder levels introduce considerable diagnostic challenges. To illustrate differential diagnosis, this section focuses on distinguishing between MDD and GAD, which are both indicative of high NA.

DSM-IV-TR (APA, 2000) diagnostic criteria define MDD as characterized by the occurrence of at least one major depressive episode, which includes at least five symptoms at least nearly every day over the course of a 2-week period. One of the symptoms must be either (1) reduced interest or pleasure in activities, or (2) depressed or irritable mood (for youth). The remaining symptoms may include significant weight fluctuations, sleep difficulties, fatigue, psychomotor agitation or retardation, feelings of worthlessness or guilt, concentration difficulties, and recurrent thoughts about death or suicide. To warrant diagnosis, such symptoms must cause significant distress or impairment in school, social, or other areas of functioning.

According to DSM-IV-TR (APA, 2000), GAD is characterized by excessive (i.e., disproportionate to the situation) and difficult-to-control anxiety or worry occurring more days than not for at least 6 months and accompanied by at least one (for youth) physiological symptom (i.e., restlessness, fatigue, sleep difficulties, muscle tension, concentration difficulties, and irritability). Such worries or concomitant symptoms cause significant distress or functional impairment. Additionally, the worries are not exclusively the focus of another Axis I disorder (e.g., being contaminated, as in OCD).

It is apparent from the diagnostic criteria that symptom presentation and course can provide useful information regarding the assignment of one diagnosis over another. First, MDD and GAD both have diagnostic criteria specifying minimum duration, with MDD requiring 2 weeks of symptoms and GAD, requiring 6 months. Second, the number of symptoms required differs for the diagnosis of MDD (depressed mood or anhedonia plus at least four more symptoms) and GAD (worrying plus at least one additional symptom). Finally, although clients may present with symptoms of both GAD and MDD, both diagnoses cannot be assigned unless the symptoms of GAD precede those of MDD by at least 6 months.

With some clients, symptom presentation and course are clear, and differential diagnosis is straightforward. With others, however, questions arise regarding the duration and course of symptoms, whether symptoms reflect clinical or subclinical difficulties, and whether they indicate anxiety or depression, thereby making differential diagnosis more difficult. In such instances, therefore, it is useful to consider the contemporary evidence on additional factors that may inform differential diagnostic decisions.

Biological Factors

FAMILY HISTORY AND GENETICS

A substantial literature examines the extent to which anxiety and depression run in families (e.g., Albano et al., 2003; Hammen & Rudolph, 2003). Frequently, however, it is difficult to parse the relative contributions of genetics and environment to the intergenerational transmission of emotional disorders, although twin and adoption studies provide greater opportunities to do so than do family studies. Research suggests that GAD aggregates in families, such that offspring of individuals with anxiety disorders are at greater risk for developing an anxiety disorder themselves, and it appears that genetics makes a major contribution to the development of GAD (Kendler, Neale, Kessler, Heath, & Eaves, 1992; Roy, Neale, Pedersen, Mathe, & Kendler, 1995). A recent meta-analysis of family and twin studies determined that individuals with GAD are six times more likely to have a first-degree relative with GAD than are individuals without GAD, with genetics accounting for approximately 32% of the variance in vulnerability for the disorder (Hettema, Neale, & Kendler, 2001). Additionally, research consistently indicates similarities in the heritability of GAD for males and females (Hettema, Prescott, & Kendler, 2001).

Parental depression is one of the most significant risk factors for depression in children (Beardslee et al., 1996; Kessler et al., 2001), with estimates of three times the risk for offspring compared to those without family histories of MDD (Williamson et al., 2004). Familial risk is most often apparent in individuals with recurrent MDD (Kendler, Gardner, & Prescott, 1999), although research suggests that early-onset depression may also be related to family history (Williamson et al., 1995), which suggests a stronger genetic component in early- compared with late-onset depression (Kovacs, Devlin, Pollock, Richards, & Mukerji, 1997). Twin and adoption studies estimate the heritability of MDD to be between 31 and 66% (Kendler & Prescott, 1999; Sullivan, Neale, & Kendler, 2000).

Despite such findings, the evidence from genetics offers little direct help as to differential diagnosis in this context, because no specific gene has been identified for either MDD or GAD. In fact, research has demonstrated that GAD and MDD share 100% of their genetic factors (Kendler et al., 1992), thereby lending importance to the identification of the unique environmental influences on the disorders. The collective evidence paints a picture suggesting that temperamental risk (i.e., NA) is the heritable component of GAD and MDD, and whether one develops one, the other, or both disorders is probably due to unique life circumstances.

TEMPERAMENT

Although there are varying conceptualizations of temperament (e.g., Buss & Plomin, 1984; Goldsmith & Campos, 1982; Rothbart, 1989; Thomas & Chess, 1985), temperament generally reflects stable and enduring tendencies that underlie behavior, emotions, reactivity, and sociability (Goldsmith et al., 1987). Because temperamental traits appear early in life, they are not only thought to have strong biological underpinnings but are also believed to be influenced by environmental factors throughout an individual's development (Goldsmith et al., 1987).

Two dimensions have endured from early to contemporary models of temperament: Eysenck's "neuroticism" and "extraversion." Neuroticism contrasts with "emotional stability" and reflects emotional reactivity, as indicated by anxiety, depression, self-criticism, and oversensitivity, whereas extraversion reflects positive emotionality in terms of sociability, high energy, and excitement seeking (Watson, Clark, & Harkness, 1994). Within the tripartite model (Mineka et al., 1998), neuroticism is analogous to NA, the general distress factor shared by anxiety and depression. Extraversion is indicated by the temperamental component unique to depression, PA. Although the third component of the tripartite model, PH, is uniquely associated with some anxiety disorders (most notably panic disorder), it is not clear at this time whether PH reflects a temperamental trait (Clark, Watson, & Mineka, 1994; Lonigan & Phillips, 2001).

NA reflects sensitivity to negative stimuli (Clark et al., 1994; Tellegen, 1985). Research suggests that high NA increases the risk of the development of anxiety and/or depression (e.g., Hirschfeld et al., 1989), whereas NA levels that are below normal may reflect an invulnerability to disorder, at least for depression (Clark et al., 1994). Additionally, NA influences the course of the disorder, such that high NA may indicate poor prognosis (Duggan, Lee, & Murray, 1990). Along the same lines, PA also influences the course of depression, such that high PA is related to better developmental outcomes (e.g., Hirschfeld et al., 1989). At this point, due to the paucity of prospective studies in the field, it is unclear whether low premorbid levels of PA increase an individual's vulnerability to developing depression (Clark et al., 1994).

It would seem that within the tripartite model, the temperamental component of PA is the most helpful in the differential diagnosis of anxiety and depression (e.g., Chorpita & Daleiden, 2002). Unfortunately, the measurement of PA is relatively underdeveloped in children. For example, well-validated PA scales have not been normed in children; thus, there are no absolute standards for designations of "high" or "low" PA. Multiple scores from a single individual may be useful as one indicator of treatment progress, yet they are currently of limited value to diagnosis.

Psychosocial Factors

FAMILY ENVIRONMENT

Just as parental psychopathology may indicate direct genetic vulnerability for disorders related to NA, it may also have indirect effects through socialization processes. Because children first learn about emotion and emotion regulation from their parents, children of anxious or depressed parents are apt to display anxious or depressogenic emotions, cognitions, and behaviors modeled by their parents (Muris, Steerneman, Merckelbach, & Meesters, 1996; Seligman et al., 1984). Depressed parents may also experience difficulty responding consistently and contingently to their children, and may exhibit less PA during interactions with their children (Field, 1995), which, over time, may be perceived as parental rejection (Whitbeck et al., 1992). Compared with parents without anxiety disorders, anxious parents tend to overprotect, discourage children's autonomy, and inhibit their children's involvement in "risky" play activities that are a normal part of child development (Chorpita & Barlow, 1998; Hirshfeld, Biederman, Brody, Faraone, & Rosenbaum, 1997; Siqueland, Kendall, & Steinberg, 1996). Anxious or depressed parents may also inadvertently reinforce their children's avoidant or depressive coping behaviors by selectively attending to anxious and depressive symptoms

(Chorpita, Albano, & Barlow, 1996; Dadds & Roth, 2001). Certainly, parents not suffering from psychopathology who engage in the parenting behaviors just described may also increase the vulnerability of their children to developing an emotional disorder. Despite a considerable body of research, at present, limited information is available that speaks to differences in family environment that would allow for the discrimination between GAD and MDD in a child.

LIFE EVENTS

Although a large literature supports the idea that life events and stressors are related to depression and anxiety (e.g., Boer et al., 2002; Spence, Namjan, Bor, O'Callaghan, & Williams, 2002), some researchers have emphasized the objective degree of distress associated with such events (e.g., Holmes & Rahe, 1967), whereas others have emphasized the psychological response in defining stressful life events (e.g., Johnson, 1982). Although it is somewhat tempting to imagine strong content specificity for the relationship of life events to anxiety and depression (e.g., early separation experiences leading to separation anxiety), there is limited evidence for such a pattern. Indeed, the majority of research suggests that life events appear to exert an influence on overall propensity for anxiety or depression (e.g., Spence et al., 2002), in a manner consistent with developmental theory (Chorpita, 2001). Thus, differential diagnosis for anxiety and depression is best focused on other dimensions we outlined earlier, such as symptom constellation and temperamental differences (e.g., positive affectivity).

Psychological Factors: Perceived Control and Cognitive Biases

One dimension on which anxiety and depression are proposed to differ is an individual's perception of control, or the ability to influence events in one's environment through behavioral contingencies that result in positive or negative outcomes (Alloy, Kelly, Mineka, & Clements, 1990). Specifically, an anxious state occurs in the context of uncertainty about one's ability to control the outcomes of a situation (i.e., "uncertain helplessness"). Affect characterized as mixed anxiety–depression develops as the lack of control increases (i.e., "certain helplessness"). Depressed affect occurs when an individual's perception of control is entirely reduced and a negative outcome is certain (i.e., "hopelessness"; Alloy et al., 1990; Chorpita, 2001; Chorpita & Barlow, 1998). Although anxiety and depression may potentially be distinguished by the level of perceived control, it is important to note that perceived control is a common element to both anxiety and depression, thereby highlighting the similarities of these states of NA and the progression of anxiety into depression (Alloy et al., 1990; Chorpita & Barlow, 1998). Differences then, are a matter of degree, not of the presence or absence of low perceived control.

Just as the perception of loss of control can immediately result in NA within a particular situation, so too can an individual's historical experiences with perception of low control increase the vulnerability for long-term anxiety or depression (Chorpita & Barlow, 1998). For example, a child who has repeated experiences during childhood that allow her to understand the relationship between her behavior on the one hand, and the attainment of rewards and avoidance of punishment on the other, develops a sense of mastery over her environment. In contrast, a child whose rewards and punishment are not contingent on his behavior may develop a sense of diminished control and the expectation of negative outcomes regardless of his behavior. In future situations with the potential for negative outcomes, the first child is likely to realize the potential for control, thereby decreasing the likelihood that she will experience anxiety or depression, whereas the second child is likely to feel anxious or depressed as a result of his expectation of a negative outcome that he is unable to avoid. In terms of differentiating between anxiety and depression, the matter of a history of control-related experiences again appears to be one of degree, with depression involving a greater perceived lack of control relative to GAD.

Other research that has evaluated the different cognitive manifestations of anxiety and depression has focused specifically on rumination and worry. Rumination is characteristic of depression and has been found to be negatively valenced and focused on past events, whereas worry—characteristic of anxiety—has been shown to be negatively valenced but focused more on future events (e.g., Segerstrom, Tsao, Alden, & Craske, 2000). A recent study with adult women that replicated these findings with respect to temporal orientation also found that worry had greater chronicity, unpleasantness, and feelings of insecurity, whereas rumination was felt to be more realistic in nature. Less is known about such differences in children, and the research on the specificity of content in children's cognitions across anxiety and depression has shown somewhat mixed findings (e.g., Ronan & Kendall, 1997).

In summary, when a child's symptom presentation and course are clear, differential diagnosis may be straightforward. In other cases, however, the quality of the assessment protocol is integral in determining differential diagnosis and developing the most appropriate treatment plan. In general, symptom patterns and the degree of PA and perceived control appear to be among the best domains by which differential diagnostic decisions between anxiety and depression may be informed.

CASE FORMULATION: CONCEPTUAL MODEL OF ASSESSMENT AND TREATMENT

Case Presentation

Erin was a 14-year-old girl referred to the University of Hawaii Child and Adolescent Stress and Anxiety Program by school staff for difficulties with emotional functioning and absenteeism. Erin and her mother attended the diagnostic intake interview. At the time of the assessment, Erin lived with her parents, her 18-year-old sister, and her 5-year-old brother. Erin reported that she got along "OK" with her father and had an especially close relationship with her mother, with whom she often spent her free time. She indicated, however, that her parents occasionally argued, and that she worried that they would get divorced.

At the time of the assessment, Erin was a ninth-grade student. Erin reported that she did not enjoy attending school, indicating that the classes were difficult and other students were "mean." Although her grades during earlier school years consisted of mostly B's, Erin and her mother reported that after entering high school, her grades dropped to D's and F's. Erin's mother indicated that Erin's grades declined as a result of her inconsistent school attendance. Erin's teachers were concerned because Erin rarely participated in class, did not socialize with other students, and often refused to turn in her schoolwork to be graded and to take exams. Her school counselor indicated that Erin's attendance had decreased to the point that "seeing her 2 days a week at school was a good week." More concerning, however, was that Erin recently had been hospitalized overnight following a "nervous breakdown," as her mother described it. Specifically, Erin had become inconsolably distraught following an incident in which she tripped and fell at school in front of a group of older students who then laughed at her. Erin's mother indicated that she had allowed Erin to stay home from school for a few days following this incident, and that she was having significant difficulty getting Erin to return to school. Erin had not attended school at all in the 2 weeks prior to the assessment.

Erin, her mother, and her school counselor all reported that Erin had a best friend, but overall had fewer friends than other youth her age and experienced difficulty initiating friendships because she worried what other people thought of her. Erin reported that she often felt tongue-tied in social situations, and that she had stopped eating lunch at school following an incident in which a boy teased her about her weight. Erin's mother indicated that Erin had been "shy" since early childhood, had always preferred to remain close to home, and had been diagnosed with and successfully treated for SAD when she was in elementary school. Erin indicated that she preferred staying home from school because she did not have to face the other students and she could babysit her brother. Erin's mother noted that Erin had also begun "acting out," and she recounted a recent incident during which Erin locked herself in her room when her mother was having company.

Erin and her mother also reported that Erin had recently begun experiencing frequent feelings of sadness. Specifically, both indicated that Erin had felt sad every day for the 9 days prior to the assessment. Both Erin and her mother indicated that Erin's feelings of sadness started after she told her best friend's secret to a classmate, who then revealed to the best friend that Erin had broken her confidence. Erin reported that this incident had caused her to become distressed to the point that she had cried uncontrollably at home for an extended period of time and could not stop thinking about the situation. Erin's mother reported that Erin believed "everyone hated her."

Erin's case provided a number of areas of consideration for differential diagnosis. In terms of general areas of concern, Erin's behavior suggested possible difficulties with oppositionality (e.g., school truancy, refusing to turn in schoolwork and take exams, and locking herself in her room when company arrived), anxiety (e.g., discomfort with eating lunch at school, not participating in class, feeling tongue-tied, several areas of worry), and depression (e.g., recent sadness, rumination). Oppositional defiant disorder was an unlikely diagnosis, however, because Erin's oppositionality was not pervasive and characterized by anger; rather, it seemed to occur in response to anxiety-provoking situations.

With regard to anxiety, it was important to consider whether Erin's feelings and behavior were normal. Erin had recently entered high school, where the schoolwork was difficult and she had to meet new people, at least one of whom had teased her. Anxiety in such a situation might be considered normal, although Erin exhibited behaviors that appeared excessive (e.g., completely avoiding lunch out of embarrassment and extreme distress following her tripping incident, and being teased about her weight). Additional information regarding Erin's temperament and past history with anxiety, however, suggested that her symptoms were chronic, pervasive, and clinically significant, but more detailed information was required to determine which anxiety disorder best characterized Erin's difficulties. Erin's feelings of sadness, however, were not necessarily excessive in light of her discord with her best friend, especially because she did not have many other friends. Additionally, her sadness had persisted less than the 2-week period required for a depressive disorder diagnosis, and she reported no concomitant symptoms directly related to her sadness; therefore, a depressive disorder was not diagnosed at the time. During treatment for anxiety, however, it would be important to monitor these symptoms and intervene if they did not improve.

Assessment

Diagnostic Interviews

Structured and semistructured interviews can be particularly useful in the early phases of assessment, because they provide a general survey of difficulties and may elucidate difficulties other than the client's presenting problem. The structured diagnostic interview is considered the current "gold standard" for clinical diagnosis (Edelbrock & Costello, 1990; Matarazzo, 1983). Compared with unstructured interviews, structured diagnostic interviews offer superior reliability through clear specification of the diagnostic areas to be assessed and their use of a standard format to reduce interviewer bias (DiNardo, O'Brien, Barlow, Waddell, & Blanchard, 1983; Edelbrock & Costello, 1990). These properties are important given the particularly differentiated nature of anxiety disorders and the increasingly explicit diagnostic criteria in recent DSM revisions (e.g., DSM-IV-TR; APA, 2000).

One of the most commonly used structured interviews for childhood anxiety disorders is the Anxiety Disorders Interview Schedule for DSM-IV, Child and Parent Versions (ADIS-IV-C/P; Silverman & Albano, 1996), which are structured clinical interviews for children and parents designed specifically for DSM-IV diagnoses of childhood anxiety disorders, mood disorders, and selected behavior disorders. A particular strength of the ADIS-IV-C/P is its detail with respect to multiple parameters of anxiety disorders. For example, it often directs the interviewer to inquire about the severity, intensity, interference, avoidance, or uncontrollability of fear and anxiety, both at symptom and syndrome levels with each diagnosis. Separate diagnostic profiles are derived from separate parent and child interviews, which are combined to form a consensus diagnosis (Silverman & Albano, 1996). Good to excellent interrater reliability has been demonstrated for the ADIS-IV-C/P (Silverman, Saavedra, & Pina, 2001).

One of the main limitations of the ADIS-IV-C/P is its lengthy administration time, with interviews for children and parents totaling approximately 4–5 hours, not including scoring, interpretation, or report writing. Given this potential challenge, some practitioners might choose to administer only portions of the structured interview that seem relevant. Such an approach could base the selection of interview sections on those disorders that appear to be likely candidates based on other information gathered. Few, if any, studies support this strategy of partial administration; however, this general approach to structured interviewing was outlined in some detail by Chorpita, Yim, and Tracey (2002) and showed considerable promise in Monte Carlo simulations.

Case Assessment

Accurate diagnosis of Erin's difficulties was a necessary step in establishing a treatment plan. It appeared that Erin was experiencing clinically significant difficulties with anxiety, but additional information was needed to determine the exact nature of her problems. Erin and her mother were interviewed separately by the same therapist using the ADIS-IV-C/P. The chronicity and pervasiveness of Erin's difficulties with anxiety were apparent, but the ADIS-IV-C/P interviews yielded information essential to the differential diagnosis among anxiety disorders. Erin and her mother reported that since elementary school, Erin had been extremely nervous in a number of situations, including answering questions in class, reading aloud in front of her classmates, asking teachers a question or for help, taking tests, participating in PE (physical education or "gym") class, starting or joining in on a conversation with others, eating in front of others, and speaking to adults. Erin sometimes became very agitated and refused to engage in the indicated activity (e.g., giving a speech). Additionally, both reported that Erin frequently worried what other people thought of her, and feared that others thought she was stupid. Since starting high school, Erin had also begun to worry about how she was doing in school. Moreover, Erin indicated that she also worried that her parents would divorce following their occasional arguments. This information suggested two possible diagnoses: social phobia and GAD. Erin was diagnosed with social phobia based on her fear of social and evaluative situations that had persisted for at least 6 months. With regard to GAD, Erin indicated that she worried about the stability of her parents' relationship only on those occasions when they argued, and that she was able to alleviate her anxiety about the possibility of divorce after she witnessed her parents make up, thereby indicating her ability to control her worry in this domain. It appeared that Erin's worry, therefore, was primarily confined to social situations, and was thus subsumed under a social phobia diagnosis. Her recent worry regarding her academic progress appeared to be appropriate given that she was failing, and her worry had neither persisted the 6 months required for a GAD diagnosis nor was it accompanied by somatic complaints; therefore, a GAD diagnosis was not warranted in Erin's case.

Self-Report Measures

Self-report of anxiety and depression is one of the best and most efficient ways to gauge the nature and intensity of a youth's difficulties, and self-report instruments complement structured interviews within an assessment battery. One of the benefits to using self-report measures is their easy administration. This may allow for the administration to several individuals who know the child (e.g., parents, teachers, etc.), thereby providing information about the child's behaviors from different perspectives and in different contexts. Additionally, self-report instruments are easily administered across multiple occasions (e.g., pre- and postintervention), thereby providing a baseline against which change may be measured. A second advantage is that sometimes clients feel less self-conscious about reporting their difficulties on paper, as opposed to a face-to-face interview.

Self-report measures generally take the form of written rating scales and may survey a broad array of behaviors (broad-band), or they may be more circumscribed in focus (narrow-band). Broad-band measures are those that index an entire domain, typically offering multiple scales that tap relatively different dimensions of anxiety or depression. The advantage is that they provide information regarding different aspects of anxiety or depression across a broad range of dimensions. Disadvantages are that they may provide comparatively less information about each specific dimension than might be found using narrow-band measures, and that they may involve more items and a longer administration time.

Narrow-band measures are those that focus their assessment on a particular dimension within the anxiety or depression domain. For example, a narrow-band instrument might measure depression, social anxiety, worry, or separation anxiety only. Such scales can still have multiple dimensions or subscales, but these all load on the single, narrow dimension of interest. Narrow-band measures may be useful for getting lots of information about a specific area, but they are less useful when there is interest in multiple areas of anxiety or depression. An alternative to the use of domain measures is to administer many different narrow-band measures, although administration time can be prohibitive.

One broad-band measure, the Revised Child Anxiety and Depression Scales (RCADS; Chorpita, Yim, Moffitt, Umemoto, & Francis, 2000) is a 47-item, self-report questionnaire for children and adolescents ages 8–18, with six subscales corresponding to SAD, Social Phobia, GAD, Panic Disorder, OCD, and MDD. The RCADS requires respondents to rate how true each item is with respect to their usual feelings (e.g., "I worry when I think I have done poorly at something" and "Nothing is much fun anymore"). In a series of studies in both clinical and community samples, the RCADS has demonstrated excellent psychometric properties (Chorpita, Moffitt, & Gray, 2005; Chorpita, Yim, et al., 2000; De Ross, Gullone, & Chorpita, 2002). Two particular strengths are that this measure contains scales corresponding to a large number of anxiety diagnostic syndromes, which can be helpful for determining the focus of intervention, and a brief scale to assess the presence of depression. Extensive normative data are also available.

In contrast, the Penn State Worry Questionnaire for Children (PSWQ-C; Chorpita, Tracey, Brown, Collica, & Barlow, 1997), a narrow-band measure of worry in youth ages 7–17, most commonly is used to assess the dimension of generalized anxiety only. This 14-item, self-report questionnaire measures both the frequency and controllability of worry (e.g., "Many things make me worry"). The PSWQ-C has shown good psychometric properties with respect to clinical worry and GAD in youth. For example, the PSWQ-C has discriminated children with GAD from children with other anxiety disorders, and from nonclinical controls (Chorpita et al., 1997).

As mentioned earlier, anxiety and mood disorders appear to be connected by the underlying influence of NA. Understanding this tendency to react to situations with negative emotions is at the core of the intervention program; thus, the assessment of NA is of considerable importance. Assessment of NA can help the clinician with inferences about things such as the likelihood of co-occurring anxiety disorders, the propensity for the current anxiety problem to be long-lasting, and the probability of new anxiety foci emerging over development. Another affective dimension specifically inversely related to depression is that of PA (Clark et al., 1994). Measuring PA can be helpful as well, particularly in terms of identifying the presence of depression or determining which youth are at risk of becoming depressed in the future. In that sense, PA is one of the dimensions that best discriminates between youth with anxiety and those with depression (e.g., Chorpita & Daleiden, 2002; Lonigan, Carey, & Finch, 1994). At present, the two best-evaluated measures of these dimensions in youth are the Affect and Arousal Scales (Chorpita, Daleiden, Moffitt, Yim, & Umemoto, 2000) and the Positive and Negative Affect Schedule for Children (Laurent et al., 1999), which are summarized below.

The Affect and Arousal Scale (AFARS) is a 27-item, self-report questionnaire for youth designed to measure PA and NA, along with the dimension of PH. The PH scale measures the presence of autonomic symptoms, such as breathlessness, rapid heartbeat, and sweating. As mentioned previously, PH has been found to be associated with some anxiety disorders in youth, most notably panic disorder (Chorpita, 2001; Chorpita, Plummer, et al., 2000). The AFARS asks respondents to endorse how true items are (e.g., "I get upset easily," I have fun at school," "My mouth gets dry"). The psychometric properties of the AFARS have been found to be favorable in several studies (Chorpita & Daleiden, 2002; Chorpita, Daleiden, et al., 2000; Daleiden, Chorpita, & Lu, 2000).

The Positive and Negative Affect Schedule for Children (PANAS-C; Laurent et al., 1999) is another well-researched measure of affect in youth. Unlike the AFARS, the PANAS-C asks children to rate 27 individual adjectives (e.g., "sad," "blue") with respect to how often they felt that way in the past few weeks. Laurent et al. reported favorable psychometrics for this measure. In a series of comparative analyses in clinical sample, Chorpita and Daleiden (2002) found that the NA subscales of the PANAS-C and AFARS were both associated with measures of anxiety, with the PANAS-C NA subscale showing slightly higher validity coefficients. In that same study, the PANAS-C PA subscale demonstrated a clear advantage in its association with depression, although it showed some problems with discriminant validity by yielding significant correlations with measures of NA, worry, and panic.

As part of an assessment research protocol, Erin was administered the RCADS, PSWQ-C, AFARS, and PANAS-C. Erin's scores on these instruments generally converged with her reported concerns of anxiety. On the RCADS, Erin scored in the clinical range of the Social Phobia and SAD subscales. The lack of elevated scores on the GAD subscale of the RCADS and the PSWQ-C suggested that Erin's worrying was not clinically significant at the time of the assessment. Erin's scores on the NA scales of the AFARS and PANAS-C were elevated, and she obtained low scores on the PA scales of both instruments. Her score on the PH scale was not elevated. Overall, these scores converged with reports on the ADIS-IV-C/P that indicated Erin was experiencing difficulty with anxiety and depression.

Behavioral Observations and Tests

The information obtained from structured interviews and self- and parent-report instruments is often sufficient to determine whether a youth's difficulties reflect normatively extreme manifestations of NA, or whether an anxiety or depressive disorder diagnosis is warranted. In some cases, however, the clinician is challenged to synthesize different information based on informant perspectives. When oral reports from multiple informants fail to yield a clear picture of the problem, behavioral observation may be extremely useful. Because observation procedures typically are more costly and demanding than self-report methods, observation is best used when it is expected to provide important new information about the child's problem that is not available by other means. Additionally, observation may yield detailed information that is valuable to developing the treatment plan and monitoring treatment progress.

BEHAVIOR AVOIDANCE TEST

A classic procedure for behavioral observation of fear or anxiety is the behavioral avoidance test (BAT), in which an individual is observed encountering a feared stimulus (e.g., Melamed & Siegel, 1975). With such a procedure, the youth is gradually brought into increasingly closer contact with the stimulus and is usually asked to provide subjective ratings of fear. For example, a child might be asked to rate his or her level of fear on a 1- to 10-point scale every minute or so during the test. Other variables obtained include length of time to approach the stimulus, distance traveled toward the stimulus, or time in contact with the object or time spent in a feared situation (Strauss, 1993). BATs can be conducted in laboratory or naturalistic settings and have been used to assess a variety of fears, including fear of heights (Van Hasselt, Hersen, Bellack, Rosenblum, & Lamparski, 1979), blood (Van Hasselt et al., 1979), and animals (Evans & Harmon, 1981).

The benefits are that such procedures may be designed specifically for the treated youth (e.g., with a highly specific stimulus that best approximates the presenting anxiety problem), and that they allow for assessment of multiple responses, such as physiological reactivity, avoidance strategies, or social skills. For example, in a social anxiety behavior test, a youth might asked to give a brief speech to three peers. The assessor could not only take fear ratings but also observe or even code the social performance of the youth (e.g., was there good eye contact; was the voice clear and slow?), using these results to provide feedback for improvement. Overall, the BAT is one of the best methods for determining frequency and severity of behaviors and symptoms, but again, its use must always be weighed against its cost and inconvenience.

BEHAVIORAL OBSERVATION

Behavioral observation is important when the purpose of the assessment is to identify functional relations or contingencies related to the maintenance of a particular behavior (Haynes & O'Brien, 2000). For example, behavioral observation is well-suited to examining the environmental contingencies of a child's school refusal behavior but less informative regarding an individual's particular diagnosis. Behavioral observations can occur in natural or analogue settings, the latter of which are purposefully manipulated to test hypotheses regarding factors potentially related to the behavior. Ideally, behavioral observations should be conducted in situations to which the child is frequently exposed, and should be performed on multiple occasions. As with the BAT, benefits of the information derived from behavioral observation must be considered in relation to its cost and inconvenience. If behavioral observation is not feasible, there exist multiple measures that can help to illuminate motivation and contingencies for behavior, including the Motivation Assessment Scale (Durand & Crimmins, 1988) and the School Refusal Assessment Scale (Kearney, 1995).

In Erin's case, it was apparent from the information obtained from the interview and questionnaires that because Erin feared social situations, the benefit of conducting behavioral observations of Erin in social situations would be minimal. At the same time, Erin's school avoidance was a significant problem that needed to be addressed early in treatment rather than after an entire procession of exposure exercises. The assessor conducted behavioral observations to gather more information about Erin's absenteeism. Three days in a row, the assessor went to Erin's house in the morning, before she was supposed to leave for school. On the first day, Erin woke up late, and her mother implored her to hurry so she could drop Erin at school before leaving for work. Erin, however, hit her "snooze" button for an hour, after which her exasperated mother left for work without taking Erin to school. In this situation, Erin's delay in getting out of bed resulted in staying home from school. Because Erin preferred staying home over going to school, her behavior appeared to function as an escape or avoidance tactic. On the second day, Erin's mother told her that if she got up and went to school, then they would go to the movies that night. Again, Erin's mother left for work before Erin got out of bed. In this situation, it appeared that the reward for getting ready for school was not immediate or attractive enough to Erin to provide an adequate incentive for Erin to endure the unpleasantness of school. On the third day, Erin's mother closely supervised her daughter's morning routine, and Erin made it to school a half-hour late. At lunchtime, however, after receiving a distressing call from her daughter, Erin's mother picked her up from school and took her home. These three situations provided the assessor with important information regarding the environmental contingencies of Erin's anxiety that needed to be addressed to promote her school attendance.

Monitoring

Monitoring entails having individuals complete observation forms that help them collect information about problem behaviors, as well as antecedents and consequences, over a specified time period. Monitoring is relatively easy to conduct with multiple people across multiple occasions. Additionally, it illuminates discrepancies between what people say they do and what they observe themselves doing, thereby potentially increasing the reliability of the assessment information. For example, parents may say they ensure that their child complies with a task demand, but monitoring may indicate that if the child has a tantrum or sulks enough, than he or she escapes the demand. Two drawbacks to monitoring, however, are the tendency of people to forget to complete the forms and the possibility that monitoring may result in a behavior change as self-awareness is increased.

At one point during treatment, when it appeared that Erin's depressive symptoms were worsening, her therapist asked her to keep a log of her moods and activities for one week. Specifically, every 2 hours, Erin rated her mood and noted the activity in which she was involved. Additionally, Erin indicated what, if anything, she was able to do to improve her mood. After reviewing this information, the therapist was able to identify some evident patterns in the logs, such as an improvement in mood when Erin spent time with her best friend, and a worsening of mood when she was home alone watching television. With this information in hand, the therapist was able to incorporate brief behavioral interventions aimed at improving Erin's mood within the larger context of the intervention for her anxiety.

Link between Assessment and Treatment

Proper assessment is of primary importance in the delivery of interventions for youth seeking treatment for anxiety and depression difficulties. An assessment approach targeting multiple domains—as outlined earlier—allows for the development of an integrated clinical formulation, which in turn determines the course of action in treatment.

Although there exist multiple models for case formulation (e.g., Haynes & O'Brien, 2000; Linehan, 1993; Nezu & Nezu, 1989; Persons, 1989), they share components that provide clinicians with strategies useful to making treatment-related decisions. The first step generally entails the identification and specification of a youth's difficulties, as well as their relative importance to each other (Haynes & O'Brien, 2000). Relative importance may be determined in part by the impairment in functioning or degree of distress that the problem causes for the youth. The second step involves the recognition of important environmental or contextual influences that may contribute to the onset or maintenance of a youth's difficulties. The third step requires the identification of the best intervention strategy to target a youth's difficulties.

It is important to remember that case formulations are dynamic; thus, it is imperative to conduct ongoing assessments to evaluate the effects of an intervention. With the exception of the ADIS-IV-C/P, the measures described in the assessment section of this chapter may be given regularly and at low cost, and index the degree of impairment or intensity of symptoms particularly well suited for treatment evaluation. Given an intervention program that explicitly *does not* define a fixed duration, intensity, or frequency of therapy for youth, it is all the more important that measures be taken at the outset and along the way to ensure that the structure and content of the intervention is an appropriate fit for the youth's problem. With regard to anxiety and depression, weekly assessment of the youth's fear or mood ratings is an explicit part of the treatment protocol; thus, the assessment measures outlined earlier are designed to substantiate and extend these data, which serve as the primary index of clinical progress.

Interventions vary in the degree to which they are standardized versus individualized. Recent developments in cognitive-behavioral protocols have emphasized the need for increased individualization and flexibility. Although manualization has brought with it many advantages for standardization, training, and dissemination, some argue that the ability to individualize interventions according to basic cognitive-behavioral principles has been challenged (Chorpita, 1997; Persons, 1992; Wolpe, 1989). There is not uniform support for the idea that flexibility of this nature enhances treatment effects (e.g., Schulte, 1992), and debate has continued on both sides of the flexibility controversy (e.g., Persons, 1992; Wilson, 1996; Wolpe, 1989). It does seem clear that some time or effort to maintain the integrity of core strategies is related to positive outcomes, whether the intervention is flexible or not (e.g., Schoenwald & Henggeler, 2003). Ideally, interventions should strike a balance, whereby each treatment technique is outlined with specific instructions for its proper administration, but selection and ordering of techniques have some degree of latitude to accommodate individual differences in case presentations. A prime example of an intervention program that blends standardized and individualized approaches is exposure for anxiety. Because of its efficacy in treating anxiety, exposure is widely used with anxious clients; however, the foci of exposure, as well as other treatment components, such as psychoeducation, modeling, and reinforcement, may differ considerably across and within individuals over time.

The therapist identified social phobia as Erin's primary difficulty, with some symptoms of depressed mood. Evidence for the relative importance of Erin's social phobia over her sadness was provided by the course of Erin's difficulties, such that her nervousness in social situations was chronic and pervasive, whereas her depressed mood had a more recent onset and was mildly significant. Additionally, it appeared that Erin's social anxiety created significant impairment for her by escalating the importance of the incident with her best friend, exacerbating her absenteeism, and interfering with her participation in social activities. The therapist also noted that out of sympathy for her daughter, Erin's mother permitted her to miss school, which served to maintain Erin's absenteeism, thereby alleviating her school-related worries on a daily basis but sustaining her anxiety in the long run. With this information, the therapist selected an intervention that prioritized Erin's social phobia, required the involvement of Erin's mother, and elected to reassess the need for intervention for Erin's depression after her anxiety improved.

Treatment

Preview

The ultimate goal of an intervention for anxiety or depression is to provide a youth with the tools he or she needs to demonstrate short-term and maintain long-term improvement of symptoms. The premise of the treatment approach outlined here, and of cognitive-behavioral therapy in general, is that thoughts and behaviors are related to emotions. Although the collective evidence on anxiety and depression suggests that a similar set of biological, psychological, and social influences operates on the youth and likely involves the general temperamental risk factor of NA (Albano et al., 2003; Barlow, Chorpita, & Turovsky, 1996), the cognitive-behavioral strategies used to address anxiety and depression differ. Currently, no single intervention targets NA in general; rather, efficacious interventions are based on the underlying syndrome of either anxiety or depression.

At the same time, to the extent that NA disorders are characterized by negatively biased thought and avoidance/withdrawal, the treatment methods for NA collectively encourage objective reappraisal of objects and events and approach/engagement with the environment. For example, consider activity scheduling, a technique commonly incorporated in treatment of depression, and exposure, primarily used to address anxiety. Activity scheduling involves the introduction of mood-enhancing activities into a youth's day (Weisz, Thurber, Sweeney, Proffitt, & Le Gagnoux, 1997), and exposure involves a youth's contact with anxiety-provoking situations (Chorpita & Southam-Gerow, 2006). Activity scheduling and exposure are actually more similar than they are different. Both involve doing things that the client believes will be emotionally unpleasant due to cognitive misinterpretation, and both serve as behavioral experiments to allow for corrective emotional learning and changes in reinforcement. Specifically, activity scheduling provides an individual with evidence for the relationship between positive activities and feeling good, and serves to increase positive reinforcement, thereby improving mood, because low rates of positive reinforcement have been hypothesized to be an antecedent of unipolar depression (Lewinsohn, Biglan, & Zeiss, 1976). Similarly, exposure provides the evidence needed for a youth to reassess the threat involved in a feared situation, and promotes successful anxiety management as the reinforced behavior rather than avoidance. In the adult NA disorders literature, work is currently underway to identify core underlying features of NA disorders, such as negatively biased thought and avoidance described earlier, to be targeted by a unifying treatment (e.g., Barlow, Allen, & Choate, 2004).

As noted earlier, based on information obtained from the assessment, the therapist selected an intervention that prioritized Erin's social phobia and elected to reassess the need for intervention targeting Erin's depression after her anxiety improved. Therefore, the therapist selected a manualized intervention that satisfied three conditions:

1. The intervention would address Erin's misperceptions of threat and decrease her anxiety. By learning new skills with which to evaluate scary situations, Erin would be able to distinguish real from imagined threat ("false alarms") and identify when her anxiety was unnecessary.

2. The selected intervention was designed to generalize to other anxiety-based difficulties not necessarily related to social situations. By focusing on the core common features across all anxiety disorders, it would be possible to address other anxiety-based difficulties during treatment (e.g., worry or separation anxiety) with the use of a single manual.

3. The treatment program was a flexible protocol that permitted the development of an individualized treatment plan selected from a collection of established techniques for disorders related to NA. This type of intervention allowed the therapist to match the intervention components and strategies to Erin's specific difficulties. (For a detailed illustration of modularity, please see Chorpita, Daleiden, & Weisz, 2005b.)

Treatment Process

Use of a set of evidence-based techniques provides a strong foundation for successful treatment. At the same time, however, other facets of therapy for the therapist to consider at the beginning and throughout the intervention—therapy process—include youth and family engagement, and unexpected circumstances, attention to which can set the stage for positive treatment outcomes.

YOUTH ENGAGEMENT

"Engagement," defined as the youth's and the family's active and collaborative participation in the intervention, is essential to the long-term success of the therapeutic process. As such, at the outset of treatment, rapport-building exercises are an important part of any good cognitive-behavioral therapy (CBT) approach. Because no single activity appeals to all youth, it is important for the clinician to be creative, drawing on his or her own best skills in connecting with a client, and to remember that although the relationship may be critical in creating a safe environment for learning those skills that ultimately reduce symptoms, the therapeutic relationship itself does not reduce NA, nor is it the primary goal of therapy. For that reason, it is advisable to make the purpose of therapy clear from the very beginning, and always to connect activities back to that central theme.

Keeping in mind that Erin experienced anxiety regarding her social impressions, the therapist designed an age-appropriate, rapport-building exercise designed to elicit some moderately personal information. Both the therapist and Erin wrote down their favorite books, movies, and food, as well as who each would like to be, if she could be someone else. When the therapist named "Harry Potter" as the person she would like to be, Erin glanced at her in surprise and chuckled, because she had not expected an adult to be so familiar with a teenage character. As Erin shared her favorites, the therapist expressed interest and initiated additional conversation on each topic. In the end, the exercise was successful, because it helped the therapist to establish rapport with her client and also connected back to a primary goal of treatment: to allow Erin to experience success in a social situation.

FAMILY ENGAGEMENT

Treatment progress is often bolstered by the involvement of caregivers, so it is necessary to monitor family engagement in therapy. Although there is a scarcity of well-designed research on engagement for treatment of internalizing disorders (for strategies to increase engagement in treatment for externalizing disorders, see Nock & Kazdin, 2005), research has identified that attrition (premature termination of therapy) in the context of other treatments can be predicted by certain demographics (i.e., low socioeconomic status, membership in a minority group, having a single-parent family, being on public assistance, and adverse child-rearing practices) and perceived barriers (i.e., perceived family stressors and obstacles, perceived treatment relevance, and relationship with the therapist; e.g., Kazdin, Holland, & Crowley, 1997).

It is important to implement strategies to improve engagement as soon as the therapist recognizes a problem. Families challenged by divorce, poverty, transportation issues, and the like, are often perceived to be continually in "crisis mode." Such families may benefit from involvement in problem-solving exercises to map their priorities and identify the steps to achieve them (e.g., Nock & Kazdin, 2005). A skilled therapist can introduce a plan—which may or may not prioritize the obstacle as a short-term target for intervention—that will clarify the next steps the family must take if the youth's treatment program is to have the best chance for success.

Frequently, though, even without major obstacles, families experience a burden when a child is involved in therapy, because their already busy lives are filled with competing demands. These families may or may not be at risk for attrition, or their engagement difficulties may be manifest as impaired collaboration (participation in some aspects of the intervention program, without proper performance of particular critical aspects, such as homework assignments, role plays, etc.). Providing information about the challenges of therapy may remedy this issue. Families should be told that CBT requires practice, and usually at least some minimal observation or documentation of feelings, thoughts, or behaviors. Therapists can emphasize that this is a short-term–long-term trade-off; whereas the work and stress in the short term might increase, the advantage is that the problems in the long run should be minimized. In many instances, providing this knowledge up front inoculates the family by making the challenges predictable and time-limited. Additionally, it may be necessary to simplify the procedures of therapy or to reduce the demand of the paperwork or monitoring associated with CBT to allow therapy to fit better into the context of busy daily lives.

Furthermore, some families do not recognize the relevance of CBT in addressing their child's difficulties. For many families, therapists need to focus on making the success of the child as obvious and dramatic as possible. Frequent praise and review serve to highlight the advantages and the benefits of staying with the program. Sometimes it helps to go after the high-priority targets first (i.e., those fears that have the greatest effect in impressing the family or alleviating their own worries).

At the initial treatment session, the therapist explained the importance of Erin's mother's involvement in therapy. Erin's mother expressed interest in participating in therapy but indicated that she worked two jobs, which precluded her attendance at many of the treatment sessions. Rather than holding treatment sessions at the clinic, the therapist offered to hold sessions at a location in the family's neighborhood, so that Erin's mother could attend at the end of the workday. This not only provided a convenient solution to a potential engagement obstacle but it also decreased the social distance of the therapist, thereby increasing her relevance and credibility with the family. On days when Erin's mother absolutely could not attend the session, she and the therapist agreed to discuss the session's content and Erin's progress by phone.

In some cases, despite a clinician's best efforts, it is nearly impossible to engage a youth and family to participate fully at all times. Under such circumstances, it is nevertheless possible to achieve a positive outcome. For example, in the investigation by Chorpita, Taylor, Francis, Moffitt, and Austin (2004), one of the participants had no parent willing to see or talk with the therapist. Nevertheless, a positive outcome was achieved. Such families should be told that there are costs to minimizing parent participation, and that the expected outcome for CBT without including parents tends to be less positive.

UNANTICIPATED EVENTS

Any good clinician knows that no matter how well laid out a plan, there is always a chance that the unanticipated or unfathomable will occur. Such situations may include grief related to the loss of a pet or family member, child abuse, parental psychopathology, managing academics, hospitalization, and family vacations, among a multitude of other situations. In our experience, almost every case involves at least one session devoted to troubleshooting. This "macro-level" troubleshooting involves larger and often idiosyncratic issues that seem to challenge the therapist's ability to move forward with the therapy altogether. Practicing therapists are encouraged to discuss with supervisors, colleagues, or peers (1) whether a significant issue has arisen that warrants direct attention and time away from the core clinical strategies, and (2) how that issue should be addressed in the context of the case formulation, such that the youth and family can eventually get back on track with the core procedures. Except under exceedingly rare circumstances (e.g., the emergence of a medical disorder, psychosis, the precedence of serious legal issues), the goal is to resolve the issue or incorporate it into the therapy program, such that the child can continue to engage in successful treatment for NA.

Description of Treatment Components

There exists in clinical psychology a movement toward empirically supported treatments (ESTs) that advocates the evaluation of treatments based on the empirical evidence of their efficacy in randomized controlled trials (RCTs). RCTs have provided empirical support for numerous CBT manuals for NA-related disorders (Barrett, 1998; Clarke, Rohde, Lewinsohn, Hops, & Seeley, 1999; Kendall, 1994; Pediatric OCD Study Team, 2004; Weisz et al., 1997), many of which incorporate similar treatment components in various combinations. A novel approach to thinking about commonalities across treatment protocols, recently outlined in the distillation and matching model (DMM; Chorpita, Daleiden, et al., 2005a), involves identifying the specific treatment techniques or "practice elements" (e.g., "relaxation training" or "exposure") that comprise intervention protocols to identify commonalities across successful treatment programs. In a simple example, reviews of the literature that used the DMM procedure indicated that 100% of the efficacious treatments for specific phobia involved exposure, whereas approximately 30% involved psychoeducation for the youth (Chorpita, Daleiden, et al., 2005a). A clinician presented with a client with a specific phobia can use this information to develop a treatment plan involving exposure, but perhaps omitting psychoeducation. The practice element profile for depression differs from that of anxiety, in that no element is present in all efficacious treatments. Relaxation has been present in approximately 80% of successful depression interventions, but elements such as problem solving and activity scheduling are also present in at least half of the successful interventions reviewed (Chorpita, Daleiden, et al., 2005a). At present, the DMM procedure can provide information about the frequency with which particular practice elements are present within treatment protocols and for specific populations; more research is needed to determine the extent to which practice elements are necessary and sufficient for treatment progress.

The therapeutic practice elements described in this and the following sections represent those most often present in treatments successfully targeting the negatively biased thoughts and withdrawal/avoidance behaviors of youth struggling with NA disorders (Chorpita, Daleiden, et al., 2005a). Specifically, these practice elements for anxiety (i.e., psychoeducation, exposure, self-monitoring, and cognitive restructuring) and depression (i.e., activity scheduling, problem solving, and relaxation) collectively encourage objective reappraisal of objects and events, and approach/engagement with the environment, forming the basis for Erin's treatment.

PSYCHOEDUCATION

The purpose of psychoeducation is to provide information to youth and their parents about the nature of NA difficulties and the rationale for intervention.

Additionally, psychoeducation normalizes children's difficulties and illustrates individual differences in behavior and emotions, thereby minimizing the stigma of treatment and encouraging youth participation and parental involvement in the intervention.

EXPOSURE

Based on the model that some aspects of anxiety are learned and, therefore, may be unlearned, the goal of exposure is to provide for anxious youth the skills to manage anxiety successfully through contact with anxiety-provoking situations, while decreasing avoidance of feared situations. Exposure is a gradual process that begins with identifying the feared situation and breaking it down into smaller steps, so that the youth can practice coping skills to manage anxiety successfully before attempting to approach more difficult situations. For example, exposure involving a youth who is afraid of dogs may begin with the youth looking at pictures of dogs and progress over many steps to the youth imagining petting a dog and actually standing in a room with and touching a dog. Successful anxiety management during exposure is indicated when the child exhibits habituation (levels of decreased anxiety sustained over time) to the situation. In some instances, habituation occurs quickly within a single session; in other instances, the same situation must be practiced over multiple sessions to achieve habituation. Habituation may be determined by various means, including the therapist's observation of the child's behavioral approach/avoidance and the child's quantitative rating of fear (e.g., 0, *Not at all afraid*; 10, *Extremely afraid*).

SELF-MONITORING

Self-monitoring involves the repeated collection and recording of information regarding one's behavior or emotions. During treatment, self-monitoring can illuminate areas of concern and provide important information about treatment progress.

Self-monitoring begins with identification of the target behavior or emotion that is to be monitored, such as "fear" in the case of anxiety. After a target has been identified, it is necessary to define it (e.g., a fear rating greater than 2 during exposure homework exercises indicates "fear") to increase the accuracy of the observations. Following identification and definition of the behavior, a recording procedure must be created. This entails devising a recording form and determining when (e.g., during exposure exercises) and how often (e.g., daily) monitoring will occur and what information about the behavior will be recorded (e.g., type of exposure exercise and fear ratings [0, *Not at all afraid*; 10, *Extremely afraid*]). Over time, a decrease in fear ratings regarding a targeted feared situation provides evidence of treatment progress.

COGNITIVE RESTRUCTURING

The objective is to introduce cognitive restructuring as a technique to correct negative thinking. This approach is typically used with older youth who appear to have overly negative or pessimistic ideas. This technique is particularly important if the negative or pessimistic ideas appear to be interfering with a youth's ability to engage in or benefit from other parts of the therapy program.

Cognitive restructuring often targets two types of negative thinking: probability overestimation and catastrophic thinking. "Probability overestimation" is the tendency for a youth to expect that things will go badly, when in reality, a negative outcome is unlikely. For example, some children may avoid being outside during a storm for fear that they will be struck by lightning. To counter this type of negative bias, they are taught to think of alternative outcomes to the situation (e.g., being outside and not being struck by lightning) and to estimate the likelihood of each event based on facts about the situation (e.g., number of people struck by lightning each year) and their own experiences (e.g., never having been struck or having known anyone who was struck by lightning).

"Catastrophic thinking" is the tendency for some children to expect a much worse outcome than would really occur, and to think that they would be unable to cope with the outcome. For example, a youth may fear that if he dropped the ball during a baseball game, everyone would blame him if the team lost the game. Cognitive restructuring for catastrophic thinking may include addressing both probability overestimation (e.g., how likely it is that he would blamed for the loss) and the youth's ability to cope with the feared outcome (e.g., "Is there any evidence suggesting that you would be able to cope with it, that you have coped with something similar in the past, or that the situation would not last forever?")

In summary, cognitive restructuring includes training the youth to identify thoughts, often by using a thought record or other-self monitoring tool. These thoughts are then reviewed for their accuracy, and alternatives are generated and rehearsed.

ACTIVITY SCHEDULING

Activity scheduling involves the introduction of enjoyable scheduled activities into the youth's day. This technique serves multiple purposes. First, it helps the youth understand the link between positive activities and feeling good, as well as the link between a passive, withdrawn lifestyle and feeling depressed (Reynolds & Coats, 1986; Weisz et al., 1997). Second, activity scheduling keeps a youth too busy to feel bad, because activities serve to distract the youth from negative thinking (Weisz et al., 1997). Third, activity scheduling can promote both improved mood and social relationships when a youth participates in activities with someone whom he or she likes, or activities that help others (Clarke, Lewinsohn, & Hops, 1990; Weisz et al., 1997). Last, activity scheduling can promote a youth's skills development in a certain activity (Clarke et al., 1990).

The first step in activity scheduling entails the identification of mood-enhancing activities. In addition to being designed to improve the youth's mood, it is important for the activities to be simple, free, and easily accessible almost anytime (e.g., walking a dog, calling a friend, looking through a photo album). The formality of activity scheduling for the youth can vary from choosing appropriate activities from a written list to an hour-by-hour, daily schedule of pleasant and necessary (e.g., homework, chores) activities. It is often helpful to identify social, as opposed to solitary, activities to decrease a youth's social isolation. To that end, it is useful to identify specific individuals with whom the youth enjoys spending time and participating in pleasant activities. The identification of competence-enhancing activities may improve mood by helping a youth to experience success at a task. Activity scheduling may be paired with a self-monitoring exercise, whereby the child records his or her activities and a mood rating before and after each activity to emphasize the relationship between activity and mood.

PROBLEM SOLVING

The goal of problem solving is to provide for youth a systematic way to negotiate problems that arise in everyday life (Beck, Rush, Shaw, & Emery, 1979; Weisz et al., 1997). This skill is an important one for youth with a variety of difficulties, because it provides a process by which youth can consider alternative solutions to situations. Problem solving may help youth to consider solutions of which they were unaware, to gain a sense of mastery over their environment, and to minimize the impact of a negative situation. Problem-solving strategies also help counteract cognitive biases that lead depressed and anxious youth to assume that a situation will not work out for them.

Problem-solving strategies, which are designed to address the everyday and interpersonal difficulties youth face, begin with a clear definition of the problem. First, it is necessary to identify the problem explicitly, so that youth have a concrete definition of the problem. The second step is to generate possible solutions *without* evaluating them (a process that occurs later), because youth often believe that nothing will work. The third step is to examine the possible outcomes, both positive and negative, of each solution. Following this, youth select and implement the solution that is most likely to achieve the desired outcome. The final step is to evaluate the actual effectiveness of the solution. In cases in which the desired outcome is not achieved, youth are encouraged to reconsider the alternative solutions.

RELAXATION

The first goal of relaxation training is to demonstrate what relaxation feels like to a youth who has difficulty relaxing. The second goal is to increase a youth's awareness about his or her own tension, so that relaxation exercises can be implemented. The third goal is to reduce a youth's tension just before a tension-provoking situation. When practiced regularly, relaxation exercises can also reduce general tension.

Relaxation procedures can take the form of full deep-muscle relaxation (lasting between 10 and 20 minutes; e.g., Clarke et al., 1990) or a brief "secret calming" (Weisz et al., 1997; covert and lasting just a few minutes). Deep-muscle relaxation is most often used as a general relaxation strategy, whereas secret calming techniques are well-suited to tense situations. Before beginning deep-muscle relaxation, it is important for the youth to find a quiet place and a quiet time of day to engage fully in the relaxation techniques. Deep-muscle relaxation often follows a script, with the first step calling for the youth to get into a comfortable position, with closed eyes and deep breathing. The youth is then prompted to tense progressively and relax various muscles groups, until the session ends with the youth feeling relaxed. The shorter, secret calming techniques do not require a quiet location and time of day; rather, they are designed to be done anytime and anyplace the youth feels the need to reduce tension but cannot participate in deep-muscle relaxation. After the youth is comfortably seated, secret calming may entail looking down or repeating a key word or phrase (e.g., "relax") as a cue for relaxation. Deep breathing, rather than tensing and relaxing muscle groups, is the key to relaxation in secret calming. The youth is instructed to take very deep breaths and to exhale slowly to relax. Imagery may also be incorporated into both relaxation techniques if a youth is instructed to imagine a serene place.

TROUBLESHOOTING

Troubleshooting the application of specific clinical strategies is a common therapeutic exercise. For example, a frequent complaint among youth who receive the detailed psychoeducation portion of the protocol is that the interaction with the therapist "feels like school." Because psychoeducation is one of the earliest strategies covered, too much lecturing may potentially interfere with rapport or motivation. In terms of troubleshooting, one option is to leave out much of the extra detail about how anxiety and depression work, and how emotions, thoughts, and behaviors are related. The therapist should attempt to gauge the level of the child's aptitude and curiosity and simply cover material in an appropriate way. The therapist should also use interactive activities to make sure the child is having fun. Frequent praise, high-fives, and other social reinforcers may help to keep the child focused on learning. Finally, strategies may be covered across multiple sessions. If a child appears to be learning the material and enjoying it, but time is still running short, then it is best to spread this psychoeducation over more than one session.

Another instance of the need for troubleshooting often arises in the context of implementing cognitive procedures. For example, some children appear to have difficulty distinguishing between thoughts and emotions; that is, when asked about an anxious thought, they might offer the example "I am afraid," which is simply a description of an emotional state at the time. This creates some problems for training youth in cognitive restructuring, because the initial step involves identifying unrealistically negative predictions about the outcome(s) of the feared situation. The therapist's job is to use the statement "I am afraid" as a starting point to help youth articulate a feared outcome that can be used in cognitive exercises.

THE PROCESS OF TREATMENT: STEP-BY-STEP GUIDELINES

Session 1: Building Rapport

Erin and her mother came to the clinic to meet the therapist, Kate Smith. Kate briefly described the format of the first session, the goals of which were to get acquainted and to provide a treatment overview. Following this explanation, Kate and Erin spent some time alone together engaging in various rapport-building exercises, such as those described previously. After these activities, Kate provided Erin with an overview of the treatment program, explaining that they would work together to reduce Erin's anxiety in challenging social situations by focusing on how Erin responds to her anxiety and how she thinks about things. Kate stressed the importance of in-session practice, homework, and regular attendance. To avoid overwhelming Erin, Kate provided only a general overview; more detail would be provided during upcoming sessions. Kate also introduced the fear thermometer, a 0- to 10-point scale that Erin would use to monitor her anxiety. To ensure that Erin understood how to use the rating scale, Kate asked Erin to rate her fear of various situations, such as "watching your favorite movie," "spending time with your best friend," and "seeing a shark while swimming in the ocean." Kate encouraged Erin to ask questions by saying, "Your participation in treatment is very important to me. When other teens have come to our clinic, the treatment we provide is often very different from what they have tried in the past, and it doesn't always make sense at first, so they have questions. You will probably have thoughts or questions too, and I would like to hear them." At the end of the session, Erin's mother jointed them and was given a brief synopsis of what Kate and Erin had discussed. The session ended with confirmation of their next scheduled session and a fun, rapport-building exercise involving Kate, Erin, and Erin's mother.

Session 2: Construction of the Fear Hierarchy

Kate met with Erin alone and told her that the session would be spent gathering more information about the types of social situations that make Erin anxious. Kate said, "Let's try to think of as many situations as possible that make you scared or nervous. This is a very important task, and the better we do on this, the more successful we'll be at helping your anxiety go away." Kate wrote each situation Erin generated on an index card. At one point, Erin had difficulty thinking of more situations, so Kate selected one that Erin had already noted, "starting a conversation," and created two additional situations after Erin indicated that she would feel anxious starting a conversation "with a teacher" and "with a group of students." After Erin had come up with 12 fear-provoking situations, she rated her anxiety in each situation, using the fear thermometer Kate had introduced the previous week. Kate sorted the situations in order of their fear ratings, making sure that at least one situation was rated for each scale level from 1 to 10 to have a range of items with different intensity levels, because these situations would form the basis for Erin's gradual exposure. After Erin left, Kate used these situations to create Erin's fear ladder (see Figure 5.2).

FEAR LADDER

Date: _____

Please give a rating for how scary each of these things is today. Remember to use the scale from 0 to 10.

Filled out by: (✓) child ( ) parent ( ) other _____

Speaking (answer/reading) questions in front of my class	10
Making a mistake while writing on the chalkboard	10
Starting a conversation with a group of students	9
Eating in front of others	8
Starting a conversation with a teacher	7
Starting a conversation with the nicest person in class	7
Walking in the hallways at school	6
Asking a store clerk a question	5
Sitting in the counselor's office at school	4
Eating in front of my best friend	3
Being on campus while school is not in session	2
Talking to my mom on the phone	1

FIGURE 5.2. Fear ladder hierarchy completed by Erin at the intake assessment. Instrument adapted by permission from Chorpita (2007). Copyright 2007 by The Guilford Press.

Sessions 3 and 4: Psychoeducation

Sessions 3 and 4 entailed providing psychoeducation to Erin and her mother separately to inform them about the nature of Erin's difficulties and to introduce the framework and rationale for treatment.

Kate began by explaining that anxiety has three parts: behavior, thoughts, and feelings. With assistance from Kate, Erin gave examples of how she behaved (e.g., avoided reading aloud in class), what she thought (e.g., "Everyone will laugh if I make a mistake and I won't be able to cope with it"), and how her body felt (e.g., butterflies in her stomach) when she was anxious. Through these exercises, Erin began to understand that what she thought and did, and how she felt when anxious served to increase her anxiety over time. For example, when Erin avoided an anxiety-provoking situation, her anxiety decreased in the short run, thereby reinforcing avoidance as a coping strategy. With continued avoidance over time, however, her anxiety regarding that situation actually increased, because she never had the opportunity to learn whether she could successfully handle the situation.

Kate normalized Erin's experience of anxiety by pointing out that everyone feels anxious at times, and that anxiety can alert us to danger, thereby acting as an alarm. She also explained that anxiety may sometimes be a false alarm that makes a nonthreatening situation appear scary. Collectively, this information increased Erin's awareness of cues about her anxiety and provided the foundation for intervention strategies such as exposure and cognitive restructuring. Although she was skeptical, Erin learned that CBT involving exposure would allow her to practice new behaviors (e.g., reading aloud in a small group) to change how she felt (e.g., relaxed) and thought (e.g., "No one will laugh if I make a mistake and even if someone does laugh, I can handle it"), thereby decreasing her anxiety. Although psychoeducation was the focus of Session 3, Kate reminded Erin about these principles of anxiety frequently throughout treatment. At the end of the session, she praised Erin for her attention and participation.

Providing psychoeducation to Erin's mother was very important, because she had become increasingly frustrated with Erin's behavior. Additionally, at times, she unwittingly reinforced Erin's avoidance of feared situations. Psychoeducation was provided to Erin's mother in a format similar to that provided for Erin. When Kate explained the rationale for CBT involving exposure, Erin's mother said that it would be too difficult for Erin to engage in exposure. Kate explained that exposure was a gradual process that began with identifying the feared situation and breaking it down into smaller steps to allow Erin to practice coping skills to manage her anxiety successfully before attempting to approach more difficult situations. At the end of the session, Erin's mother revealed that she looked forward to trying these new strategies, because she had gone back and forth between her own strategies of "tough love" and being "overprotective," and that neither had been effective in decreasing Erin's fears.

Session 5: Exposure

Kate met Erin and her mother in a private room at a local community center and had them each complete anxiety ratings of Erin's fear ladder items. Fear ladder ratings completed at the beginning of each session would provide self- and parent-monitoring data about Erin's treatment progress. After that, Kate and Erin met alone and discussed the practice that would take place in this and upcoming sessions to help Erin develop the skills she needed to cope with her anxiety. They reviewed Erin's fear ladder ratings, and Kate reminded Erin that exposure was a gradual process that at the start was relatively easy, and became progressively more challenging as Erin succeeded in managing her anxiety. Together, they decided to begin exposure by practicing Erin's easiest item, "talking to my mom on the phone." Kate explained that they would monitor Erin's anxiety throughout the phone call by having Erin provide anxiety ratings on the 0- to 10-point scale they had been using. "How anxious are you to call your mom?" asked Kate. Erin replied, "Four, because you are watching me and that is weird." Kate suggested that they set a goal of decreasing Erin's anxiety until it was minimal, as indicated by a rating of 0, 1, or 2. Erin called her mom, who was in another room, and approximately every minute, she provided an anxiety rating, which Kate wrote down. After 5 minutes, Kate signaled to Erin to end the conversation and provide a final rating. They reviewed the ratings—4 (before calling), 4, 3, 3, 2, 2, 1—and Erin realized that her anxiety had decreased over time as a result of practicing. "Erin, you did a great job! I think you are ready to practice something else. What can you practice that is similar to calling your mom but a little more difficult?" asked Kate. "I could call my best friend," replied Erin. "She knows I am here today, but I would still feel a little funny calling her with you sitting here." For the rest of the session, Erin practiced calling her best friend and other family members, while providing anxiety ratings during each call. At the end of the session, Erin understood that practicing helped to decrease her anxiety, and that each phone call she made had been easier than the previous call. Kate and Erin reconvened with Erin's mother and told her what Erin had accomplished during the session. They also agreed that Erin's homework would be to call family and friends on the phone, while Erin's mother sat in front of her. Finally, they made arrangements to meet at Erin's school the following weekend, so that they could practice with no one around.

Session 6: School-Based Exposure

Kate and Erin met at Erin's school on a Saturday afternoon when no one was around. They sat at a picnic table near the main office. Kate and Erin began the session by discussing Erin's homework. Erin indicated that she had practiced calling family and friends almost every night, and that over time the calls had become easier and "boring." Kate praised Erin's hard work and pointed out that her boredom was evidence that her anxiety over talking on the phone to people had decreased. After Erin completed her anxiety ratings on her fear ladder, Kate noted that Erin's anxiety rating for being on campus at that moment was 2. She asked Erin what they could do to practice something a little more anxiety provoking while on campus. Erin noted that there were many places on campus where she felt very anxious, so Kate and Erin conducted exposure exercises by going to these different locations and taking Erin's fear ratings. For example, when they approached Erin's math classroom, Erin indicated that her anxiety level was 5, because she had particular difficulty with the subject. They remained outside the classroom door taking anxiety ratings approximately every minute, until Erin reported her anxiety to be a 2. Other locations at which they conducted exposures were the cafeteria, the principal's office, and the gymnasium. Overall, Erin's exposure practice at school was very successful, but Erin downplayed her success, indicating that it was "no big deal" to come to school when no one was there. Kate praised Erin for her hard work and pointed out that although it might not seem like a big deal, Erin had just taken a big step toward managing her anxiety. Erin and Kate agreed that Erin's homework would be to practice the following day (Sunday), then to meet Kate Monday morning at the front entrance to her school for another session.

Session 7: School-Based Exposure Continued

Because Erin's social anxiety interfered significantly with her school attendance and academic achievement, Kate's plan was to get Erin back on campus as early in treatment as possible. Kate had laid the groundwork for the success of her plan by fostering rapport with Erin through warmth and praise, continually demonstrating that she respected Erin's opinion and encouraging her input with regard to exposure practice, and by helping Erin achieve early success through exposure. Although capitalizing on Erin's treatment momentum, Kate needed to ensure that exposure sessions at school were only moderately challenging so as not to overwhelm Erin.

The designated appointment time came and went, with no sign of Erin. Kate called Erin's house, and Erin's mother told her that Erin was upset and did not want to meet her at school. Kate spoke to Erin on the phone and asked her to report her thoughts as she envisioned walking onto the school campus in the morning. Erin said, "I am nervous," to which Kate responded, "You are feeling nervous. What thought is going through your mind?" Erin replied, "I am thinking that I am scared." Realizing that Erin was having difficulty distinguishing between her thoughts and her emotions, Kate asked, "What are you afraid might happen if you come to school?" Framed to elicit a "guess" about the feared consequence, this question had the intended effect when Erin answered, "I think everyone will stare at me and wonder why I haven't been in school for a while."

Kate replied, "Hmm . . . Erin, you know, I am wondering how well *you* are able to keep track of *other* people's attendance."

Erin chuckled and said, "Not well. I am always worried about what other people are thinking of me and how I am doing in school."

Kate capitalized on her response, asking, "Do you think other students also might have their own concerns?" After Erin responded in the affirmative, Kate asked, "How many people do you think would actually stare at you and wonder why you haven't been in school?"

"Probably just one or two, if they were in my class, I guess," said Erin.

Kate queried, "And if a couple people looked at you and even asked you why you haven't been in school, do you think if we came up with some responses that you could handle it?"

Following this exchange, Erin agreed to meet Kate. Kate's use of cognitive techniques helped Erin realize that what she had feared originally was unlikely to occur, and that even if something anxiety-provoking did occur, she would be able to handle it. Erin's thoughts also provided ample substance for subsequent cognitive restructuring and exposure exercises.

Upon Erin's arrival on campus, Kate praised her bravery. They spent the majority of the session taking Erin's fear ratings near the front entrance, then near the counselor's office, until Erin's anxiety was minimal in these locations. Although Erin initially intended to go home after the session, she agreed to remain inside the counselor's office until the end of the school day. This was a huge step forward for Erin, who had not attended school in 2 weeks.

Sessions 8–11: School-Based Exposure Continued

Kate planned to use multiple exposure sessions in a row to help decrease Erin's school avoidance; thus, she and Erin agreed to meet at the front entrance before school each morning that week. Erin was able to make it to school without incident each morning. Over the course of the week, Kate and Erin conducted exposure exercises in the various locations that Erin had indicated on Saturday were fear provoking, such as her math classroom. Although Erin was not ready to go inside her classroom, she was able to practice standing outside her classroom until her anxiety ratings were minimal. Erin was demonstrating both in-session and between-session habituation to her feared situations.

While Erin experienced success with exposure therapy, Kate also worked with Erin's mother to develop several strategies, based on the observations conducted during the assessment, to encourage Erin to get ready in the morning on her own. For example, Erin's mother woke Erin up instead of allowing Erin to use the alarm and hit "snooze" repeatedly. If Erin was ready on time, her mother rewarded her with a ride to school, whereas if Erin was late, she would need to take the bus. Additionally, Erin's mother told her that if she were able to attend school again every day of the following week (which she did, without Kate), they would do the fun activity of Erin's choice over the next weekend. By changing one factor contributing to Erin's absenteeism (namely, her alarm clock) and incorporating both short- and long-term rewards, Erin's mother was able to support her daughter's success.

Sessions 21–25: Addressing Therapeutic Complications

After Session 11, Erin was able to get to school on her own, where she sat in the counselor's office each day. Kate met her after school every day the following week (Sessions 12–16) to conduct exposure exercises that involved moderately challenging situations, such as sitting in empty classrooms and eating in an empty cafeteria, as well as situations that Erin had considered very difficult at the beginning of treatment, such as starting a conversation and eating in front of one or two people. Sessions 17 through 20 were held twice a week (Sessions 17 and 18 one week and 19 and 20 the next) and consisted of Erin sitting inside her classrooms during class. Kate was thrilled with Erin's progress, but Erin did not seem proud of herself. On days when she did not have a session with Kate, Erin began skipping school. Eventually, she skipped several sessions in a row with Kate.

To complicate matters, although initially engaged in treatment and continually expressing interest in being involved, Erin's mother had difficulty supporting her daughter's treatment. Kate frequently was unable to reach her by phone to talk about Erin's treatment, and Erin's mother no longer assisted her daughter with therapy homework. Kate arranged to meet Erin's mother alone to discuss engagement obstacles and to develop a plan for increasing her involvement. Erin's mother indicated that Erin had told her that therapy was not working; thus, Erin's mother reverted to strategies that had seemed to work to improve Erin's mood and decrease her anxiety in the past, such as allowing Erin to stay home from school and buying Erin material goods when she was feeling especially distressed. Understanding the underlying issue, Kate highlighted Erin's successes at that point in treatment, while providing the reference point of Erin's chronic absenteeism earlier in the school year. Kate addressed each of Erin's mother's concerns by providing additional information regarding the known long-term success of CBT for anxiety and depression, relative to the short-term and questionable success of the strategies employed by Erin's mother. By handling these issues directly, Kate assisted Erin's mother in appreciating Erin's progress and the potential for even greater improvement because of her involvement in Erin's treatment.

Addressing Erin's mother's concerns was only half the battle. Kate needed to address Erin's thoughts and concerns too. She told Kate, "I feel so dumb. I can't even go to school by myself like a normal person. Everyone must think I'm a baby."

Because it appeared that Erin's depressive symptoms were worsening, Kate asked her to self-monitor by keeping a log of her moods and activities for 1 week. Specifically, Erin rated her mood and noted the activity in which she was involved every 2 hours. Additionally, Erin indicated whether she was able to do anything to improve her mood. After reviewing this information, Kate was able to identify some patterns, evident in the logs, such as improved mood when Erin spent time with her best friend and a worsening mood when she was home alone watching television. With this information in hand, Kate was able to introduce brief behavioral interventions during each session, aimed at improving Erin's mood within the larger context of the intervention for Erin's anxiety. For example, Kate introduced the idea of activity scheduling, and she and Erin developed a list of activities that Erin enjoyed, such as hanging out with her best friend, riding her bike with her mother, and playing with her brother. Because Erin had had difficulty coping with distressing peer situations in the past, Kate taught her relaxation techniques that she could use to calm herself when at home alone and in distressing situations. Finally, Kate also taught Erin problem-solving strategies that would help her select a course of action, so that she could proactively handle distressing situations, thereby allowing her to maintain control and reduce her feelings of helplessness and hopelessness. In the end, while they continued exposure exercises during treatment sessions, Kate monitored Erin's depressive symptoms, and Erin practiced activity scheduling, relaxation, and problem solving as needed to improve her mood.

Session 35: Therapeutic Breakthrough

By this point in treatment, Erin had engaged in numerous exposure sessions with Kate. She was attending school on a regular basis, and her teachers had noted tremendous improvement in her attitude and participation in class, but there was still more practice to be done. Kate and Erin had agreed to meet one afternoon at school, but Erin did not show up. Kate was concerned by Erin's absence and was determined to address whatever issue may have arisen before it interfered with Erin's treatment. Later that day, she spoke with Erin on the phone. Erin told her that over the weekend she had been hired to work in a movie theater taking tickets, and that she had been anxious about her first day of work and had completely forgotten about her session with Kate. Kate was delighted: Not only had Erin applied for a job in a public place, but she had done it all on her own, without Kate's help. Kate praised Erin for her accomplishments and knew that this was a turning point in treatment.

Session 42: Maintenance and Relapse Prevention

The goal of this session was to demonstrate to Erin the gains she had made throughout treatment and to discuss ways she could continue practicing her skills after treatment ended, so that she could continue to improve. Kate and Erin met, and always, Erin completed her anxiety ratings on her fear ladder. Kate showed Erin a graph she had developed to plot Erin's average fear ratings across each treatment session. Whereas Erin's ratings on her initial fear ladder ranged from 1 to 10, with an average of 6, only one of the items on Erin's current fear ladder was rated above a 2: Reading–speaking in front of the class was rated as a 3. Kate asked Erin why she thought her fear ratings had gone down during treatment and Erin replied, "Because I practiced each situation until I wasn't really scared anymore." Kate praised Erin for all of her hard work during sessions. "Erin, you did a terrific job practicing by yourself too, when we were not in session. Do you think that practicing will be something that you will be able to do on your own in the future?" After Erin agreed, Kate emphasized that continued practice would keep Erin's skills sharp, much the same way that a skilled basketball player would need to keep practicing his free throws and a musician would need to keep practicing her instrument to maintain their skills levels. Together, they brainstormed situations in which Erin would be able to practice, such as talking to patrons at the movie theater, talking and reading in class, and eating in public places. Kate provided further encouragement.

> "You have made tremendous gains in your ability to manage your anxiety and your feelings of sadness. There may be times, however, when you feel very anxious or sad. This is normal and we wouldn't expect that you will never have bad feelings again. The important thing is not to become overwhelmed and upset, thinking you are back to square one. Instead, you will need to use the skills we've worked on to make yourself feel better. The difference will be that when you feel bad in the future, you will have more control over those feelings and can make yourself feel better faster."

This led to a review of strategies, such as exposure, cognitive restructuring, activity scheduling, relaxation, and problem solving, that Erin had found effective in countering her anxiety and depression during treatment.

Case Summary

Erin demonstrated considerable improvement across 47 treatment sessions with Kate. Treatment sessions had been scaled back to every other week following Session 42, and Erin required no booster or follow-up sessions.

The groundwork for successful treatment was provided by a thorough assessment of not only the symptoms comprising Erin's primary diagnosis but also other difficulties, such as worry and sadness, absenteeism, and psychosocial influences (e.g., environmental contingencies). Kate demonstrated her solid therapeutic skills by engaging Erin in treatment and maintaining strong rapport. Additionally, she not only encouraged Erin's participation in exposure but also her involvement in treatment decisions, such as what to practice. Furthermore, Kate effectively addressed therapeutic complications involving Erin and her mother. Kate's flexible application of core strategies targeting the negative thinking and avoidance common to NA disorders allowed her to individualize Erin's treatment plan within the context of effective interventions for anxiety and depression (Chorpita, 2007). What began as a set of strategies that Erin used primarily during treatment sessions developed into a personal repertoire of skills that Erin relied on in her daily life.

CONCLUSIONS

A growing body of evidence supports the tripartite model of emotion (Clark & Watson, 1991; Mineka et al., 1998), indicating that anxiety and depression appear to share a common influence (NA; Brown et al., 1998; Chorpita, 2002; Lonigan et al., 2003; Watson, Clark, et al., 1995; Watson, Weber, et al., 1995). NA accounts in part for symptom overlap among anxiety and depressive disorders. Whereas there are common cognitive, behavioral, and physiological symptoms among anxiety and depressive syndromes, there also exist differences. However, the differences appear to be a matter of degree rather than of type. Although each anxiety and depressive syndrome appears to be related to NA, the strength of the association and the specific manifestation (e.g., worry, shyness, panic, sadness) of NA differ across the syndromes, such that each anxiety and depressive disorder has its own key features (Barlow, 2002; Mineka et al., 1998).

Given that anxiety and depression share so many components, it follows that youth with anxiety or depression are almost always at risk for both, if they do not already exhibit anxiety–depression comorbidity. Thus, a therapist's skills set for addressing disorders related to NA should involve consideration of the full set of tools or elements that draw from the evidence base for anxiety and depressive disorders. A thorough assessment targeting multiple domains—as described earlier—allows for the development of an integrated clinical formulation that will determine the best course of treatment.

The overarching goal of treatment for anxiety and depression is to provide the youth with the tools he or she needs to demonstrate short-term and maintain long-term improvement. Currently, efficacious interventions are designed to target symptoms at the disorder level (i.e., anxiety or depression), rather than targeting NA in general. At the same time, however, the treatment methods for anxiety and depression collectively address the negatively biased thought and the avoidance/withdrawal characteristic of anxiety and depressive disorders. Specifically, the most common practice elements for anxiety (i.e., psychoeducation, exposure, self-monitoring, and cognitive restructuring) and depression (i.e., activity scheduling, problem solving, and relaxation) encourage objective reappraisal of objects and events and approach/engagement with the environment.

Although data are preliminary, there is some evidence to suggest that flexible, guided application of the specific CBT techniques described in this chapter may be efficacious for youth (e.g., Chorpita et al., 2004). Knowledge of what skills to apply when, and what clinical targets to prioritize, draws from a thorough, evidence-based, and theory-driven assessment. As protocols continue to be developed for these syndromes/disorders, continuing investigation and implementation of integrated or modular approaches will be important (Barlow et al., 2004; Chorpita, Daleiden, et al., 2005b).

REFERENCES

Achenbach, T. M. (1991a). *Manual for the Child Behavior Checklist/4–18 and 1991 profile*. Burlington: University of Vermont, Department of Psychiatry.

Achenbach, T. M. (1991b). *Manual for the Teacher's Report Form and 1991 profile*. Burlington: University of Vermont, Department of Psychiatry.

Albano, A. M., Chorpita, B. F., & Barlow, D. H. (2003). Childhood anxiety disorders. In E. J. Mash & R. A. Barkley (Eds.), *Child psychopathology* (pp. 279–329). New York: Guilford Press.

Alloy, L. B., Kelly, K. A., Mineka, S., & Clements, C. M. (1990). Comorbidity of anxiety and depressive disorders: A helplessness–hopelessness perspective. In J. D. Maser & C. R. Cloninger (Eds.), *Comorbidity of mood and anxiety disorders* (pp. 499–543). Washington, DC: American Psychiatric Association.

American Psychiatric Association (APA). (2000). *Diagnostic and statistical manual of mental disorders* (4th ed., text rev.). Washington, DC: Author.

Avenevoli, S., Stolar, M., Li, J., Dierker, S., & Merikangas, K. R. (2001). Comorbidity of depression in children and adolescents: Models and evidence from a prospective high-risk family study. *Biological Psychiatry, 49*, 1071–1081.

Barlow, D. H. (1988). *Anxiety and its disorders: The nature and treatment of anxiety and panic*. New York: Guilford Press.

Barlow, D. H. (2002). *Anxiety and its disorders: The nature and treatment of anxiety and panic* (2nd ed.). New York: Guilford Press.

Barlow, D. H., Allen, L. B., & Choate, M. L. (2004). Toward a unified treatment for emotional disorders. *Behavior Therapy, 35*, 205–230.

Barlow, D. H., Chorpita, B. F., & Turovsky, J. (1996). Fear, panic, anxiety, and disorders of emotion. In D. A. Hope (Ed.), *Nebraska Symposium on Motivation, 1995: Perspectives on anxiety, panic, and fear* (pp. 251–328). Lincoln: University of Nebraska Press.

Barrett, P. M. (1998). Evaluation of cognitive-behavioral group treatments for childhood anxiety disorders. *Journal of Clinical Child Psychology, 27*, 459–468.

Beardslee, W. R., Keller, M. B., Seifer, R., Lavori, P. W., Staley, J., Podorefsky, D., et al. (1996). Prediction of adolescent affective disorder: Effects of prior parental affective disorders and child psychopathology. *Journal of the American Academy of Child and Adolescent Psychiatry, 35*, 279–288.

Beck, A. T., Rush, A. J., Shaw, B. F., & Emery, G. (1979). *Cognitive therapy of depression*. New York: Guilford Press.

Bell-Dolan, D., & Brazeal, T. J. (1993). Separation anxiety disorder, overanxious disorder, and school refusal. *Child and Adolescent Psychiatric Clinics of North America, 2*, 563–580.

Bell-Dolan, D. J., Last, C. G., & Strauss, C. C. (1990). Symptoms of anxiety disorders in normal children. *Journal of the American Academy of Child and Adolescent Psychiatry, 29*, 759–765.

Biederman, J., Faraone, S., Mick, E., & Lelon, E. (1995). Psychiatric comorbidity among referred juveniles with major depression: Fact or artifact? *Journal of the American Academy of Child and Adolescent Psychiatry, 34*, 579–590.

Birmaher, B., Ryan, N. D., Williamson, D. E., Brent, D. A., Kaufman, J., Dahl, R. E., et al. (1996). Childhood and adolescent depression: A review of the past 10 years: Part I. *Journal of the American Academy of Child and Adolescent Psychiatry, 35*, 1427–1439.

Blanchard, J. J., Mueser, K. T., & Bellack, A. S. (1998). Anhedonia, positive and negative affect, and social functioning in schizophrenia. *Schizophrenia Bulletin, 24,* 413–424.

Boer, F., Markus, M. T., Maingay, R., Lindhout, I. E., Borst, S. R., & Hoogendijk, T. (2002). Negative life events of anxiety disordered children: Bad fortune, vulnerability or reporter bias? *Child Psychiatry and Human Development, 32,* 87–199.

Brady, E. U., & Kendall, P. C. (1992). Comorbidity of anxiety and depression in children and adolescents. *Psychological Bulletin, 111,* 244–255.

Brent, D. A., Kolko, D. J., Birmaher, B., Baugher, M., Bridge, J., Roth, C., et al. (1998). Predictors of treatment efficacy in a clinical trial of three psychosocial treatments for adolescent depression. *Journal of the American Academy of Child and Adolescent Psychiatry, 37,* 906–914.

Brown, T. A., & Barlow, D. H. (2005). Dimensional versus categorical classification of mental disorders in the fifth edition of the *Diagnostic and Statistical Manual of Mental Disorders* and beyond: Comment on the Special Section [Special issue: Toward a Dimensionally Based Taxonomy of Psychopathology]. *Journal of Abnormal Psychology, 114,* 551–556.

Brown, T. A., Chorpita, B. F., & Barlow, D. H. (1998). Structural relationships among dimensions of the DSM-IV anxiety and mood disorders and dimensions of negative affect, positive affect, and autonomic arousal. *Journal of Abnormal Psychology, 107,* 179–192.

Buss, A. H., & Plomin, R. (1984). *Temperament: Early developing personality traits.* Hillsdale, NJ: Erlbaum.

Campos, J. J., Campos, R. G., & Barrett, K. C. (1989). Emergent themes in the study of emotional development and emotion regulation. *Developmental Psychology, 25,* 394–402.

Chorpita, B. F. (1997). Since the operant chamber: Is behavior therapy still thinking in boxes? *Behavior Therapy, 28,* 577–583.

Chorpita, B. F. (2001). Control and the development of negative emotion. In M. W. Vasey & M. R. Dadds (Eds.), *The developmental psychopathology of anxiety* (pp. 112–142). New York: Oxford University Press.

Chorpita, B. F. (2002). The tripartite model and dimensions of anxiety and depression: An examination of structure in a large school sample. *Journal of Abnormal Child Psychology, 30,* 177–190.

Chorpita, B. F. (2007). *Modular cognitive behavior therapy for childhood anxiety.* New York: Guilford Press.

Chorpita, B. F., Albano, A. M., & Barlow, D. H. (1996). Cognitive processing in children: Relation to anxiety and family influences. *Journal of Clinical Child Psychology, 25,* 170–176.

Chorpita, B. F., Albano, A. M., & Barlow, D. H. (1998). The structure of negative emotions in a clinical sample of children and adolescents. *Journal of Abnormal Psychology, 107,* 74–85.

Chorpita, B. F., & Barlow, D. H. (1998). The development of anxiety: The role of control in the early environment. *Psychological Bulletin, 124,* 3–21.

Chorpita, B. F., & Daleiden, E. L. (2002). Tripartite dimensions of emotion in a child clinical sample: Measurement strategies and implications for clinical utility. *Journal of Consulting and Clinical Psychology, 70,* 1150–1160.

Chorpita, B. F., Daleiden, E. L., Moffitt, C., Yim, L., & Umemoto, L. A. (2000). Assessment of tripartite factors of emotion in children and adolescents: I. Structural validity and normative data of an Affect and Arousal Scale. *Journal of Psychopathology and Behavioral Assessment, 22,* 141–160.

Chorpita, B. F., Daleiden, E., & Weisz, J. R. (2005a). Identifying and selecting the common elements of evidence based interventions: A distillation and matching model. *Mental Health Services Research, 7,* 5–20.

Chorpita, B. F., Daleiden, E., & Weisz, J. R. (2005b). Modularity in the design and application of therapeutic interventions. *Applied and Preventive Psychology, 11,* 141–156.

Chorpita, B. F., Moffitt, C. E., & Gray, J. (2005). Psychometric properties of the Revised Child Anxiety and Depression Scale in a clinical sample. *Behaviour Research and Therapy, 43,* 309–322.

Chorpita, B. F., Plummer, C. M., & Moffitt, C. E. (2000). Relations of tripartite dimensions of emotion to childhood anxiety and mood disorders. *Journal of Abnormal Child Psychology, 28,* 299–310.

Chorpita, B. F., & Southam-Gerow, M. (2006). Fears and anxieties. In E. J. Mash & R. A. Barkley (Eds.), *Treatment of child disorders* (3rd ed., pp. 271–335). New York: Guilford Press.

Chorpita, B. F., Taylor, A. A., Francis, S. E., Moffitt, C. E., & Austin, A. A. (2004). Efficacy of modular cognitive behavior therapy for childhood anxiety disorders. *Behavior Therapy, 35,* 263–287.

Chorpita, B. F., Tracey, S. A., Brown, T. A., Collica, T. J., & Barlow, D. H. (1997). Assessment of worry in children and adolescents: An adaptation of the Penn State Worry Questionnaire. *Behaviour Research and Therapy, 35,* 569–581.

Chorpita, B. F., Yim, L. M., Moffitt, C. E., Umemoto, L. A., & Francis, S. E. (2000). Assessment of symptoms of DSM-IV anxiety and depression in children: A revised child anxiety and depression scale. *Behaviour Research and Therapy, 38,* 835–855.

Chorpita, B. F., Yim, L. M., & Tracey, S. A. (2002). Feasibility of a simplified and dynamic Bayesian system for use in structured diagnostic interviews. *Journal of Psychopathology and Behavioral Assessment, 24,* 13–23.

Cicchetti, D., & Toth, S. L. (1998). The development of depression in children and adolescents. *American Psychologist, 53,* 221–241.

Clark, L. A., & Watson, D. (1991). Tripartite model of anxiety and depression: Psychometric evidence and taxonomic implications. *Journal of Abnormal Psychology, 100,* 316–336.

Clark, L. A., Watson, D., & Mineka, S. (1994). Temperament, personality, and the mood and anxiety disorders. *Journal of Abnormal Psychology, 103,* 103–116.

Clarke, G. N., Lewinsohn, P. M., & Hops, H. (1990). *Leader's manual for adolescent groups: Adolescent Coping with Depression course.* Eugene, OR: Castalia.

Clarke, G. N., Rohde, P., Lewinsohn, P. M., Hops, H., & Seeley, J. R. (1999). Cognitive-behavioral treatment of adolescent depression: Efficacy of acute group treatment and booster sessions. *Journal of the American Academy of Child and Adolescent Psychiatry, 38,* 272–279.

Cole, D. A., & Turner, J. E. (1993). Models of cognitive mediation and moderation in child depression. *Journal of Abnormal Psychology, 102,* 271–281.

Costello, E. J., Mustillo, S., Erkanli, A., Keeler, G., & Angold, A. (2003). Prevalence and development of psychiatric disorders in childhood and adolescence. *Archives of General Psychiatry, 60,* 837–844.

Dadds, M. R., & Roth, J. H. (2001). Family processes in the development of anxiety problems. In M. W. Vasey & M. R. Dadds (Eds.), *The developmental psycho-pathology of anxiety* (pp. 278–303). New York: Oxford University Press.

Daleiden, E., Chorpita, B. F., & Lu, W. (2000). Assessment of tripartite factors of emotion in children and adolescents: II. Concurrent validity of the Affect and Arousal Scales for Children. *Journal of Psychopathology and Behavioral Assessment, 22*, 161–182.

De Ross, R., Gullone, E., & Chorpita, B. F. (2002). The Revised Child Anxiety and Depression Scale: A psychometric investigation with Australian youth. *Behaviour Change, 19*, 90–101.

Dienstbier, R. A. (1989). Arousal and physiological toughness: Implications for mental and physical health. *Psychological Review, 96*, 84–100.

DiNardo, P. A., O'Brien, G. T., Barlow, D. H., Waddell, M. T., & Blanchard, E. H. (1983). Reliability of DSM-III anxiety disorders categories using a new structured interview. *Archives of General Psychiatry, 40*, 1070–1074.

Duggan, C. F., Lee, A. S., & Murray, R. M. (1990). Does personality predict long-term outcome in depression? *British Journal of Psychiatry, 157*, 19–24.

Durand, V. M., & Crimmins, D. B. (1988). Identifying variables maintaining self-injurious behavior. *Journal of Autism and Developmental Disorders, 18*, 99–117.

Edelbrock, C., & Costello, A. J. (1990). Structured interviews for children and adolescents. In G. Goldstein & M. Hersen (Eds.), *Handbook of psychological assessment* (2nd ed., pp. 308–323). Elmsford, NY: Pergamon Press.

Egger, H. L., Costello, E. J., Erkanli, A., & Angold, A. (1999). Somatic complaints and psychopathology in children and adolescents: Stomach aches, musculoskeletal pains, and headaches. *Journal of the American Academy of Child and Adolescent Psychiatry, 38*, 852–860.

Evans, P. D., & Harmon, G. (1981). Children's self-initiated approach to spiders. *Behaviour Research and Therapy, 19*, 543–546.

Fennig, S., Geva, K., Zalzman, G., Weitzman, A., Fennig, S., & Apter, A. (2005). Effect of gender on suicide attempters versus nonattempters in an adolescent inpatient unit. *Comprehensive Psychiatry, 46*, 90–97.

Field, T. (1995). Infants of depressed mothers. *Infant Behavior and Development, 18*, 1–13.

Flannery-Schroeder, E., Suveg, C., Safford, S., Kendall, P. C., & Webb, A. (2004). Comorbid externalising disorders and child anxiety treatment outcomes. *Behaviour Change, 21*, 14–25.

Fombonne, E., Wostear, G., Cooper, V., Harrington, R., & Rutter, M. (2001a). The Maudsley long-term follow-up of child and adolescent depression: 1. Psychiatric outcomes in adulthood. *British Journal of Psychiatry, 179*, 210–217.

Fombonne, E., Wostear, G., Cooper, V., Harrington, R., & Rutter, M. (2001b). The Maudsley long-term follow-up of child and adolescent depression: 2. Suicidality, criminality, and social dysfunction in adulthood. *British Journal of Psychiatry, 179*, 218–223.

Goldsmith, H. H., Buss, A., Plomin, R., Rothbart, M. K., Thomas, A., Chess, S., et al. (1987). Roundtable: What is temperament?: Four approaches. *Child Development, 58*, 505–529.

Goldsmith, H. H., & Campos, J. J. (1982). Toward a theory of infant temperament. In R. N. Emde & R. J. Harmon (Eds.), *The development of attachment and affiliative systems* (pp. 161–193). New York: Plenum Press.

Goodman, S. H., Schwab-Stone, M., Lahey, B., Shaffer, D., & Jensen, P. S. (2000).

Major depression and dysthymia in children and adolescents: Discriminant validity and differential consequences in a community sample. *Journal of the American Academy of Child and Adolescent Psychiatry, 39,* 761–770.

Goodwin, R. D., Fergusson, D. M., & Horwood, L. J. (2004). Early anxious/withdrawn behaviours predict later internalizing disorders. *Journal of Child Psychology and Psychiatry and Allied Disciplines, 45,* 874–883.

Gullone, E., King, N. J., & Ollendick, T. H. (2001). Self-reported anxiety in children and adolescents: A three-year follow-up study. *Journal of Genetic Psychology, 162,* 5–19.

Gunnar, M. R. (2001). The role of glucocorticoids in anxiety disorders: A critical analysis. In M. W. Vasey & M. R. Dadds (Eds.), *The developmental psychopathology of anxiety* (pp. 143–159). New York: Oxford University Press.

Gurley, D., Cohen, P., Pine, D. S., & Brook, J. (1996). Discriminating depression and anxiety in youth: A role for diagnostic criteria. *Journal of Affective Disorders, 39,* 191–200.

Hammen, C., & Rudolph, K. D. (2003). Childhood mood disorders. In E. J. Mash & R. A. Barkley (Eds.), *Child psychopathology* (2nd ed., pp. 233–278). New York: Guilford Press.

Haynes, S. N., & O'Brien, W. H. (2000). *Principles and practice of behavioral assessment.* New York: Kluwer.

Hettema, J. M., Neale, M. C., & Kendler, K. S. (2001). A review and meta-analysis of the genetic epidemiology of anxiety disorders. *American Journal of Psychiatry, 158,* 1568–1578.

Hettema, J. M., Prescott, C. A., & Kendler, K. S. (2001). A population-based twin study of generalized anxiety disorder in men and women. *Journal of Nervous and Mental Disease, 189,* 413–420.

Hirshfeld, D. R., Biederman, J., Brody, L., Faraone, S. V., & Rosenbaum, J. F. (1997). Expressed emotion toward children with behavioral inhibition: Associations with maternal anxiety disorder. *Journal of the American Academy of Child and Adolescent Psychiatry, 36,* 910–917.

Hirschfeld, R. M., Klerman, G. L., Lavori, P., Keller, M. B., Griffith, P., & Coryell, W. (1989). Premorbid personality assessments of first onset of major depression. *Archives of General Psychiatry, 46,* 345–350.

Holmes, T. H., & Rahe, R. H. (1967). The Social Readjustment Rating Scale. *Journal of Psychosomatic Research, 11,* 213–218.

Johnson, J. H. (1982). Life events as stressors in childhood and adolescents. In B. B. Lahey & A. E. Kazdin (Eds.), *Advances in clinical child psychology* (Vol. 5, pp. 219–253). New York: Plenum Press.

Joiner, T. E., Jr., Catanzaro, S. J., & Laurent, J. (1996). Tripartite structure of positive and negative affect, depression, and anxiety in child and adolescent psychiatric inpatients. *Journal of Abnormal Psychology, 105,* 401–409.

Joiner, T. E., Jr., & Lonigan, C. J. (2000). Tripartite model of depression and anxiety in youth psychiatric inpatients: Relations with diagnostic status and future symptoms. *Journal of Clinical Child Psychology, 29,* 372–382.

Kasius, M. C., Ferdinand, R. F., van den Berg, H., & Verhulst, F. C. (1997). Associations between different diagnostic approaches for child and adolescent psychopathology. *Journal of Child Psychology and Psychiatry and Allied Disciplines, 38,* 625–632.

Kazdin, A. E., Holland, L., & Crowley, M. (1997). Family experience of barriers to treatment and premature termination from child therapy. *Journal of Consulting and Clinical Psychology, 65*, 453–463.

Kearney, C. A. (1995). School refusal behavior. In A. R. Eisen, C. A. Kearney, & C. E. Schaefer (Eds.), *Clinical handbook of anxiety disorders in children and adolescents* (pp. 251–281). Northvale, NJ: Aronson.

Kearney, C. A. (2001). *School refusal behavior in youth: A functional approach to assessment and treatment.* Washington, DC: American Psychological Association.

Kearney, C. A., Sims, K. E., Pursell, C. R., & Tillotson, C. A. (2003). Separation anxiety disorder in young children: A longitudinal and family analysis. *Journal of Clinical Child and Adolescent Psychology, 32*, 592–598.

Kendall, P. C. (1994). Treating anxiety disorders in children: Results of a randomized clinical trial. *Journal of Consulting and Clinical Psychology, 62*, 100–110.

Kendler, K. S., Gardner, C. O., & Prescott, C. A. (1999). Clinical characteristics of major depression that predict risk of depression in relatives. *Archives of General Psychiatry, 56*, 322–327.

Kendler, K. S., Neale, M. C., Kessler, R. C., Heath, A. C., & Eaves, L. J. (1992). Major depression and generalized anxiety disorder: Same genes, (partly) different environments? *Archives of General Psychiatry, 49*, 716–722.

Kendler, K. S., & Prescott, C. A. (1999). A population-based twin study of lifetime major depression in men and women. *Archives of General Psychiatry, 56*, 39–44.

Kessler, R. C., Avenevoli, S., & Merikangas, K. R. (2001). Mood disorders in children and adolescents: An epidemiologic perspective. *Biological Psychiatry, 49*, 1002–1014.

Kessler, R. C., McGonagle, K. A., Zhao, S., Nelson, C. B., Hughes, M., Eshleman, S., et al. (1994). Lifetime and 12-month prevalence of DSM-III-R psychiatric disorders in the United States: Results from the National Comorbidity Study. *Archives of General Psychiatry, 51*, 8–19.

Kessler, R. C., & Walters, E. E. (1998). Epidemiology of DSM-III-R major depression and minor depression among adolescents and young adults in the National Comorbidity Survey. *Depression and Anxiety, 7*, 3–14.

Kovacs, M., Akiskal, H. S., Gatsonis, C., & Parrone, P. L. (1994). Childhood-onset dysthymic disorder: Clinical features and prospective naturalistic outcome. *Archives of General Psychiatry, 51*, 365–374.

Kovacs, M., Devlin, B., Pollock, M., Richards, C., & Mukerji, P. (1997). A controlled family history study of childhood-onset depressive disorder. *Archives of General Psychiatry, 54*, 613–623.

Kovacs, M., Gatsonis, C., Paulauskas, S. L., & Richards, C. (1989). Depressive disorders in childhood: IV. A longitudinal study of comorbidity with and risk for anxiety disorders. *Archives of General Psychiatry, 46*, 776–782.

Last, C. G., Hansen, C., & Franco, N. (1997). Anxious children in adulthood: A prospective study of adjustment. *Journal of the American Academy of Child and Adolescent Psychiatry, 36*, 645–652.

Last, C. G., Hersen, M., Kazdin, A. E., Finkelstein, R., & Strauss, C. (1987). Comparison of DSM-III separation anxiety and overanxious disorders: Demographic characteristics and patterns of comorbidity. *Journal of the American Academy of Child and Adolescent Psychiatry, 26*, 527–531.

Last, C. G., Strauss, C. C., & Francis, G. (1987). Comorbidity among childhood anxiety disorders. *Journal of Nervous and Mental Disease, 175*, 726–730.

Laurent, J., Catanzaro, S. J., Joiner, T. E., Rudolph, K. D., Potter, K. I., Lambert, S., et al. (1999). A measure of positive and negative affect for children: Scale development and preliminary validation. *Psychological Assessment, 11,* 326–338.

Leon, G. R., Fulkerson, J. A., Perry, C. L., Keel, P. K., & Klump, K. L. (1999). Three to four year prospective evaluation of personality and behavioral risk factors for later disordered eating in adolescent girls and boys. *Journal of Youth and Adolescence, 28,* 181–196.

Lewinsohn, P. M., Biglan, T., & Zeiss, A. (1976). Behavioral treatment of depression. In P. Davidson (Ed.), *Behavioral management of anxiety, depression, and pain* (pp. 91–146). New York: Brunner/Mazel.

Lewinsohn, P. M., Rohde, P., Seeley, J. R., & Hops, H. (1991). Comorbidity of unipolar depression: I. Major depression with dysthymia. *Journal of Abnormal Psychology, 100,* 205–213.

Lewinsohn, P. M., Rohde, P., Seeley, J. R., Klein, D. N., & Gotlib, I. H. (2000). Natural course of adolescent major depressive disorder in a community sample: Predictors of recurrence in adults. *American Journal of Psychiatry, 157,* 1584–1591.

Lewinsohn, P. M., Zinbarg, R., Seeley, J. R., Lewinsohn, M., & Sack, W. H. (1997). Lifetime comorbidity among anxiety disorders and between anxiety disorders and other mental disorders in adolescents. *Journal of Anxiety Disorders, 11,* 377–394.

Linehan, M. M. (1993). *Cognitive-behavioral treatment of borderline personality disorder.* New York: Guilford Press.

Lonigan, C. J., Carey, M. P., & Finch, A. J. (1994). Anxiety and depression in children and adolescents: Negative affectivity and the utility of self-reports. *Journal of Consulting and Clinical Psychology, 62,* 1000–1008.

Lonigan, C. J., Hooe, E. S., David, C. F., & Kistner, J. A. (1999). Positive and negative affectivity in children: Confirmatory factor analysis of a two-factor model and its relation to symptoms of anxiety and depression. *Journal of Consulting and Clinical Psychology, 67,* 374–386.

Lonigan, C. J., & Phillips, B. M. (2001). Temperamental influences on the development of anxiety disorders. In M. W. Vasey & M. R. Dadds (Eds.), *The developmental psychopathology of anxiety* (pp. 60–91). New York: Oxford University Press.

Lonigan, C. J., Phillips, B. M., & Hooe, E. S. (2003). Relations of positive and negative affectivity to anxiety and depression in children: Evidence from a latent variable longitudinal study. *Journal of Consulting and Clinical Psychology, 71,* 465–481.

Matarazzo, J. D. (1983). The reliability of psychiatric and psychological diagnosis. *Clinical Psychology Review, 3,* 103–145.

McBurnett, K., Raine, A., Stouthamer-Loeber, M., Loeber, R., Kumar, A. M., Kumar, M., et al. (2005). Mood and hormone responses to psychological challenge in adolescent males with conduct problems. *Biological Psychiatry, 57,* 1109–1116.

Melamed, B. G., & Siegel, L. J. (1975). Reduction of anxiety in children facing hospitalization and surgery by use of filmed modeling. *Journal of Consulting and Clinical Psychology, 43,* 511–521.

Mineka, S., Watson, D., & Clark, L. A. (1998). Comorbidity of anxiety and unipolar mood disorders. *Annual Review of Psychology, 49,* 377–412.

Muris, P., Merckelbach, H., Gadet, B., & Moulaert, V. (2000). Fears, worries, and scary dreams in 4- to 12-year-old children: Their content, developmental pattern, and origins. *Journal of Clinical Child Psychology, 29,* 43–52.

Muris, P., Steerneman, P., Merckelbach, H., & Meesters, C. (1996). The role of parental fearfulness and modeling in children's fear. *Behaviour Research and Therapy*, *34*, 265–268.

Nezu, A. M., & Nezu, C. M. (1989). Identifying and selecting target problems for clinical interventions: A problem-solving model. *Psychological Assessment*, *5*, 254–263.

Nilzon, K. R., & Palmerus, K. (1998). Anxiety and withdrawal of depressed 9–11 year olds three years later: A longitudinal study. *School Psychology International*, *19*, 341–349.

Nock, M. K., & Kazdin, A. E. (2005). Randomized controlled trial of a brief intervention for increasing participation in parent management training. *Journal of Consulting and Clinical Psychology*, *73*, 872–879.

Pardini, D., Lochman, J., & Wells, K. (2004). Negative emotions and alcohol use initiation in high-risk boys: The moderating effect of good inhibitory control. *Journal of Abnormal Child Psychology*, *32*, 505–518.

Pediatric OCD Study Team. (2004). Cognitive-behavior therapy, sertraline, and their combination for children and adolescents with obsessive–compulsive disorder: The Pediatric OCD Treatment Study (POTS) randomized controlled trial. *Journal of the American Medical Association*, *292*, 1969–1976.

Persons, J. B. (1989). *Cognitive therapy in practice: A case formulation approach*. New York: Norton.

Persons, J. B. (1992). The patient with multiple problems. In A. Freeman & F. M. Dattilio (Eds.), *Comprehensive casebook of cognitive therapy* (pp. 241–247). New York: Plenum Press.

Rapee, R. M. (2003). The influence of comorbidity on treatment outcome for children and adolescents with anxiety disorders. *Behaviour Research and Therapy*, *41*, 105–112.

Reynolds, W. M., & Coats, K. I. (1986). A comparison of cognitive-behavioral therapy and relaxation training for the treatment of depression in adolescents. *Journal of Consulting and Clinical Psychology*, *54*, 653–660.

Ronan, K. R., & Kendall, P. C. (1997). Self-talk in distressed youth: States-of-mind and content specificity. *Journal of Clinical Child Psychology*, *26*, 330–337.

Rothbart, M. K. (1989). Temperament and development. In G. A. Kohnstamm, J. E. Bates, & M. K. Rothbart (Eds.), *Temperament in childhood* (pp. 187–247). New York: Wiley.

Roy, M. A., Neale, M. C., Pedersen, N. L., Mathe, A. A., & Kendler, K. S. (1995). A twin study of generalized anxiety disorder and major depression. *Psychological Medicine*, *25*, 1037–1049.

Schniering, C. A., & Rapee, R. M. (2004). The relationship between automatic thoughts and negative emotions in children and adolescents: A test of the cognitive content–specificity hypothesis. *Journal of Abnormal Psychology*, *113*, 464–470.

Schoenwald, S. K., & Henggeler, S. W. (2003). Current strategies for moving evidence-based interventions into clinical practice: Introductory comments. *Cognitive and Behavioral Practice*, *10*, 275–277.

Schulte, D. (1992). Criteria of treatment selection in behaviour therapy. *European Journal of Psychological Assessment*, *8*, 157–162.

Segerstrom, S. C., Tsao, J. C. I., Alden, L. E., & Craske, M. G. (2000). Worry and rumination: Repetitive thought as a concomitant and predictor of negative mood. *Cognitive Therapy and Research*, *24*, 671–688.

Seligman, M. E., Peterson, C., Kaslow, N. J., Tanenbaum, R. L., Alloy, L. B., & Abramson, L. Y. (1984). Attributional style and depressive symptoms among children. *Journal of Abnormal Psychology, 93*, 235–238.

Shaffer, D., Fisher, P., Dulcan, M., & Davies, M. (1996). The NIMH Diagnostic Interview Schedule for Children Version 2.3 (DISC-2.3): Description, acceptability, prevalence rates, and performance in the MECA study. *Journal of the American Academy of Child and Adolescent Psychiatry, 35*, 865–877.

Silverman, W. K., & Albano, A. M. (1996). *Anxiety Disorders Interview Schedule for Children-IV, Child and Parent Versions.* San Antonio, TX: Psychological Corporation.

Silverman, W. K., Saavedra, L. M., & Pina, A. A. (2001). Test–retest reliability of anxiety symptoms and diagnoses with Anxiety Disorders Interview Schedule for DSM-IV: Child and Parent versions. *Journal of the American Academy of Child and Adolescent Psychiatry, 40*, 937–944.

Siqueland, L., Kendall, P. C., & Steinberg, L. (1996). Anxiety in children: Perceived family environments and observed family interactions. *Journal of Clinical Child Psychology, 25*, 225–237.

Spence, S. H., Namjan, J. M., Bor, W., O'Callaghan, M. J., & Williams, G. M. (2002). Maternal anxiety and depression, poverty and marital relationship factors during early childhood as predictors of anxiety and depressive symptoms in adolescence. *Journal of Child Psychology and Psychiatry, 43*, 457–469.

Spence, S. H., Rapee, R., McDonald, C., & Ingram, M. (2001). The structure of anxiety symptoms among preschoolers. *Behaviour Research and Therapy, 39*, 1293–1316.

Strauss, C. C. (1993). Anxiety disorders. In T. H. Ollendick & M. Hersen (Eds.), *Handbook of child and adolescent assessment* (pp. 239–250). Needham Heights, MA: Allyn & Bacon.

Strauss, C. C., Last, C. G., Hersen, M., & Kazdin, A. E. (1988). Association between anxiety and depression in children and adolescents with anxiety disorders. *Journal of Abnormal Child Psychology, 16*, 57–68.

Sullivan, P. F., Neale, M. C., & Kendler, K. S. (2000). Genetic epidemiology of major depression: Review and meta-analysis. *American Journal of Psychiatry, 157*, 1552–1562.

Tellegen, A. (1985). Structures of mood and personality and their relevance to assessing anxiety, with an emphasis on self-report. In A. H. Tuma & J. D. Maser (Eds.), *Anxiety and the anxiety disorders* (pp. 681–706). Hillsdale, NJ: Erlbaum.

Thomas, A., & Chess, S. (1985). The behavioral study of temperament. In J. Strelau & F. H. Farley (Eds.), *The biological bases of personality and behavior: Vol. 1. Theories, measurement techniques, and development* (pp. 213–225). Washington, DC: Harper & Row.

Thomsen, P. H., & Mikkelsen, H. U. (1995). Course of obsessive–compulsive disorder in children and adolescents: A prospective follow-up study of 23 Danish cases. *Journal of the American Academy of Child and Adolescent Psychiatry, 34*, 1432–1440.

Thwaites, R., & Freeston, M. H. (2005). Safety-seeking behaviours: Fact or function?: How can we clinically differentiate between safety behaviours and adaptive coping strategies across anxiety disorders? *Behavioural and Cognitive Psychotherapy, 33*, 177–188.

Van Hasselt, V. B., Hersen, M., Bellack, A. S., Rosenblum, N., & Lamparski, D.

(1979). Tripartite assessment of the effects of systematic desensitization in a multiphobic child: An experimental analysis. *Journal of Behavior Therapy and Experimental Psychiatry, 10,* 51–56.

Watson, D., Clark, L. A., & Harkness, A. R. (1994). Structures of personality and their relevance to psychopathology. *Journal of Abnormal Psychology, 103,* 18–31.

Watson, D., Clark, L. A., Weber, K., Assenheimer, J. S., Strauss, M. E., & McCormick, R. A. (1995). Testing a tripartite model: II. Exploring the symptom structure of anxiety and depression in student, adult, and patient samples. *Journal of Abnormal Psychology, 104,* 15–25.

Watson, D., Weber, K., Assenheimer, J. S., Clark, L. A., Strauss, M. E., & McCormick, R. A. (1995). Testing a tripartite model: I. Evaluating the convergent and discriminant validity of anxiety and depression symptom scales. *Journal of Abnormal Psychology, 104,* 3–14.

Weisz, J. R., Thurber, C. A., Sweeney, L., Proffitt, V. D., & Le Gagnoux, G. L. (1997). Brief treatment of mild-to-moderate child depression using primary and secondary control enhancement training. *Journal of Consulting and Clinical Psychology, 65,* 703–707.

Whitbeck, L. B., Hoyt, D. R., Simons, R. L., Conger, R. D., Elder, G. H., Lorenz, F. O., et al. (1992). Intergenerational continuity of parental rejection and depressed affect. *Journal of Personality and Social Psychology, 63,* 1036–1045.

Williamson, D., Birmaher, B., Axelson, D. A., Ryan, N. D., & Dahl, R. E. (2004). First episode of depression in children at low and high familial risk for depression. *Journal of the American Academy of Child and Adolescent Psychiatry, 43,* 291–297.

Williamson, D., Ryan, N. D., Birmaher, B., Dahl, R. E., Kaufman, J., Rao, U., et al. (1995). A case–control family history study of depression in adolescents. *Journal of the American Academy of Child and Adolescent Psychiatry, 34,* 1596–1607.

Wilson, G. T. (1996). Manual-based treatments: The clinical application of research findings. *Behaviour Research and Therapy, 34,* 295–315.

Wolpe, J. (1989). The derailment of behavior therapy: A tale of conceptual misdirection. *Journal of Behavior Therapy and Experimental Psychiatry, 20,* 3–15.

Woodward, L. J., & Fergusson, D. M. (2001). Life course outcomes of young people with anxiety disorders in adolescence. *Journal of the American Academy of Child and Adolescent Psychiatry, 40,* 1086–1093.

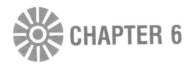 CHAPTER 6

Moodiness

Kristen Davidson and Mary A. Fristad

Bipolar disorder (BPD) is a serious and potentially incapacitating disorder that can have long-term ramifications for children and their families. Diagnosing BPD in youth is a most challenging and controversial enterprise. Clinicians and researchers continue to debate the appropriateness of the diagnostic criteria for classifying youth. Children with BPD are more likely to experience mood lability and irritability rather than the classic symptoms of mania typically observed in adults. In this chapter, the authors help us understand the symptom dimensions of moodiness and their relationship to mood and other disruptive behavior disorders. Through the case of "Jane" and her family, the authors describe their multifamily psychoeducation group (MFPG) therapy program, one of the most promising adjunctive interventions for childhood BPD. Integration with practitioners' own approaches will greatly facilitate positive treatment outcomes for this very distressed population of children and their families.—A. R. E.

INTRODUCTION

In recent decades, mood disorders in children and adolescents have increasingly gained the attention and recognition of clinicians, researchers, and the public. However, bipolar disorder (BPD) and major depressive disorder remain difficult to diagnose in this population for a number of reasons. One such difficulty is in differentiating between the "typical" moodiness and behavioral challenges that are present in children and adolescents and those that constitute a true mood disorder and require professional assessment and treatment. In addition, there is evidence that mood disorders look different in children compared to adults. Finally, the high degree of overlap between symptoms of mood disorders and other psychiatric disorders makes differential diagnosis difficult.

The challenges and controversies associated with childhood mood disorders make many professionals reluctant to diagnose them in youngsters. In this chapter, we discuss the symptom dimensions of moodiness, and their relationship to mood and other disorders as defined by the *Diagnostic and Statistical Manual of Mental Disorders* fourth edition, text revision (DSM-IV-TR; American Psychiatric Association, 2000). We also describe in detail the assessment, diagnosis, and treatment of childhood BPD using a case example.

Nature of Symptom Dimensions

Affective, behavioral, and cognitive symptom dimensions are associated with mood disorders in children and adolescents. These include affective instability, behavioral instability, and cognitive changes. Affective instability may include vacillation between periods of euphoria (i.e., intense periods of happiness or excitement), dysphoria (i.e., sadness), and/or intense irritability, and periods of euthymia (i.e., stable mood). Behavioral instability may include changes in energy level from hyperactivity (as evidenced by increased energy and restlessness, and overactive motor activity) to hypoactivity (i.e., psychomotor retardation, as evidenced by slowed motoric movements and decreased energy level). Cognitive changes may range from decreased concentration to an impulsive cognitive style. Based on how these dimensions combine, children with mood disorders may demonstrate inappropriate rage responses (i.e., a combination of irritable mood, hyperactive behavior, and impulsive cognitive style) that may be difficult to differentiate from disruptive behavior disorders, unless a careful longitudinal assessment procedure is used, as we describe below.

Relationship between Symptom Dimensions and DSM-IV-TR Diagnoses

Aspects of the symptom dimensions discussed earlier are hallmark features of a number of behavior, anxiety, or mood disorders, as defined by DSM-IV-TR. In the following section, we discuss the relationship between these symptom dimensions and DSM-IV-TR diagnoses of mood disorders. We also provide data regarding lifetime prevalence, onset, and course of mood disorders, as well as comorbidity with other psychiatric disorders.

Bipolar Disorder

DSM-IV-TR describes four types of BPD. Bipolar I disorder (BP-I) is characterized by the presence of one or more manic episodes or mixed episodes. A "manic episode" is defined by DSM-IV-TR as a distinct period of abnormally elevated, expansive, or irritable mood that lasts at least 1 week (or any duration, if hospitalization is necessary). Three or more of the following symptoms must accompany the period of mood disturbance: inflated self-esteem or grandiosity, decreased need for sleep, more talkative than usual, flight of ideas or racing thoughts, distractibility, increase in goal-directed activity or psycho-motor agitation, and excessive involvement in pleasurable activities that are likely to have negative consequences (APA, 2000). To meet criteria for a manic episode, the mood disturbance must cause marked impairment in func-tioning and must not be due to the effects of a substance or a general medica-tion condition. A "mixed episode" occurs when an individual meets criteria both for a manic episode and for a major depressive episode nearly every day during a 1-week period. Again, this mood disturbance is severe enough to cause marked impairment in functioning and is not due to the effects of a sub-stance or general medical condition. Individuals with BP-I have also usually had one or more major depressive episodes, though this is not required for a diagnosis.

Bipolar II disorder (BP-II) is diagnosed when a person experiences one or more major depressive episodes accompanied by at least one episode of hypomania. Hypomania refers to a distinct period, lasting at least 4 days, dur-ing which a person demonstrates an abnormally and persistently elevated, expansive, or irritable mood (APA, 2000). This mood disturbance must be fol-lowed by at least three (four, if the mood disturbance is irritability) of the fol-lowing symptoms: inflated self-esteem/grandiosity, decreased need for sleep, increased or pressured speech, flight of ideas, distractibility, increase in goal-directed activity, and/or excessive involvement in pleasurable activities with a high potential for painful consequences. The major distinction between hypomania and mania is that symptoms of hypomania are not severe enough to cause impairment in social or occupational functioning, or to necessitate hospitalization. Also, psychotic features are not present in a hypomanic epi-sode.

Cyclothymia is a chronic disorder (2 or more years in adults, 1 or more years in children) in which a person's mood fluctuates between periods of hypomanic symptoms and minor depressive symptoms, with no more than a 2-month period free of these mood vacillations. Finally, bipolar disorder not otherwise specified (BP NOS) includes disorders with bipolar features that do not meet criteria for BP-I, BP-II, or cyclothmia. Individuals who fall into this category include people who alternate rapidly (i.e., over several days) between manic and depressive symptoms; those whose symptoms are severe when pres-ent but do not last the requisite number of days (i.e., 4–7 days for hypomania, 7 or more days for mania); or those, for example, who fall one symptom short of meeting diagnostic criteria for BP-I or BP-II.

Researchers and clinicians continue to debate over the appropriateness of DSM-IV-TR criteria for classifying BPD in children and young adolescents (Biederman et al., 2000; Kowatch et al., 2005). Specifically, because the crite-ria for mania were developed for adults, they are frequently difficult to apply to children. Therefore, identifying the onset and offset of manic and depressive episodes may be difficult, because many children present with mixed or dysphoric mood states, with frequent periods of intense mood lability and irritability rather than classic euphoric mania as described in adult case studies of BPD (Findling et al., 2001; Geller, Zimerman, Williams, Bolhofner, Craney, & DelBello, 2000; Wozniak, Biederman, Mundy, Mennin, & Faraone, 1995). Thus, because few children meet DSM-IV-TR diagnostic criteria for BP-I or BP-II they are often placed into the BP NOS category.

Evidence also suggests that due to childhood developmental stages, symptoms of mania present differently in children compared to adults (Geller et al., 2002b; Kowatch et al., 2005). For example, whereas a hypersexual adult may have many extramarital affairs, a hypersexual 9-year-old might draw pictures of naked women or make inappropriate sexual comments to classmates.

According to Lewinsohn, Klein, and Seeley (1995), the lifetime prevalence of BPD (BP-I, BP-II, and cyclothymia) in a community sample of 1,709 older adolescents was approximately 1%, with a point prevalence of 0.53–0.64%. Additionally, 5.7% of adolescents in the sample reported core symptoms of mania that did not meet full diagnostic criteria (Lewinsohn, Klein, & Seeley, 1995). Of note, whereas parental information is considered important in making this diagnosis (Youngstrom et al., 2004), no parental information was used to derive these prevalence rates. Although BPD is not common in preadolescents, Wozniak et al. (1995) found that 16% of a sample of 262 children referred to a psychiatric clinic met DSM-III-R criteria for mania.

Misdiagnosis, including both overdiagnosis and underdiagnosis, may be common in this age group. The reluctance of some clinicians to diagnose early-onset BPD (Carlson, 1996; Weller, Weller, & Fristad, 1995) may lead to underdiagnosis. Overdiagnosis may occur due to the complex nature of differential diagnosis in children presenting with extreme irritability. Irritability is to child psychopathology what fever is to children's physical illness. Each indicates something is wrong, and in each case, it is the diagnostician's job to determine what that is. Thus, although irritability is a common feature of childhood BPD, BPD is not the most common explanation for irritability in childhood.

Major Depressive Disorder

Affective instability, behavioral instability, and cognitive changes are also consistent with a diagnosis of major depressive disorder (MDD). The hallmark feature of this disorder is the presence of one or more major depressive episodes (MDEs) in the absence of manic, mixed, or hypomanic episodes. To meet criteria for an MDE, a child or adolescent must exhibit at least five of the following symptoms during the same 2-week period: depressed or irritable mood, anhedonia, appetite changes, insomnia or hypersomnia, psychomotor agitation, fatigue or loss of energy, feelings of worthlessness or excessive guilt, difficulty concentrating, and/or recurrent thoughts of death or suicide. Estimates suggest that approximately 1% of preschool children in the general population meet diagnostic criteria for depression, with a ranges of 1–4% in clinic-referred populations (Kashani & Carlson, 1987; Kashani, Holcomb, & Orvaschel, 1986; Kashani, Ray, & Carlson, 1984). In the general population, estimates range from 0.4 to 2.5% for children and 0.4 to 8.3% for adolescents (Fleming & Offord, 1990). In clinical samples, rates have been found to range from 13 to 57% for children and 18 to 27% for adolescents (Kashani, Cantwell, Shekim, & Reid, 1982; Petersen et al., 1993; Poznanski & Mokros, 1994).

Dysthymic Disorder

Affective and behavioral instability may also suggest a diagnosis of dysthymic disorder (DD), which in children is characterized by a chronically depressed or irritable mood that occurs for most of the day, more days than not, for at least 1 year. This differs from the duration criterion for adults, which is 2 years. During periods of depressed or irritable mood, at least two of the following symptoms must also be present: appetite change, sleep disturbance, low energy or fatigue, low self-esteem, poor concentration or difficulty in making decisions, and/or feelings of hopelessness. Research has demonstrated rates ranging from 0.6 to 1.7% for children and 1.6 to 8% for adolescents (Birmaher et al., 1996; Kashani et al., 1987; Lewinsohn, Clarke, Seeley, & Rohde, 1994; Lewinsohn, Hops, Roberts, Seeley, & Andrews, 1993).

Mood Disorder Not Otherwise Specified

As defined by the DSM-IV-TR, this category includes disorders with mood symptoms that do not meet the criteria for any specific mood disorder, and for which it is difficult to choose between depressive disorder not otherwise specified and BP NOS.

Differential Diagnosis

Because, by their nature, symptoms of mania and depression wax and wane, children with mood disorders present differently at different points in time. Thus, cross-sectional snapshots of behavior are not adequate for diagnosing mood disorders in children. Instead, a clinician must conduct a longitudinal assessment of a child's symptoms, gathering information about the child's behavior throughout his or her lifetime (i.e., from birth to present) and in different settings (i.e., at home, at school, with peers). This is best done through a comprehensive evaluation that involves collecting data regarding the child's social, emotional, physical, and cognitive development from multiple sources (e.g., parents, child, teachers, other treatment providers). A number of factors should be considered in assessment for a mood disorder, including historical antecedents, biological factors, psychological and psychosocial factors, and treatment issues. These factors are briefly described below and discussed in greater detail later in the chapter, in the context of our case example.

When children or adolescents present for evaluation, it is important to gather information about their development up to that point to understand presenting symptoms within the larger context. A developmental history should include information about prenatal and perinatal health of the mother and baby; attainment of developmental milestones; academic/school history; history of medical illnesses and their treatments, hospitalizations, or surgeries; changes in family composition (e.g., birth of siblings, parental separations, deaths); psychosocial stressors, including neglect, abuse, and changes in domicile and/or caregivers; and the child's previous mental health history. We have found that it best to gather this information in the form of a developmental time line, in which information is gathered about the child's development and associated mood symptoms for each year of his or her life. The use of this time line is demonstrated in the case presentation format of this chapter.

It is also important to gather information from parents about family history of mental illness. Mental health history should be gathered for biological parents, siblings, and all second-degree relatives (aunts, uncles, grandparents). This can be accomplished in a number of ways. In our research studies, we obtain family mental health history through a structured interview, though it can also be accomplished by using a less structured interview format. However, to ensure accurate reporting, it is important to create with the family a three-generational genogram that includes the child, his or her siblings, parents, and the parents' parents and siblings. After doing this, the interviewer can ask parents the general question "How was growing up for you?"—with follow-up prompts, as needed, to determine the general quality of parents' home lives while growing up, their educational attainment, and the quality of their current relationship. The interviewer can then begin with a general question about whether any family member represented on the genogram has ever received mental health care or a diagnosis, and follow up with specific questions about the presence or absence of symptoms of mood, anxiety, substance abuse and other disorders in family members (e.g., "Has anyone in your family exhibited periods when he or she felt sad or down for a period of time?").

Although we diagnose children, not their family histories, knowing family mental health history is important for many reasons. First, it may provide the clinician with important information about the family environment. In addition, research has demonstrated that family history of BPD is a risk factor for the development of this disorder in children (Birmaher et al., 1996). Thus, knowing the family history provides information about the child's genetic risk for developing the disorder. Genetic research has suggested that BPD is one of the most highly heritable mental disorders. Twin studies have shown an increased concordance of affective illness among monozygotic compared to dizygotic twins (Allen, 1976; Kendler, Pederson, Neale, & Mathe, 1993). When narrow diagnostic criteria are used, the likelihood of a person with BPD having a monozygotic twin with BPD ranges from 50 to 67% compared to a 17 to 24% chance of a dyzygotic twin also having BPD. When broad diagnostic criteria are used for the second twin, the concordance rates range from 70 to 87% for monozygotic twins and 35 to 37% for dizygotic twins (Badner, 2003). Additional support for the role of genetics is found in research on the relationship between parents with mood disorders and the likelihood that their child will have a mood disorder. Chang, Steiner, and Ketter (2000) found that parents with BPD and a childhood history of attention-deficit/hyperactivity disorders (ADHD) were more likely to have a child with BPD. Similarly, Wozniak et al. (1995) found an increased rate of BPD, ADHD, and unipolar depression in relatives of individuals with BPD compared to controls.

To date, only one study has examined the role of temperament in pediatric BPD. Tillman and colleagues (2003) examined temperamental differences among children with BPD, children with ADHD, and community controls. They found that children with BPD and ADHD scored significantly higher in the domain of novelty-seeking compared to community controls. In addition, children with BPD and ADHD scored lower with regard to reward dependence, persistence, self-direction, and cooperativeness than children in the community control group. The only temperamental differences between children with BPD and ADHD were found with regard to parent-reported cooperativeness, which was lower for children with BPD compared to those with ADHD.

Childhood mood disorders are associated with a number of psychosocial consequences, including strained family relations, poor academic performance, and negative peer interactions (Kowatch & Fristad, 2006). Research has documented that caregivers of children with BPD experience a wide range of stressors (Hellander, Sisson, & Fristad, 2003). In a survey of parents conducted through the Child and Adolescent Bipolar Foundation (CABF), an online support, information, and advocacy group, Hellander and colleagues found that parents reported the highest levels of stress related to the following: caring for their high-needs child, advocating for their child's educational needs, worry about the future, physical illnesses, financial strain, isolation, stigma, guilt, and blame.

Family factors such as expressed emotion (EE) have been found to be associated with childhood psychopathology. EE is defined as the amount of criticism, hostility, and emotional overinvolvement displayed by family members toward a patient (Brown, Birley, & Wing, 1972). Research has indicated that high rates of parental EE predict child depression (Asarnow, Goldstein, Tompson, & Guthrie, 1993) and BPD (Miklowitz, 2005). Studies also have found a predictive relationship between high parental EE and child ADHD (Peris & Baker, 2000) and behavior problems (Jarbin, Grawe, & Hansson, 2000). High rates of EE have been associated with higher rates of relapse and poorer prognosis for patients (Butzlaff & Hooley, 1998; Miklowitz et al., 1998).

Research on school functioning has found significant impairments for children with BPD compared to children with ADHD and community controls. Specifically, Geller et al. (2002a) found that children BPD were more likely than children with ADHD or community controls to have behavior problems (79, 30, and 4, respectively). Impairments were also found in academic functioning. Children with BPD had lower grades and were less likely to be in advanced classes than children with ADHD or community controls. They found that children with BPD and ADHD had similar rates of repeating grades, being placed in remedial classes, and having a learning disability, whereas none of these difficulties was found in community controls. Geller, Zimerman, et al. (2000) also found that compared to children with ADHD and community controls, children with BPD were more likely to have few or no friends and to have poor social skills. In addition, they found that children with BPD and ADHD were significantly more likely than community controls to experience teasing, to have difficulty maintaining friendships, and to have poor sibling relationships.

Certain pharmacological treatments have been linked to an increase in manic symptoms (e.g., antidepressants, stimulants). Therefore, when conducting an assessment, it is also important to obtain a detailed history of the child's medication trials, response to treatment, and side effects and how they were managed. In conceptualizing the child's difficulties and formulating a treatment plan it is also helpful to obtain a history of previous psychotherapy and how helpful parents and children found these interventions. We have developed a systematic way to record and track medication and service provider history, response to treatment, perceived helpfulness, and treatment side effects and side effect management (Davidson, Fristad, & Goldberg-Arnold, 2003), which is discussed further later in this chapter.

Because the symptom dimensions of affective instability, behavioral instability, and cognitive changes in BPD are also associated with other mental health difficulties, distinguishing between BPD and other disorders can be challenging. This is especially true for irritability, which is exhibited by children and adolescents with a variety of mental health difficulties. Also, the high degree of comorbidity between psychiatric disorders adds further complexity to a child's clinical presentation. Below we discuss guidelines for differentiating between BPD and other mental disorders based on the patient's presenting symptoms. However, when reading the following section, the reader is advised to keep in mind that it is important to make diagnostic decisions in the context of the child's developmental history, history of the presenting problem, family history, and environment.

BPD versus ADHD

Clinicians often have difficulty distinguishing between BPD and ADHD in children due to the high degree of symptom overlap along the dimension of behavioral instability (e.g., increased energy, silliness, impulsivity). To elucidate the differences between BPD and ADHD, Geller et al. (2002a) compared the prevalence of manic symptoms in children and adolescents with BPD and

ADHD, and in normal community controls. In general, they found that the symptoms that best discriminated between BPD and ADHD were elation, grandiosity, flight of ideas/racing thoughts, decreased need for sleep, and hypersexuality. On the other hand, symptoms such as irritable mood, accelerated speech, distractibility, and increased energy were found cross-sectionally in children with a diagnosis of BPD or ADHD. Thus, Geller and colleagues (2002a) concluded that these symptoms are not useful markers of BPD in children.

In addition to differentiating between the two disorders, it is also important to consider the possibility of co-occurring disorders. According to Wozniak et al. (1995), 98% of children diagnosed with mania also met diagnostic criteria for ADHD. However, the relationship between ADHD and BPD is asymmetrical, because Wozniak et al. found that only 20% of children with ADHD in their specialty clinic in the same sample also met criteria for mania.

BPD versus MDD/DD

Affective instability (e.g., irritability), behavioral instability (e.g., sleep disturbance), and cognitive instability (e.g., decreased concentration, poor academic performance) are present in individuals with BPD and in those with unipolar depression. Therefore, it is important for clinicians to have a good understanding of how these symptoms manifest themselves in children with BPD compared to those with unipolar depression. For example, because irritability is common to BPD and to unipolar depression, it is important to assess the presence–absence of other mood symptoms in a child who demonstrates a high degree of irritability. The presence of additional manic symptoms (e.g., racing thoughts, grandiosity, decreased need for sleep) along with the irritability suggests a diagnosis of BPD, whereas the presence of additional depressive symptoms (e.g., anhedonia, low self-esteem, hopelessness, fatigue) suggest a diagnosis of MDD or DD.

Sleep disturbances are also present in individuals with BPD and those with MDD. However, there are differences in how sleep problems are manifested in these two disorders. A person who is depressed may evidence sleep disturbance in the following ways: initial insomnia (i.e., having trouble falling asleep), middle insomnia (i.e., waking in the middle of the night), early morning insomnia (i.e., waking at 4 A.M. and being unable to go back to sleep), or hypersomnia (i.e., sleeping too much). On the other hand, a child with BPD may exhibit a decreased need for sleep (i.e., a child who typically needs 8 hours of sleep now sleeps only 4 hours and feels rested afterward). In the case of a child who is depressed, the parent or child often reports that he or she is extremely tired but unable to fall asleep or stay asleep. Conversely, a child with BPD is not able to go to sleep or remain asleep due to excess energy. Furthermore, when a child with depression experiences sleep disturbance, he or she will report feeling tired the next day. As a result, the child may take a nap during the day or fall asleep at school. On the other hand, a child with BPD will not appear to be fatigued even though he or she may have gotten much less sleep than typically needed.

Behavioral instability is also present during periods of mania and depression, though these symptoms often fall on opposite ends of the spectrum. Children with depression often display psychomotor retardation or psychomotor agitation (e.g., wringing hands, picking at skin). On the other hand, during periods of mania, children with BPD exhibit restlessness, increased energy, and impulsive behavior. Cognitive changes, such as difficulty concentrating, are also present during both mania and depression. During periods of depression, children often express feeling as though their thoughts have slowed or are foggy. Children who are depressed may respond slowly to questions or have difficulty responding due to decreased thought content. Conversely, children with mania often report that they have racing thoughts and are unable to concentrate due to an increased number of thoughts. They may demonstrate this by responding to questions in a tangential manner, jumping from topic to topic, or exhibiting pressured or rapid speech.

Finally, the importance of a longitudinal perspective in diagnosing children cannot be overstated. A child with a bipolar spectrum disorder might present in a depressed phase of the illness. If the clinician does not ascertain the past history of mania or hypomania, he or she may make an erroneous diagnosis based on current symptom presentation.

BPD versus Oppositional Defiant Disorder

Given the high degree of behavioral instability in children with BPD (e.g., increased energy, irritability, tantrums), BPD may be misdiagnosed as oppositional defiant disorder (ODD). In fact, as with the other conditions discussed earlier, the high degree of comorbidity between ODD and BPD in children and adolescents can further complicate the assessment process (Carlson, 1996). Children with either ODD or BPD may frequently lose their temper and argue with adults. However, in a child with BPD, this behavior would have a waxing and waning pattern, consistent with periods of extreme emotional lability, decreased need for sleep, racing thoughts, pressured/increased speech, and possibly hypersexuality. By way of contrast, a child with ODD would not have these accompanying symptoms, and the oppositional behavior would vary more with environmental factors or specific dyadic interactions (e.g., will not talk back to the principal, but will talk back to the classroom teacher).

BPD versus Conduct Disorder

Behavioral instability is also a hallmark of conduct disorder (CD). Children and adolescents with BPD and/or CD may participate in illegal activities, making differential diagnosis complicated. As with other disorders discussed earlier, there is also a high degree of comorbidity between BPD and CD (Carlson, 1996). In determining whether a child's acting-out behaviors are due to BPD or CD, clinicians should assess for the presence–absence of other mood symptoms. If the acting-out behaviors occur only within the context of other symptoms of mania, and wax and wane with the mood symptoms, a diagnosis of BPD is likely more appropriate. However, if the acting-out behaviors and legal problems remain after mood symptoms have abated, or occur in the absence of mood symptoms, a diagnosis of CD, in addition to the BPD, may be appropriate.

BPD versus Intermittent Explosive Disorder

Behavioral instability in the form of rage attacks is common feature of both BPD and intermittent explosive disorder (IED). To make an appropriate diagnosis, a clinician must assess for the presence–absence of manic and depressive symptoms. If rage attacks occur in conjunction with other symptoms of mania and depression, and disappear during periods of euthymia, a diagnosis of BPD is most appropriate. However, rages that occur without other mood symptoms indicate the presence of IED.

BPD versus Acute Stress Disorder
and Posttraumatic Stress Disorder

Common features of BPD and acute stress disorder/posttraumatic stress disorder (ASD/PTSD) include sleep disturbance, irritability/anger outbursts, diminished interest in activities, restricted affect, and difficulty concentrating. In differentiating between BPD and ASD or PTSD, it is necessary to assess for the presence–absence of other symptoms. First, for a diagnosis of ASD or PTSD, the clinician should determine whether the child has experienced a traumatic event. If not, symptoms cannot be attributable to ASD or PTSD, and other diagnoses should be considered. Symptoms specific to PTSD and ASD, but not found in a child with BPD, include reexperiencing of a traumatic event, avoidance of stimuli associated with a traumatic event, and increased arousal that was not present before the trauma. The difference between PTSD and ASD is that the symptoms begin within 1 month of the traumatic event in ASD, whereas PTSD symptoms must be present for more than 1 month. Again, it is possible for a child/adolescent to have both BPD and ASD or BPD and PTSD, which highlights the importance of conducting a thorough assessment that includes a time line of symptom onset, offset, and duration to determine the most appropriate diagnosis, or set of diagnoses.

Many children with BPD display symptoms of hypersexuality. In fact, Geller et al. (2002a) found that hypersexuality is one of the symptoms that differentiates BPD from ADHD. When children present in a clinical setting with symptoms of hypersexuality, clinicians may also be concerned about the possibility of sexual abuse or exposure to sexual stimulation in the environment. Geller and colleagues found that whereas only 1.1% of pediatric bipolar subjects had a history of sexual abuse or overstimulation in their environment, 43% of children in this sample demonstrated hypersexuality. As always, in determining the appropriate diagnosis, it is important for clinicians to gather children's lifetime histories to determine the presence–absence of abuse or exposure. Also, for a diagnosis of BPD, hypersexuality should occur within the context of other mood symptoms and be associated with periods of mood lability.

BPD versus Psychotic Disorder

If a child presents with reports of auditory or visual hallucinations or delusions, then the clinician needs to assess for presence–absence of mood symptoms. If psychotic symptoms occur only in the presence of other symptoms of depression and/or mania, a diagnosis of MDD and/or BPD with psychotic features is warranted. However, if psychotic symptoms occur in the absence of mood symptoms, the diagnosis of a psychotic disorder may be more appropriate.

CASE FORMULATION:
CONCEPTUAL MODEL OF ASSESSMENT AND TREATMENT

In the following section, we use a case example to demonstrate relevant aspects of the assessment and treatment of BPD in children. The case described is a typical example of a child and family who participated in a research study on the efficacy of multifamily psychoeducation groups (MFPG) for children ages 8–12. As part of the research protocol, the initial diagnostic assessment was conducted through separate interviews with the patient and her mother. The standardized assessment battery included structured interviews, clinical rating scales, and self-report instruments. Though it may not always be possible to administer such a lengthy assessment battery in a clinical setting (e.g., due to limited personnel or economic restrictions), it is important to gather information from parents and children independently. Whereas research has demonstrated poor agreement in general between informants (Achenbach, McConaughy, & Howell, 1987; Yeh & Weisz, 2001; Tarullo, Richardson, Radke-Yarrow, & Martinez, 1995), Tillman et al. (2004) found that children reported more mania-specific symptoms than did their parents. Given reporting differences between parents and children, information should be collected from both informants to obtain the most complete clinical picture. Also, because children's behavior may differ based on their environment, data should be gathered from collateral informants (e.g., teachers, day care provider).

Case Presentation

At the time of the diagnostic assessment, Jane Smith, 8-year-old Caucasian female, was living with both biological parents and two younger siblings. According to Mrs. Smith's report, Jane began displaying oppositional and defiant behavior toward authority figures at age 4 and was diagnosed with ODD at age 5, and with ADHD at age 6. However, Mrs. Smith reported that Jane continued to display increasing anger and aggression toward siblings and peers (e.g., tripping children in her classroom), defiance toward parents, difficulty expressing feelings, and apparent emotional withdrawal from others (e.g., not responding "I love you" when her mother says she loves her), and social difficulties. Despite an IQ reportedly in the superior range, Jane had significant academic and behavioral problems at school (e.g., not turning in homework, talking out of turn, bothering classmates). Thus, when Jane entered our study, she was repeating the second grade. After an initial psychiatric evaluation when Jane was age 5, her parents took her to a number of service providers to find assistance for her ongoing behavior problems. At the time of study enrollment, Jane had had previously been diagnosed with ODD and ADHD, and prescribed several medications, with little effect until Jane finally experienced some improvement with a combination of Wellbutrin and clonidine.

Assessment

As explained earlier, given the cyclical nature of mood disorders, assessment should have a longitudinal focus and include information about the child's development within multiple contexts. Given that the affective instability, behavioral instability, and cognitive changes associated with BPD in children are also present in other disorders, clinicians also must gather detailed and specific information about the child's presenting symptoms to rule in or out a diagnosis of BPD. Kowatch et al. (2005) recommended that clinicians use the FIND (frequency, intensity, number duration) strategy to ascertain the presence–absence of manic symptoms. These guidelines for the diagnosis of BPD include (1) *frequency*: symptoms occur most days in a week; (2) *intensity*: symptoms are severe enough to cause extreme disturbance in one domain or moderate disturbance in two or more domains, (3) *number*: symptoms occur three or four times a day; (4) *duration*: symptoms occur 4 or more hours a day (not necessarily continuous).

Kowatch and colleagues (2005) provided the following examples to explain the importance of assessment with the FIND strategy. First, they explain that although a child who is silly to a noticeable and bothersome degree for 30 minutes twice a week does display some unusual behavior, this behavior likely does not warrant a BPD diagnosis based on FIND criteria. However, a child may have crossed the FIND threshold if he or she is "too cheerful" for several hours a day during most school days and every day after school, and this behavior has caused marked impairment in relationships with teachers, parents, and peers (Kowatch et al., 2005).

When determining whether a behavior is a symptom or is within normal limits, it is also important to consider the context in which the behavior occurs. On the one hand, elation during a trip to Disney World is considered normal and nonimpairing. On the other hand, equally elated, silly behaviors in other contexts (e.g., church, school) are considered pathological. As discussed earlier, it is also important to recognize differences between adult and child manifestations of mania (for examples of manifestations of prepubertal mania, see Geller et al., 2002b).

As mentioned earlier, the comprehensive diagnostic assessment outlined in this case presentation was conducted as part of a larger treatment study and included semistructured parent and child interviews, clinical rating scales, and self-report measures. In the following section, we discuss the instruments used in our assessments and their relationship to Jane's case. As will become apparent, the information below is separated into independent responses provided by Jane and her mother, and there are discrepancies between parent and child reports. Discrepancies in informant reporting are not a new problem and have been discussed extensively in research literature. Though researchers have attempted to determine whether there is an optimal informant, they have not reached consensus regarding this issue. Some have suggested that parents are better informants of externalizing symptoms, whereas children are better informants of internalizing symptoms (Herjanic & Reich, 1982), but Tillman and colleagues (2004) demonstrated that children are better informants of their own manic symptoms than are parents. The way we reconcile differences between parent and child reports is to consider a symptom present if it was reported by at least one informant.

Time Line

When assessing for any psychiatric disorder, it is important to gather historical information about the child's symptoms and level of functioning. Thus, we begin each assessment by creating a time line that includes information about the child, using each year of his or her life as a reference point. Relevant information includes pregnancy and birth history, child care/school placements, overall level of functioning, appearance of symptoms, relevant family changes (e.g., births, deaths, marriage, divorce), psychosocial stressors, educational functioning, social functioning, and any treatment sought.

On Jane's time line (see Figure 6.1), her mother denied problems with pregnancy or delivery and noted no postnatal medical problems. At 6 months, Jane started in day care, where Mrs. Smith described her as being "strong-willed" and "ornery." At age 3, Jane started preschool, where she displayed social problems and defiance. Jane's parents decided to withdraw her from preschool after 6 months because, she complained daily about having to attend. Later that year, Jane and her family moved out of state, and Mrs. Smith described Jane as having a difficult adjustment and missing her friends. At age 4, Jane again started preschool, this time at a private school. Mrs.

Timeline (ages 0–9):

0–1: Pregnancy and delivery unremarkable. Full-term baby, vaginal delivery. No postnatal problems. Mother working full time, Jane in day care.

1–3: Developmental milestones met within normal limits.

~2–3: "Ornery" and strong-willed.

3: Starts preschool—"So unhappy there," so stops going in spring.

3: Social problems, increased defiance, and behavior problems.

4: Family moves, mother changes jobs. Brother born. Enrolled in Catholic preschool, does pretty well.

4: Difficult adjustment to move. Unhappy, misses friends. Described as "immature." Some social problems.

5: Starts kindergarten in same school with same teacher. Mother working long hours, father providing child care ("military style").

5: Jealous of brother. Attentional difficulties. Cognitive evaluation reveals abilities in superior range. Continued problems with peers. Evaluated by psychologist and diagnosed with ODD.

6: Family moves again. Jane enrolled in private all girls' school for first grade.

6: A lot of school problems. Increased mood and behavior problems. Saw psychiatrist who prescribed Prozac and Paxil to address mood symptoms. Little improvement noted by Mrs. Smith. Jane diagnosed with ADHD and prescribed Ritalin. Trial stopped after 2 days, due to increased agitation and aggression.

7: Sister born. Starts second grade in new school. Understanding teacher is able to manage difficulties.

8: Start of the "worst" time. Hit counselor at summer camp, "horrible" summer. Episodic anger and irritability, increased energy, decreased need for sleep. Horrible aggression, angry even on family vacation. Hospitalized for emergency stabilization twice. Prescribed Depakote with little effect. Prescribed clonidine with much positive effect, especially with regard to sleep.

8–9: Repeats summer camp, much better behaviorally. Starts Montessori school, repeating second grade.

9: Prescribed Wellbutrin with positive effect. Things going "OK."

FIGURE 6.1. Time line as reported by Mrs. Smith.

Smith described this experience as better than the first, though Jane displayed some social problems and immaturity. For kindergarten, Jane remained at the same school with the same teacher. During this year, Mrs. Smith indicated that she was working a lot, and much of the child care was provided by Mr. Smith, whom she described as using a "military style" to address behavior problems. Mrs. Smith reported that Jane had trouble completing class work and increased problems with peers. Given her academic difficulties, the school administered a psychoeducational evaluation that according to Jane's parents revealed her cognitive abilities to be in the superior range. It was at this point that Jane was evaluated by a psychologist and diagnosed with ODD. After two therapy sessions, however, Jane and her family moved out of state and treatment was discontinued.

At age 6, Jane was enrolled in first grade at a private school. Mrs. Smith reported continued school problems (academic and social) during this year. Due to these difficulties, an individualized education plan (IEP) was created to address specific concerns and to provide support for Jane. During this year, Jane also began seeing a psychiatrist who prescribed trials of Prozac and Paxil, with little effectiveness. Jane also began taking Ritalin, which was discontinued after 2 days due to an increase in her aggressive behavior. Mrs. Smith described the summer after first grade until the end of second grade as the time when Jane's symptoms were the worst. During the summer, Mrs. Smith was pregnant with her third child. Jane was enrolled in a summer camp, where she demonstrated much aggression (e.g., hitting a counselor). According to Mrs. Smith, Jane was "angry all the time," even during the family vacation. Furthermore, Jane was highly active and had a decreased need for sleep. Due to concerns for her safety, Jane was placed in emergency hospitalization twice that summer. Given these difficulties, Jane was prescribed another medication, Depakote, again with little effect.

For the third time in 3 years, Jane enrolled in a new school for second grade. This time she was enrolled in a public school, where Mrs. Smith described continued academic and social difficulties, though she did note minor improvement in these areas. During second grade, Depakote was discontinued and clonidine was prescribed for Jane. Mrs. Smith reported "much improvement" with start of the clonidine, especially with regard to reducing Jane's sleep problems. The summer after second grade, Jane again attended summer camp with a much better result than the previous year. The next fall, she changed schools and repeated second grade. At the time of the initial assessment, Jane has been in school for 2 months, and Mrs. Smith described things as being "OK."

Family History

A three-generation genogram was constructed with Mrs. Smith, then the Family History–Research Diagnostic Criteria (FH-RDC) interview was administered to Mrs. Smith to gather information about family history of psychiatric

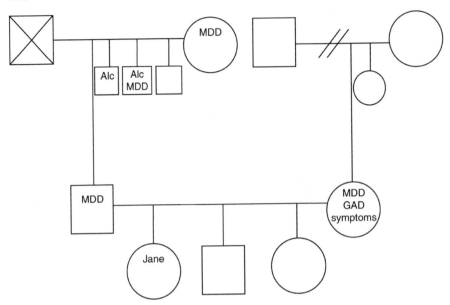

FIGURE 6.2. Genogram: Family history.

illness (see Figure 6.2). Jane's family history was remarkable for MDD (father, mother, paternal uncle, paternal grandmother), alcoholism (two paternal uncles), and symptoms of generalized anxiety disorder (mother).

Child and Parent Semistructured Interviews

CHILDREN'S INTERVIEW FOR PSYCHIATRIC SYNDROMES

Jane and her mother were interviewed independently with child and parent versions of the Children's Interview for Psychiatric Syndromes (ChIPS/P-ChIPS; Weller, Weller, Fristad, Rooney, & Schecter, 2000; Weller, Weller, Rooney, & Fristad, 1999). The ChIPS and P-ChIPS are structured psychiatric interviews that use DSM-IV criteria to assess psychopathology in children and adolescents ages 6–18 years (Fristad et al., 1998; Teare, Fristad, Weller, Weller, & Salmon, 1998a, 1998b). These instruments assess 20 behavioral, anxiety, mood, and other syndromes, as well as psychosocial stressors that the child might have experienced. Symptoms are assessed using a "yes–no" question format. Within each diagnostic section, cardinal questions are asked, and a multiple "skip" procedure is used. If a child answers "no" to a certain number of questions, the rest of the questions can be skipped. Information about onset, offset, and duration gathered for each disorder.

Based on Mrs. Smith's responses to the P-ChIPS, Jane met criteria for the following diagnoses: ADHD (onset, age 5); ODD (onset, age 4); MDD (onset, age 7); and mania (onset, age 7). Jane's mother also endorsed some symptoms of dysthymia for Jane. Current psychosocial stressors endorsed on the P-ChIPS included fighting between siblings, parent–child fighting, and minor elective surgery of a family member. Mrs. Smith reported that a past stressor was the hospitalization of a family member.

In her interview, Jane's endorsed a diagnosis of ODD (onset, age 6) and symptoms of MDD and mania. Psychosocial stressors endorsed by Jane included a history of being spanked and the death of a great-grandparent.

CHILDREN'S DEPRESSION RATING SCALE—REVISED

The Children's Depression Rating Scale—Revised (CDRS-R) was administered to Jane and her mother to evaluate the presence and severity of Jane's depressive symptoms currently (i.e., in the past 2 weeks) and during her worst period of depression. The CDRS-R is a 17-item, clinician-rated severity scale for depression in children ages 6–17 (Poznanski et al., 1984). Each item is rated on a 1- to 5-point or 1- to 7-point scale in the direction of increasing severity. Total scores range from 17 to 113. The CDRS-R total score has been found to correlate significantly with clinical global ratings of depression and to differentiate between clinically defined groups of children who differ in depression severity. Interrater reliability is adequate ($r = .86$), as is test–retest reliability over a 4-week period ($r = .81$; Poznanski et al., 1984).

Though this scale itself is not sufficient for diagnosing depression, in conjunction with data from a structured interview, it allows clinicians to further evaluate and better understand the patient's specific symptoms of depression. When interpreted in the context of other assessment tools (e.g., a structured interview such as the ChIPS), it provides valuable information regarding differential diagnosis.

Jane's total score of 31 for her "worst" period on the CDRS-R suggested a history of mild depressive symptoms. Mrs. Smith's "worst" rating of indicated a history of depressive symptoms of moderate severity. Ratings for each symptom endorsed by Jane and her mother and a description of the symptoms are provided in Table 6.1.

MANIA RATING SCALE

To assess the presence and severity of her manic symptoms currently (i.e., in the past 2 weeks) and during her worst period of manic symptoms, Jane and her mother were administered the Mania Rating Scale (MRS), an 11-item clinical rating scale for manic symptoms (Young, Biggs, Ziegler, & Meyer, 1978). Items are rated either from 0 to 4 or 0 to 8, depending on item weighting, in the direction of increasing severity. The total score can range from 0 (*No mania*) to 60 (*Severe mania*). Fristad, Weller, and Weller (1992) demonstrated that the MRS may be used to assess mania in children and suggested this scale

TABLE 6.1. Jane and Mrs. Smith's Report of Her Worst Period of Depressive Symptoms on the Children's Depression Rating Scale—Revised (CDRS-R)

Symptom	Rating based on Jane's report	Rating based on Mrs. Smith's report
Dysphoric feelings	3—A few times a week, Jane got sad for no reason. This mood lasts a few hours.	3—Jane was often sad and had a "negative outlook" on life.
Depressed affect	2—Became less responsive as interview progressed.	3—When unhappy, Jane often looked sad.
Capacity to have fun	2—Did not initiate social interactions and frequently "spoiled" opportunities.	4—Jane displayed decreased interest in her usual activities, though she occasionally engaged in some pleasurable activities.
Irritability	2—Fleeting signs of irritation while being interviewed.	7—Jane was constantly irritable and often had "explosions" when very angry.
Weeping	1—No symptoms reported.	7—Mrs. Smith reported that Jane cried almost every day.
Social withdrawal/ peer problems	3—When she felt sad, Jane "just wanted to be left alone." She did not actively approach friends to play with her, but would accept an invitation to play with a friend.	5—Jane was often aggressive when interacting with peers and therefore was often rejected by others. She had limited social relationships.
Sleep	1—No symptoms reported.	5—Prior to beginning Clonidine, Jane had nightly difficulty falling asleep. Though she went to bed around 8 P.M., she often did not fall asleep until 11:30 P.M.
Appetite	1—No symptoms reported.	1—No symptoms reported.
Hypoactivity	1—No symptoms reported.	1—No symptoms reported.
Tempo of language	2—Speech was somewhat slow during interview.	1—No symptoms reported.
Guilt	1—No symptoms reported.	1—No symptoms reported.
Schoolwork	1—No symptoms reported.	4—Jane had difficulty concentrating when she was sad or irritable. This difficulty was present both at home and at school.
Excessive fatigue	3—When sad, Jane felt more tired and wanted to rest or take naps more than when she was not sad.	1—No symptoms reported.
Physical complaints	3—Jane reported having stomachaches approximately once a week.	1—No symptoms reported.
Self-esteem	1—No symptoms reported.	1—No symptoms reported.
Morbid ideation	3—Thought a lot about great grandparents, whom she did not know.	1—No symptoms reported.
Suicidal ideation	1—No symptoms reported.	3—Mrs. Smith indicated that Jane threatened to jump out of a moving car when she was very angry during a family vacation.

may help to differentiate between mania and ADHD. Furthermore, Fristad and colleagues demonstrated that the MRS has adequate internal consistency, and convergent, and divergent validity when used with prepubertal children with BPD (Fristad et al., 1995).

Jane's total score of 16 for her "worst" period on the MRS, suggested mild manic symptoms. Mrs. Smith's "worst" rating of 34 indicated a history of moderate manic symptoms. Specific items endorsed are described in Table 6.2.

Medication/Treatment History

A history of Jane's medication trials and previous treatment was collected in a semistructured interview and recorded with the medication usage and service provider grids (Davidson, Fristad, & Goldberg-Arnold, 2004; see Figures 6.3 and 6.4). These grids are useful because they provide a user-friendly format for clinicians to record and track medication and service usage, and patient–parent satisfaction with these medications and services. In addition, the grids provide places for recording and monitoring medication side effects and reasons for addition–discontinuation of services.

Because of behavioral problems, Jane was first evaluated at age 5 in two sessions with a psychologist. However, this service was discontinued when the family moved out of the state. As demonstrated on the service grids, prior to beginning this treatment study, Jane's parents had sought help from a number of providers, including psychologists, psychiatrists, social workers, and respite services. Like many other families with whom we work, it had taken the Smiths multiple tries to find providers that were helpful and able to diagnose correctly and effectively treat Jane's difficulties.

Jane was prescribed a number of different medications prior to finding one that demonstrated a positive effect. Though her parents reported Jane's improved sleep with the use of clonidine and some improvement in symptoms with Wellbutrin, her mood swings and behavioral difficulties remained problematic.

Psychoeducational–Neuropsychological Testing

Though formal psychoeducational or neuropsychological testing was not conducted as part of the initial assessment, we obtained a brief evaluation of Jane's cognitive abilities using the Kaufman Brief Intelligence Test (K-BIT). Jane's scores were as follows: Verbal = 134; Matrices = 120; Composite = 131.

As noted earlier, Jane's parents reported that an IQ test had been given at age 5 which revealed cognitive abilities in the superior range. Though some of the academic difficulties described by Jane's parents and teachers were likely due to impairment caused by her mood symptoms, we do not have data to demonstrate whether any learning disabilities were present.

TABLE 6.2. Jane and Mrs. Smith's Reports of Her Worst Period of Manic Symptoms on the Mania Rating Scale (MRS)

Symptom	Rating based on Jane's report	Rating based on Mrs. Smith's report
Elevated mood	3—Jane stated her mood would get "too high."	0—No symptom reported.
Irritability	4—Jane got mad a few times a week for less than 1 hour.	8—Mrs. Smith stated Jane was episodically irritable and hostile to an extreme degree.
Content	0—No symptom reported.	1—Felt like she could "beat" parents and have everything her way.
Need for sleep	0—No symptom reported.	2—Three to four times a week, Jane had a lot of energy at bedtime and stayed up very late playing or reading. Even with less sleep, she was not tired the next day.
Thought disorder	1—Jane reported mild distractibility.	3—Many days, Jane's thoughts appeared to be racing. During these times she repeated herself over and over again.
Speech	0—No symptom reported. No increased rate or amount of speech noted during assessment.	4—Jane talked more episodically, though was not difficult to interrupt, and it was still possible to have a conversation with her.
Motor activity	3—Jane endorsed periods of excess energy that occurred a few times a week. During such periods, she had difficulty calming down and got into trouble at home and school.	2—When Jane was very angry she was more active (e.g., fighting with parents and siblings, hitting, kicking). Mrs. Smith denied increased activity at other times.
Sexual interest	0—No symptom reported.	0—No symptom reported.
Aggressive behavior	2—Jane sometimes fought with her brother or peers at school. She could not articulate the frequency or intensity of behaviors.	8—Several times a day, Mr. or Mrs. Smith had to restrain Jane because she was so physically aggressive. She was also restrained multiple times at school.
Appearance	0—No symptom reported. Jane was well groomed and casually dressed.	2—Mrs. Smith often had to push Jane to take care of her personal hygiene.
Insight	3—Jane did not recognize how her behavior affects others. She acknowledged that her medications were helpful but stated: "I don't want to do it, but they make me" regarding treatment.	4—Mrs. Smith reported that Jane exhibited no insight into her symptoms and did not think she needs treatment. Jane was quick to blame her difficulties on someone else rather than accepting responsibility for her actions.

Medication	Class	Dose	Length of trial	Current?	Reason for addition/change	Reason for termination	Effective	How effective?	Side effects	Side-effect management
Prozac	A		Few months	No	Mood/behavior problems	Sleep problems	2	Helped, but sleep problems	Sleep problems	Discontinued
Ritalin	B		2 days	No	Inattention	Side effects	1	Problems worsened	Increased aggression	Discontinued
Paxil	A		Few weeks	No	Mood/behavior problems	Side effects	1	Problems worsened	Increased aggression	Discontinued
Depakote	D		Few months	No	Aggression/mood problems	Side effects	1	No change	Weight gain	Discontinued
Clonidine	E	0.1 mg	1 year	Yes	Sleep problems	N/A	5	Helps sleep	Patch itched	Take liquid form
Trazadone	A		Few weeks	No	Mood symptoms	No change	1	No change	None	N/A
Wellbutrin	A	75 mg	Few months	Yes	Mood swings	N/A	3	Hard to tell if she's doing better	None	N/A

FIGURE 6.3. Medication Grid.

Mental health/ educational service or provider	Age	Length of trial	Current?	Helpful?	How helpful/unhelpful?	Reason for addition	Reason for termination
Dr. A. (psychologist)	5	2 visits	No	3	Only 2 sessions before client moved	Behavior problems	Moved
Cognitive testing	5	1 visit	No	4	Identified her intelligence	School problems	Time-limited—1 visit only
Dr. B. (psychologist)	6	Few visits	No	1	He didn't work with the school.	Behavior problems	Terminated with patient, felt he did all he could
Social worker	6	1.5 years	Yes	3	Good rapport/needs more intensive services	Behavior problems	N/A
Case management	7	1 year	Yes	3	Good rapport	Behavior problems	N/A
Dr. C. (psychiatrist)	6	Few visits	No	1	Didn't remember us at second visit. Bad experience with medication trial.	Behavior problems	Did not like provider. Negative effects of medication trial.
Dr. D. (psychiatrist)	6	1.5 years	Yes	4	Didn't help with hospitalization	Behavior problems	N/A
Respite services	7	1 week	No	4	Overnight stays helped give message that behavior not acceptable.	Severe behavior problems	Stabilized, connected with other services.
Individual Education Plan (IEP)	7	1 year	No	4	Great teacher	Academic and behavior problems	Moved to private school
Dr. E. (psychologist)	7	1 year	Yes	4	She makes sense to me	Behavior problems	N/A

FIGURE 6.4. Service Provider Grid.

Behavioral Observations

Jane presented to the assessment appropriately groomed and casually dressed. She was described as thoughtful and cooperative. However, the interviewer noted that she became fatigued as the assessment progressed, and often had difficulty responding adequately and providing detail to questions (e.g., responding "I don't know"). Her affect was described as restricted and her mood, slightly dysphoric. Furthermore, Jane's speech was somewhat slowed, causing delays in her responding.

Differential Diagnosis

During the course of the assessment, Jane and her mother reported long-standing difficulties with behavioral problems and mood instability, starting when Jane was 3 years old. Despite consultations with multiple professionals, Jane's parents did not have a good understanding of her difficulties and had reported only minor improvements in her symptoms. This is a very common experience for parents, who often are confused by conflicting information provided by various professionals. The structured interviews administered as part of this assessment suggested diagnoses of ADHD, ODD, MDD, and mania. Specific manic and depressive symptoms endorsed by Jane and Mrs. Smith on the ChIPS and P-ChIPS, respectively, appear in Table 6.3.

A diagnosis of MDD was further supported by results of the CDRS-R, as evidenced in Table 6.1. Furthermore, the diagnosis of mania was supported by Jane's and Mrs. Smith's report of symptoms on the MRS (see Table 6.2). Based on the information gathered from Jane and her mother, Jane was diagnosed with BP-II, most recent episode depressed.

Link between Assessment and Treatment

Evidence-based assessment is linked to evidence-based treatment. In the MFPG study, we attempt to carefully diagnose children using evidence-based assessment strategies prior to their participation in an efficacy study of family psychoeducation as a treatment for childhood mood disorders. In the following section, we provide detail about the eight-session MFPG therapy program. A pilot study that examined the efficacy of MFPG found that immediately following and at 4-months posttreatment, families reported greater knowledge about mood disorders and treatment options. Other benefits reported by parents included increased social support, and changes in coping skills and attitudes following participation in the intervention (Goldberg-Arnold, Fristad, & Gavazzi, 1999; Fristad, Goldberg-Arnold, & Gavazzi, 2002). The efficacy of these groups is currently being evaluated in a study of 165 families as part of a National Institute of Mental Health (NIMH) R01 research grant awarded to M. Fristad.

TABLE 6.3. Jane and Mrs. Smith's Endorsements on the ChIPS and P-ChIPS

	Jane's report	Mrs. Smith's report
Depressive symptoms		
Mood		
Dysphoric	X	X
Irritable		X
Anhedonia		X
Appetite changes		
Increased appetite		
Decreased appetite		
Sleep disturbance		
Early insomnia		X
Hypersomnia	X	
Psychomotor changes		
Low energy	X	
Guilt		
Impaired concentration		X
Ideation		
Morbid	X	
Suicidal		X
Manic symptoms		
Mood		
Elevated	X	
Discrete periods of irritability		X
Grandiosity		
Increased energy	X	X
Rapid, unstoppable speech		X
Racing thoughts		X
Impaired concentration		X
Excessive involvement in problematic behaviors		

X, endorsed; blank, not endorsed.

Treatment

Preview

The MFPG treatment program was designed to be an *adjunctive* intervention. Therefore, children who are enrolled are often receiving concurrent mental health counseling and medication management from providers in the community, in addition to support services at school. MFPG was designed for children ages 8–12. Given the family component, we require that at least one (and preferably two, when possible) parents[1] participate in the program along with

---

[1] For simplicity, the term "parent(s)" is used from this point on to refer to parents, legal guardians, and other/additional caretakers (e.g., live-in boyfriend).

their child. Groups are led by trained mental health professionals (i.e., clinical psychologist, licensed social worker). Typically, parent groups are run by one leader, whereas child groups have two leaders. Thus far, we have implemented these groups in a medical center setting, though they likely can be easily transferred to other settings as well.

Components of MFPG Treatment Groups

The MFPG program is administered in eight weekly, 90-minute sessions. Though parents and children participate in separate groups, each session begins and ends with a family component. During the middle portion of each group, when parents and children meet separately, the content of children's and parents' sessions is thematically connected. Parent groups are typically run by one leader and are relatively informal. Parents are encouraged to ask questions, request clarification, or otherwise interrupt to seek additional information about the topic at hand. Parents are provided with a workbook to follow along with the formal presentation and to make notes about the material. They also receive homework handouts at the end of each session. Parents are expected to complete these home activity projects each week and bring them to the group to be reviewed and collected the following week.

Child sessions are run by two leaders and are largely activity-based. Children are given a workbook containing information sheets reviewed during group, as well as group and home activities. Children earn points for their participation and behavior during group, which they exchange for prizes during the last group session. The end of each group includes *in vivo* social skills training. In our setting, we have access to a gym. Although not all treatment setting may have such an option, creating opportunities for *in vivo* social skills training that involve large muscle movement is recommended. During this time, children engage in different activities (e.g., soccer, tag, specified group games) and are coached by group leaders to practice the skills being reviewed during group.

Groups are scheduled to accommodate school, work, and other activity schedules so usually they are offered in the late afternoon or early evening on a weekday. We have found it helpful to provide light refreshments given the time of day and the desire to facilitate a congenial atmosphere among group members.

FRAMEWORK AND GOALS FOR PARENT GROUPS

There are three main goals for the parents' groups: (1) social support; (2) information, and (3) skills building. First, it has been our experience that parents experience considerable relief by simply looking around the room and seeing other people who can relate to the experiences they have had with their child. Second, parents are eager to receive well-organized information about their children's conditions. In addition to sessions devoted to providing infor-

mation on phenomenology, treatment, and healthy–unhealthy family responses to the disorder, parents are particularly interested in better understanding the educational and mental health systems, and how to work
effectively with each to benefit their children. Thus, a primary goal of the
MFPG program is to teach parents about the different "players" in the system, so they can learn to interact more effectively as a consumer of the health
care and educational services their children receive. Finally, homework assignments and role playing are used to concretize the information provided in
each session.

FRAMEWORK AND GOALS FOR CHILDREN'S GROUP

First, consistent with the goals of the parent group, children also have the
opportunity to meet others the same age who struggle with issues similar to
their own. This provides them with some relief in knowing they "aren't the
only one" with these problems (and that others sometimes "have it worse").
Second, group participation promotes increased awareness of symptoms,
symptom management, and the ability to complete a "cost–benefit" analysis
of treatment (e.g., "how well medicine helps me control my bad feelings" vs.
"how unpleasant it is to take"). Children frequently have questions about
their medications in particular, and appreciate the chance to ask questions
they might have in the comfortable atmosphere of the group. Third, because
children with mood disorders are frequently socially rejected or isolated from
peers and often do not fully develop age-appropriate social skills due to the
impairment caused by their mood disorder and comorbid conditions, a particular emphasis is placed on social skills training. Role playing is used extensively to practice affect recognition and response, initiating and maintaining
conversations, and becoming included in social interactions. Conflict management skills are reviewed, with particular emphasis on the application of these
skills in peer, school, and family situations. The clinician helps children
develop skills in each step of conflict management, which includes defining the
problem, brainstorming and evaluating possible solutions, then choosing and
evaluating a solution. Particular emphasis is placed on using a stop–think–
plan–do–check format, "I messages," and not blaming the other person. Conducting this treatment in a group format allows children the opportunity to
practice these skills with assistance from the group leaders. The children end
each session by rejoining the parents' group to give a brief report of their session activities.

THE PROCESS OF TREATMENT: STEP-BY-STEP GUIDELINES

In this section, we provide a brief overview of the content and process of each
parent and child session, along with examples of group exercises and home
activity projects. Readers who are interested in learning more about the spe-

cific content of MFPG groups should contact M. Fristad to obtain this information.

Session 1

The goal of the first session is to orient families to the MFPG treatment program and provide them with background information about mood disorders. During the beginning portion of the first session, when parents and children meet together, family members introduce themselves and share some common information (e.g., the child's grade in school, where they go to school, their diagnosis). Next, group leaders present an overview of what family members can expect throughout the eight sessions (e.g., structure of sessions, topics covered, home activities). Following this brief introduction, the children and their group therapists move into an adjacent room.

Parent Group: Introduction/Symptoms and Disorders

The focus of the first parent group is to provide parents with information about mood disorders and their symptoms. Group leaders review myths (e.g., "Mood-impaired kids are bad or lazy") and provide facts about mood disorders (e.g., prevalence rates, information regarding etiology, problems associated with not pursuing treatment). Parents are taught specific diagnostic criteria for each type of mood disorder, along with information about episode length, recurrence, and comorbid conditions. The first session concludes with an overview of biological, social, and psychological treatment options.

Child Group: Introduction/Symptoms

The child group begins with group members discussing and agreeing upon rules for the group. Group leaders ensure that issues regarding confidentiality and safety are addressed and incorporated into the rules. Rules are drafted on a large sheet of poster board and hung on the wall, so that members can refer to them as needed. Next, group leaders inform participants that they will earn points during group for following the rules and for active group participation. Points are also earned for completing and returning projects each week. Points may also be subtracted each week for off-task or for disruptive behavior. Points are recorded by leaders throughout each session and may be exchanged for prizes during the final group session. The remainder of the child group session is spent discussing symptoms of depression and mania. Children are provided with worksheets listing the symptoms of each. Leaders encourage members to discuss their experiences with these symptoms. Comorbid difficulties (e.g., ADHD, anxiety) are also briefly reviewed and discussed. After their *in vivo* social skills training, children return to the parent group to review the project for next week.

Family Project: "Fix-It List"

The goal of the first family project is for parents and children to identify and agree upon treatment goals. Parents and children are instructed independently to identify three problems they would like to fix in the next 8 weeks. These can be problems that occur at home, at school, or with friends, but they should be solvable over the course of the group (i.e., not too big to address within 8 weeks). After parents and children create their individual lists, they are instructed to discuss their goals and agree upon three family goals.

Jane's Fix-It List included the following: (1) Stop fighting with my brother; (2) make a new friend; and (3) have my parents listen better to me. Her parents' list for Jane included (1) stop yelling; (2) take better care of myself; and (3) Have Jane listen when we ask her to do something. After discussing these goals, they comprised their family "Fix-It List," which included (1) less arguing among siblings; (2) less yelling from parents; and (3) better communication and listening between Jane and parents.

Session 2

At the beginning of Session 2 and each subsequent session, parents and children meet together to share their project with the other members. After a brief discussion, children leave with their therapists to continue their portion separately.

Parent Group: Medication

The focus of Session 2 is to provide parents with important factual information regarding medications used to treat mood disorders and to address concerns associated with side effects, medication compliance, and adequate trial lengths. Procedures associated with taking medication (e.g., blood levels, how/when to stop medication) are briefly reviewed as well. Parents are given a medication log tracking sheet and encouraged to use this form to track their child's response to medication trials, as well as any side effects. Specific information (e.g., brand and generic names, side effects) regarding each class of medication is reviewed. Information about nutritional interventions for BPD and research associated with these interventions (e.g., omega-3 fatty acids, multivitamin–mineral complexes) is also shared. Considerable time is spent discussing with parents common ways to manage side effects. As a project, parents are asked to make a list of their children's current medications and reason for taking them, as well as any observed side effects.

Child Group: Medication

During the child portion of Session 2, leaders review commonly used medications for treating mood disorders. Children are provided with information sheets for each class of medication. These sheets contain information about the symptoms targeted by each medication, common side effects, and ways to manage side effects. Children are asked to make a list of their medications, dosages, and reason for taking the medication. If children are unable to do so, they are encouraged to discuss this with their parents to become more aware of their treatment regimen. Next, they complete as a group the "Symptom–Self" exercise (described below). After a brief period of *in vivo* social skills training, the last 10 minutes of group are spent conjointly with parents reviewing the family project.

Family Project: "Symptom–Self" Exercise

The goal of the "Symptom–Self" exercise is to help family members recognize and differentiate between the child's characteristics and the characteristics of the mood disorder (Fristad, Gavazzi, & Soldano, 1999). The worksheet is divided into two columns. Under the "Me" column, family members list characteristics of the child (e.g., funny, good with animals, caring). Under the "My Symptoms" column, family members list diagnoses, followed by symptoms that the child experiences (e.g., Depression—irritability, can't concentrate, don't want to play with friends; Mania—too much energy, talk too loud and too much, don't need to sleep, too silly). After the lists are completed, families are instructed to fold the paper so that the "Me" column is covered by the "My Symptoms" column. This illustrates how the mood disorder symptoms are covering up who the child really is, and that the goal of treatment is to manage symptoms so the child can be "rediscovered." In Jane's case, under the "Me" column, she and her parents listed the following attributes: good reader, good sense of humor, caring, intelligent, and helpful. In the "My Symptoms" column were listed anger, irritability, aggression, trouble concentrating, and problems with friends.

Session 3

Parent Group: Understanding Symptoms

The primary goal of Session 3 is to empower parents to be the best possible advocate for their child by providing them with specific, detailed information about different types of mental health providers (e.g., psychiatrist, psychologist, social worker, case manager) and services (e.g., outpatient, inpatient, residential, respite care). Examples of information provided to parents includes the necessary educational background and roles for each member of a child's treatment team, types of therapies available, and goals for each form of therapy (e.g., cognitive behavioral therapy, family therapy, medication management). After reviewing information specific to mental health treatment, the focus of the session shifts to the educational setting. Group leaders review the personnel who make up a child's education team (e.g., teachers, guidance counselor, school social worker, principal, special education coordinator), and is also define and discuss important terminology (e.g., FAPE, free and appropriate education; IEP, individual educational plan; MFE, multifactored evaluation). Parents are also instructed about requirements for special education, alternatives to regular classroom placement, and how to request special services at school. As their project, parents are asked to identify the important members of their child's treatment and educational teams.

Child Group: Feelings Management

The focus of Session 3 is on helping children learn ways to manage their mad, sad, and bad feelings. Children are asked to brainstorm triggers that cause them to feel mad, sad, and/or bad, and to list them on the provided worksheet. Next, body signals for certain feelings are discussed (e.g., stomachache, headache, clenched fists), and children identify their specific body signals by coloring the relevant sections on a cartoon picture of a body. The discussion of coping skills is framed in terms of "building a Tool Kit" to manage negative emotions. The Tool Kit comprises four categories: creative (e.g., music, art), rest and relaxation (e.g., bubble bath, watching TV), social (e.g., playing with friends, talking with a parent), and physical (e.g., running, playing a sport). Children brainstorm activities in each of these categories to help them feel better when they are upset, and write these in the provided worksheet.

THERAPIST: We have been talking the last few weeks about different feelings people can have. For example, sometimes people feel happy, and other times they feel mad or sad. What are some of the things that make you all feel mad or sad?

MEGAN: I feel sad when nobody wants to play with me at school.

THERAPIST: I wonder if anyone else has ever felt that way?

JANE: (*Raises her hand along with several other children.*) Sometimes the other kids at school are mean to me, and that makes me feel mad *and* sad.

THERAPIST: That's right! Sometimes people can have more than one feeling at the same time. When people feel upset, sometimes their body gives them certain clues, like having a stomachache. What clues do your bodies give you when you are feeling upset?

JOHN: When I get worried my heart beats really fast.

THERAPIST: Good example! That is something that I bet a lot of people experience. What other ways do your bodies let you know that you're upset?

JANE: When I get mad my face gets red and hot.

MEGAN: That happens to me, too! My mom always says that she can tell when I'm mad!

THERAPIST: So sometimes other people can tell how we are feeling based on how we look, too! When we are feeling mad or sad, it is important to recognize how we are feeling, then find a way to help ourselves feel better. Today we're going to build a Tool Kit that you can use to help yourself calm down when you are feeling mad, sad, worried, or frustrated. Who knows what a Tool Kit is?

MIKE: (*Raises his hand.*) I do! It's something that has different tools in it that you can use to fix things when they are broken.

THERAPIST: Right! People use tools to fix things that are broken. The Tool Kit we are going to build works the same way. We will brainstorm different types of things people can use to help themselves calm down. Does anyone know why it is important to have more than one tool in a Tool Kit?

JANE: Because you might need a different tool depending on the problem.

THERAPIST: That's right, Jane! (*Points to diagram on the wall.*) In our Tool Kit we have four kinds of tools: Creative, Rest and Relaxation, Physical, and Social. Let's talk a little bit about each category and different examples. Then, as your project for next week, you will each make your own Tool Kit and bring it back next week to share with the group.

Child Project: Building My "Tool Kit"

Jane's "Tool Kit" included the following tools: (1) *Creative*: write a story, color, draw; (2) *Rest and relaxation*: read, write in a journal, watch my favorite TV show, take deep breaths; (3) *Social*: talk with my parents, a friend, or the school counselor, write an e-mail to my grandmother, talk on the phone with a friend; and (4) *Physical*: go for a walk, play outside with my brother, ride my bike.

Session 4

Parent Group: Negative Family Cycles

The parent portion of Session 4 focuses on a discussion of the family struggles associated with having a child with a mood disorder (e.g., problems getting along, unpredictable behavior on the part of the child, dangerous/violent outbursts) and encourages parents to discuss their own struggles and ways they have dealt with them. Discussing parental burden normalizes these experiences and allows parents to gain support from one another.

Child Group: "Thinking, Feeling, Doing"

In a continuation of the discussion from Session 3, the child portion of Session 4 is devoted to discussing ways children can change negative thoughts, feelings, and behaviors into more positive ones. To do so, we use the "Thinking,

Feeling, Doing" paradigm (Fristad, Davidson, & Leffler, in press; Goldberg-Arnold & Fristad, 2003), which provides a context for helping children understand that they can change their mood by altering their thoughts and behaviors. The cartoon-like simplicity of the schemata is appealing to children. On the left side of the page, the child's name is written next to the outline of a person (typically a stick figure). Below the stick figure is a light switch, which signifies the event or "trigger" that led to a negative mood state. Next to the stick figure appear three shapes: a heart for recording feelings, a thought bubble for recording thoughts, and a box for behaviors. Each shape is divided into "helpful" (positive) and "hurtful" (negative) sections.

When first describing this activity, the therapists provide the children with an example of a trigger that would make somebody feel mad or sad (e.g., getting a bad grade on a test). Next, the group leaders facilitate discussion with group members about what they might be thinking in that situation (e.g., "I'm so stupid") and what hurtful behaviors they might display (e.g., "Yell at my mother when I get home from school"). Group members then brainstorm alternative, helpful thoughts and actions that would make them feel better. Finally, the leaders draw arrows between the hurtful thoughts, feelings, and behaviors to demonstrate how they cause a "vicious cycle" that makes it difficult for people to improve their mood. Alternatively, leaders discuss how changing hurtful thoughts and actions to more helpful ones can often help people improve their mood state.

THERAPIST: Now that you all have Tool Kits to help you cope with your mad, bad, and sad feelings, let's talk a little bit about how your thoughts and behaviors might affect the way you feel. Who here thinks that people's thoughts are related to the way they feel?

JANE: (*Looks thoughtful.*) I guess so. Sometimes when I'm mad I notice that I think really bad thoughts, like that I hate everyone.

THERAPIST: I wonder if anyone else has had that experience. (*Several children raise their hands.*) Let's think of an example. Say you got a bad grade on a test. How would you feel?

MIKE: I'd be pretty mad about that!

JANE: Me too!

THERAPIST: OK, so you'd be feeling mad. (*Writes this in the heart on the diagram. Points to thought bubble on diagram.*) What kinds of hurtful thoughts would you be thinking?

JANE: I'd be thinking how stupid I am.

THERAPIST: (*Writes this in the hurtful thoughts portion of the thought bubble.*) Anyone else?

MIKE: I'd be thinking about how much I hate the teacher.

THERAPIST: (*Writes this down as well.*) OK, so if you are thinking hurtful thoughts like "I am so stupid" or "I hate my teacher," how do you think you might act?

JANE: I would probably be grumpy toward people.

THERAPIST: (*Writes this in the box for hurtful behaviors.*) Ok, so we first said that we would feel mad if we got a bad grade on the test. How would you rather feel?

JOHN: Happy.

THERAPIST: (*Writes this in the "positive" half of the heart diagram.*) Now let's brainstorm some helpful thoughts that we can use to replace the hurtful thoughts. Who can think of an example?

JANE: Maybe I could think I'll do better next time.

THERAPIST: (*Writes this in the box for helpful thoughts.*) OK, good! Can anyone think of a more helpful behavior than being grumpy toward people?

MEGAN: Maybe we could ask the teacher for help on the answers we got wrong.

THERAPIST: That is a good one! (*Writes it in the box for helpful behaviors. Next, draws arrows between the negative feeling, hurtful thoughts, and hurtful behaviors. Points to the arrows.*) So, you can see that when we are feeling mad, sometimes we think and do things that are hurtful, and that can make us feel madder and even get us into trouble. (*Draws arrows between positive feelings, helpful thoughts, and helpful behaviors. Points to these arrows.*) But, when we change our hurtful thoughts to helpful thoughts, and our hurtful behaviors to helpful behaviors, this can help us to feel better.

Family Project: "Thinking, Feeling, Doing"

For their family project, the Smiths completed the "Thinking, Feeling, Doing" activity at home. Jane's trigger for that week was not getting to go to watch her favorite TV program. She reported feeling "extremely mad!" and her thoughts included "I hate Mom and Dad. They never let me do what I want!" and "I have the world's meanest parents!" Jane's actions included yelling at her parents, slamming her door, and throwing things around her bedroom. Alternative thoughts brainstormed by Jane and her parents included "Mom and Dad must have a good reason for not letting me watch TV" and "I can go do something else instead." Alternative behaviors included reading, playing outside, and talking calmly with her parents about why they would not let her watch TV. If she engaged in these alternative thoughts and behaviors, Jane predicted that she would feel calmer.

Session 5

Parent Group: Problem Solving

The goal of Session 5 is help parents develop strategies for managing behavioral difficulties (e.g., the use of empathy, positive reinforcement, structuring environments). Group leaders also discuss pitfalls to avoid, such as not allowing the child's difficulties to take over family life, not making big decisions during a mood episode, and not feeling guilty over not being able to meet all of the child's needs. Finally, problem-solving strategies are reviewed and discussed (e.g., identify the problem, identify and evaluate possible solutions, pick a solution, evaluate the result). Parents and children are asked to complete a family project addressing the use of problem solving for managing the child's symptoms.

Child Group: Problem Solving

Similarly, the child group is focused on the steps for problem-solving. Children are given a worksheet outlining the following steps: *Stop*, and use a tool from the Tool Kit to regain control; *Think* of several possible solutions; *Plan* for which solutions you will try; *Do* one of the solutions; and *Check* how well the solution worked. If it does not work, choose another solution to do. These steps are introduced to the children with an example chosen by one of the group members of a problem he or she has recently faced. Group members help to brainstorm ideas and choose a solution.

THERAPIST: Today we're going to talk about how we can solve problems. Open your folder and turn to the page on problem solving. First, let's review the steps. Who can tell me what the light switch signifies?

JANE: The trigger.

THERAPIST: Right, so the first step is to figure out what the problem is. And what do you think the stop sign means?

JOHN: Stop and think about it.

THERAPIST: Why do you think it is important to stop before you jump in and do anything about it?

JANE: So you don't do something that gets you into trouble.

THERAPIST: Right! So it is important to stop and give yourself some time to calm down. Now, that can be easier said that done, especially if your trigger is something that really bothers you. How do you think you can help yourself calm down?

KATIE: Use something from your Tool Kit.

THERAPIST: That's a good idea! Now let's talk about the next step. What do you think the light bulb stands for?

JANE: Think.

THERAPIST: Think of what?

JOHN: Think of positive things.

THERAPIST: If we're talking about a problem you're having, what do you think we specifically want you to think about?

MIKE: Probably stop and think about the problem that you're having, and think of good solutions.

THERAPIST: Yes, that's it! The next step is to do what we call brainstorming. Has anyone done brainstorming at school before? What does it mean to brainstorm?

JANE: Throw out ideas.

THERAPIST: That's right, and when we brainstorm, we want to think of all possible solutions to the problem. The next step is to Plan. What do you think that means?

MEGAN: Plan what you're going to do.

THERAPIST: Good. You're going to pick which of the solutions to try, so part of that means thinking about the pros and cons of each solution that you thought of when you were brainstorming. The next step is to Do. What do you think that is?

JANE: You pick one solution and try it out.

THERAPIST: Good. How about Check?

MIKE: Check and make sure that it is going to work.

THERAPIST: Yes, after you've picked a solution and done it, you want to check and see whether it worked. If it didn't work, you want to go back and brainstorm some more, and figure out what to do next time. Now we're going to talk about some examples. Does anyone have any problems you want the group to help with?

Child Project: Problem Solving

Children are asked to use the Stop, Think, Plan, Do, Check framework to solve a problem that occurs during the next week. Jane's problem occurred in school, when a classmate teased her during gym class. Though she initially got mad, she remembered to Stop and use deep breathing, one of the tools from her Tool Kit, to help herself calm down. Next, she thought of a few solutions for her problem, which included (1) hitting the classmate who teased her; (2) telling the teacher; or (3) calmly telling her classmate that she hurt her feelings. During the planning phase, Jane was able to recognize that Solution 1 would probably get her into more trouble. Also, though Solution 2 might be a good one, it could also make other students think she was a "tattletale." Instead, Jane decided to tell her classmate that she had hurt her feelings and asked her to stop. To Jane's surprise, her solution worked, and her classmate apologized for hurting her feelings.

Session 6

Parent Group: Communication

The focus of Session 6 is to review the communication cycle (i.e., sending and receiving messages) and highlight the importance of helpful versus hurtful communication. Parents are provided with examples of hurtful communication (e.g., name-calling, blaming, mind reading) and helpful alternatives (e.g., empathy, XYZ talk—when you X, I feel Y; I'd like you to do Z). Specific emphasis is also placed on giving parents examples of how to respond to their children when they are having difficulties.

Child Group: Nonverbal Communication

The child portion of Session 6 focuses specifically on nonverbal communication. Group leaders and members discuss the importance of communication and its components (e.g., talking, listening, verbal, nonverbal). The following five aspects of nonverbal communication are defined, discussed, and demonstrated: facial expressions, body gesture, body posture, tone of voice, personal space. Group leaders and members may practice using and interpreting nonverbal communication through activities such as playing Charades.

THERAPIST: Today we are going to talk about communication. Can anyone explain to the group what communication is?

JANE: The way we talk to each other.

THERAPIST: Right! Communication has to do with how we express our thoughts and feelings to others. People can express themselves in different ways. For example, like Jane said, sometimes people use words. Other times people communicate using body language. Today we're going to talk about body language, or nonverbal communication. One kind of nonverbal communication is facial expression. (*Makes a sad face.*) Who can tell how I am feeling right now by looking at my face?

MIKE: Sad.

THERAPIST: How can you tell?

MIKE: Because you are frowning.

THERAPIST: Good! How else?

JANE: Your eyes look sad.

THERAPIST: Let's see if we can guess how somebody is feeling by their facial expression. Who wants to go first?

JOHN: I will. (*Makes a mad face.*)

THERAPIST: Who can guess how John is feeling?

JANE: Mad, because his eyes are squinted and his teeth are clenched.

THERAPIST: Good job! So, you can see that facial expressions are an important part of communication. They can tell you a lot about how people are feeling, without them even having to say anything.

Family Project: Paying Attention to Feelings

Parents and children practice their nonverbal communication skills by using nonverbal cues to act out a feeling and see whether the other person can guess it correctly. They are provided with a worksheet listing a variety of feelings (e.g., sad, angry, scared, confused) and asked to take turns acting out each feeling, while the other tries to guess. They are also instructed to track the number of correct guesses and to bring the worksheet back with them to the next session. Jane and her parents reported that they had fun completing this family project together. Based on her worksheet, Jane was easily able to identify her parents' nonverbal cues for sad, confused, stressed, and bored, but she had more difficulty with feelings such as scared, angry, and proud. Likewise, Jane was able to get her parents to correctly guess sad, angry, confused, bored, and proud, but she had more difficulty demonstrating "stressed" using nonverbal cues.

Session 7

Parent Group: Symptom Management

In Session 7, parents are provided with practical skills for managing their child's symptoms of mania and depression. Topics reviewed include creating a safety plan, therapeutic holds, emergency phone numbers, knowing insurance coverage. Parents are also instructed on handling suicidal concerns (e.g., taking it seriously, removing available materials, knowing when to hospitalize). Typical difficulties (e.g., medication adherence, dealing with stigma, rules and expectation) are reviewed, and families spend time brainstorming possible solutions for addressing such concerns. Finally, the session includes a discussion of managing caregiver burden to help parents reduce the likelihood of becoming overwhelmed and to increase their ability to care for their child effectively.

Child Group: Verbal Communication

The child portion of Session 7 is a continuation of the discussion from the previous session regarding communication skills. Aspects of verbal communication are discussed, and children are asked to brainstorm ways to change hurtful communication (e.g., "You're stupid!") into helpful communication (e.g., "I got upset when you teased me, I wish you would stop").

THERAPIST: Sometimes when people get upset they say things that can be very hurtful. In your workbook are some examples of hurtful communications. Let's brainstorm ways to change these statements, so that they are more helpful. One way to do this is to explain how you are feeling and how you would like things to be different. For example, the first statement is "I hate you." A more helpful thing to say might be "I'm feeling mad right now; I would prefer to be alone." Who can tell us what the next statement says?

JANE: It says "Shut up!"

THERAPIST: How would you feel if somebody said that to you?

JANE: I would be mad at them.

THERAPIST: OK, so let's think of something more helpful you could say. Who can think of something?

MIKE: How about, "Can you please be quiet?"

THERAPIST: That's a good one! How would you feel if somebody said that to you?

MIKE: I would be more likely to do what they said.

THERAPIST: So when people use hurtful communication, it can make others angry and less likely to listen. But, if you change your communication style to make it more helpful, people will be more likely to listen to you and try to help you out. Let's try another example.

Family Project: "Let's Talk"

The goal of this final family project is to increase helpful communication between parents and children by having them identify their "wishes" with regard to communication. Children are asked to identify three things they would like their parents to do differently to improve parent–child communication (e.g., "Give me compliments," "Don't yell at me"). Likewise, parents are asked to identify three things they would like their children to do differently to improve their communication (e.g., "Talk quietly," "Don't interrupt"). Jane said that she would like her parents to (1) stop yelling so much; (2) tell her when she is doing something well; and (3) give her their full attention when she is speaking to them. Jane's parents wished that Jane would (1) look at them when they were talking; (2) stop interrupting when they talk; and (3) be aware of her nonverbal cues.

Session 8

Parent Group: Review

The final session is primarily an opportunity to review the information presented throughout the course of treatment (e.g., cause/course of mood disorders, ways to manage difficulties in the child and family) and allow parents to ask any questions that remain unanswered. Parents are also provided with extensive information about resources that may be helpful in managing their child's mood disorder (e.g., books, websites, local support groups).

Child Group: Review

Similarly, the final child group focuses on reviewing the previously presented material, in the form of a trivia game in which group members earn points by correctly answering questions. At the end of the group, these points are combined with the points earned throughout the group, and children are able to trade their points in for prizes.

During the trivia game, Jane was eager to demonstrate her new knowledge about BPD and the strategies she learned for managing her symptoms. When asked about the most important thing she had learned in group, Jane replied, "It helps to know that I'm not alone, and that there are other kids going through the same things I am."

Posttreatment Follow-Up

Reevaluation of Jane's symptoms of mania and depression after her participation in MFPG revealed a significant reduction in scores on the CDRS-R and MRS. Mrs. Smith's report on the CDRS-R suggested a mild level of depressive symptoms (total score of 27, compared to a pretreatment score of 47). Specifically, Mrs. Smith stated that during the 2 weeks prior to the assessment, Jane demonstrated mild anhedonia, mild difficulties with concentration at school, and a moderate level of irritability. Mrs. Smith's report of Jane's posttreatment scores on the MRS also indicated improvement in Jane's manic symptoms (total score of 11 posttreatment compared to 34 pretreatment). The only symptoms endorsed by Mrs. Smith for Jane at posttreatment were moderate irritability and moderate disruptive–aggressive behavior. All other symptoms of mania were denied.

CONCLUSIONS

BPD in children wreaks havoc on family life, school functioning, and peer relationships. Appropriate diagnosis and intervention is imperative for improving patient outcomes and minimizing later difficulties. As described in this chapter, assessment of BPD in children is complicated by a number of factors. Among these are the high degree of overlap between symptom dimensions across different psychiatric disorders; high comorbidity between BPD in children and disorders such as ADHD, ODD, and CD; and the developmental considerations in the way mania is expressed in children versus adults. Therefore, clinicians must be cognizant of these difficulties and knowledgeable about the ways mania is expressed in children and adolescents to distinguish accurately between mania and other childhood disorders, and to eliminate misdiagnosis. As described in this chapter, proper assessment of childhood BPD includes the following elements: (1) longitudinal history of the child's development and symptom expression; (2) family history of mood and other psychiatric disorders; (3) thorough assessment of symptoms using the FIND criteria (Kowatch et al., 2005); (4) behavioral observation of child; and (5) information from relevant collateral contacts. In this chapter, we have illustrated these elements using a case example of an 8-year-old girl diagnosed with BPD.

Psychosocial interventions for children with BPD are scarce (Kowatch et al., 2005). In this chapter, we have described elements of a group therapy program developed as part of a larger multifamily psychoeducation program for families of preadolescent children with mood disorders. Preliminary research has found this program to be effective for increasing parental knowledge of mood disorders and treatment options. Parents who have participated in these groups have also described how they benefit from improved social support (Goldberg-Arnold et al., 1999).

Though initial examination of MFPG suggests that it is a promising adjunctive treatment for BPD in children, much work is still needed to refine developmentally appropriate, empirically validated treatment strategies for children and adolescents with affective disturbances. Similarly, continued research is needed on the clinical presentation of mania in children and adolescents to create appropriate clinical guidelines and to ensure the accurate diagnosis of bipolar spectrum disorders in children and adolescents. Finally, also needed are valid, reliable, and developmentally appropriate assessment tools that reflect differences in the clinical presentation of mania in children and adults.

REFERENCES

Achenbach, T. M., McConaughy, S. H., & Howell, C. T. (1987). Child/adolescent behavioral and emotional problems: Implications of cross-informant correlations for situational specificity. *Psychological Bulletin, 101*(2), 213–232.

Allen, M. G. (1976). Twin studies of affective illness. *Archives of General Psychiatry, 33*(12), 1476–1478.

American Psychiatric Association (APA). (2000). *Diagnostic and statistical manual of mental disorders* (4th ed. text rev.). Washington DC: Author.

Asarnow, J. R., Goldstein, M. J., Tompson, M., & Guthrie, D. (1993) One-year outcomes of depressive disorders in child psychiatric in-patients: Evaluation of the prognostic power of a brief measure of expressed emotion. *Journal of Child Psychology and Psychiatry, 34*(2), 129–137.

Badner, J. A. (2003). The genetics of bipolar disorder. In B. Geller & M. DelBello (Eds.), *Bipolar disorder in early childhood and adolescence*. New York: Guilford Press.

Biederman, J., Mick, E., Faraone, S. V., Spencer, T., Wilens, T., & Wozniak, J. (2000). Pediatric mania: A developmental subtype of bipolar disorder? *Biological Psychiatry, 48*(6), 458–466.

Birmaher, B., Ryan, N. D., Williamson, D. E., Brent, D. A., Kaufman, J., Dahl, R. E., et al. (1996). Childhood and adolescent depression: A review of the past 10 years, Part I. *Journal of the American Academy of Child and Adolescent Psychiatry, 35*(11), 1427–1439.

Brown, G. W., Birley, J. L., & Wing, J. K. (1972). Influence of family life on the course of schizophrenic disorders: A replication. *British Journal of Psychiatry, 121*, 241–258.

Butzlaff, R. L., & Hooley, J. M. (1998). Expressed emotion and psychiatric relapse: A meta-analysis. *Archives of General Psychiatry, 55*, 547–552.

Carlson, G. A. (1996). Clinical features and pathogenesis of child and adolescent mania. In K. I. Shulman, M. Tohen, & S. P. Kutcher (Eds.), *Mood disorders across the life span* (pp. 127–147). New York: Wiley-Liss.

Chang, K. D., Steiner, H., & Ketter, T. A. (2000). Psychiatric phenomenology of child and adolescent bipolar offspring. *Journal of the American Academy of Child and Adolescent Psychiatry, 39*(4), 453–460.

Davidson, K. H., Fristad, M. A., & Goldberg-Arnold, J. S. (2003). *The medication usage and service provider grids.* Unpublished manuscript, The Ohio State University, Columbus, OH.

Findling, R. L., Gracious, B. L., McNamara, N. K., Youngstrom, E. A., Demeter, C. A., Branicky, L. A., et al. (2001). Rapid, continuous cycling and psychiatric co-morbidity in pediatric bipolar I disorder. *Bipolar Disorders, 3*, 202–210.

Fleming, J. E., & Offord, D. R. (1990). Epidemiology of childhood depressive disorders: A critical review. *Journal of the American Academy of Child and Adolescent Psychology, 29*(4), 571–580.

Fristad, M. A., Cummins, J., Verducci, J. S., Rooney, M., Teare, M., Weller, E. B., & Weller, R. A. (1998). Part IV: Children's Interview for Psychiatric Syndromes (ChIPS): Revised psychometrics for DSM-IV. *Journal of Child and Adolescent Psychopharmacology, 8*(4), 225–234.

Fristad, M. A., Davidson, K. H., & Leffler, J. (in press). Thinking–Feeling–Doing: A cognitive behavioral therapeutic approach for children and adolescents with bipolar disorder. *Journal of Family Psychotherapy.*

Fristad, M. A., Gavazzi, S. M., & Soldano, K. W. (1999). Naming the enemy: Learning to differentiate mood disorder "symptoms" from the "self" that experiences them. *Journal of Family Psychotherapy, 10*(1), 81–88.

Fristad, M. A., Glickman, A. R., Verducci, J. S., Rooney, M., Teare, M., Weller, E. B., & Weller, R. A. (1998). Part V: Children's Interview for Psychiatric Syndromes (ChIPS): Psychometrics in nonclinical samples. *Journal of Child and Adolescent Psychopharmacology, 8*(4), 235–243.

Fristad, M. A., Goldberg-Arnold, J. S., & Gavazzi, S. (2002). Multifamily psychoeducation groups (MFPG) for families of children with bipolar disorder. *Bipolar Disorders, 4*(4), 254–262.

Fristad, M. A., Rooney, M., Teare, M, Weller, E. B., Weller, R. A., & Salmon, P. (1998). Part III: Development and psychometric properties of the parent version of the Children's Interview for Psychiatric Syndromes (P-ChIPS). *Journal of Child and Adolescent Psychopharmacology, 8*(4), 219–224.

Fristad, M. A., Weller, E. B., & Weller, R. A. (1992). The Mania Rating Scale: Can it be used in children? A preliminary report. *Journal of the American Academy of Child and Adolescent Psychiatry*, 31(2), 252–257.

Fristad, M. A., Weller, R. A., & Weller, E. B. (1995). The Mania Rating Scale (MRS): Further reliability and validity studies with children. *Annals of Clinical Psychiatry*, 7(3), 127–132.

Geller, B., Bolhofner, K., Craney, J., Williams, M., DelBello, M., & Gundersen, K. (2000). Psychosocial functioning in a prepubertal and early adolescent bipolar disorder phenotype. *Journal of the American Academy of Child and Adolescent Psychiatry*, 39(12), 1543–1548.

Geller, B., Zimerman, B., Williams, M., Bolhofner, K., Craney, J., DelBello, M., et al. (2000). Diagnostic characteristics of 93 cases of a prepubertal and early adolescent bipolar disorder phenotype by gender, puberty and comorbid attention deficit hyperactivity disorder. *Journal of Child and Adolescent Psychopharmacology*, 10, 157–164.

Geller, B., Zimerman, B., Williams, M., DelBello, M., Bolhofner, K., Craney, J., et al (2002a). DSM-IV mania symptoms in a prepubertal and early adolescent bipolar disorder phenotype compared to attention-deficit hyperactive and normal controls. *Journal of Child and Adolescent Psychopharmacology*, 12, 11–25.

Geller, B., Zimerman, B., Williams, M., DelBello, M., Frazier, J., & Beringer, L. (2002b). Phenomenology of prepubertal and early adolescent bipolar disorder: Examples of elated mood, grandiose behaviors, decreased need for sleep, racing thoughts, and hypersexuality. *Journal of Child and Adolescent Psychopharmacology*, 12, 3–9.

Goldberg-Arnold, J. S., Fristad, M. A., & Gavazzi, S. (1999). Family psychoeducation: Giving families what they want and need. *Family Relations: Interdisciplinary Journal of Applied Family Studies*, 48(4), 411–417.

Goldberg-Arnold, J. S., & Fristad, M. A. (2003). Psychotherapy for children with bipolar disorder. In B. Geller & M. P. DelBello (Eds.), *Bipolar disorder in childhood and early adolescence* (pp. 272–294). New York: Guilford Press.

Hellander, M., Sisson, D. P., & Fristad, M. A. (2003). Internet support for parents of children with early-onset bipolar disorder. In B. Geller & M. DelBello (Eds.), *Bipolar disorder in childhood and early adolescence* (pp. 314–329). New York: Guilford Press.

Herjanic, B., & Reich, W. (1982). Development of a structured psychiatric interview for children: Agreement between child and parent on individual symptoms. *Journal of Abnormal Child Psychology*, 10(3), 307–324.

Jarbin, H., Grawe, R. W., & Hansson, K. (2000). Expressed emotion and prediction of relapse in adolescents with psychotic disorders. *Nordic Journal of Psychiatry*, 54(3), 201–205.

Kendler, K. S., Pedersen, N., Johnson, L., Neale, M. C., & Mathe, A. A. (1993). A pilot Swedish twin study of affective illness. *Archives of General Psychiatry*, 50(9), 699–700.

Kashani, J. H., Cantwell, D. P., Shekim, W. O., & Reid, J. C. (1982). Major depressive disorder in children admitted to an inpatient community mental health center. *American Journal of Psychiatry*, 139, 671–672.

Kashani, J. H., & Carlson, G. A. (1987). Seriously depressed preschoolers. *American Journal of Psychiatry*, 144, 348–350.

Kashani, J. H., Carlson, G. A., Beck, N. C., Hooper, E. W., Corcoran, C. M., McAllister, J. A., et al. (1987). Depression, depression symptoms, and depressed mood among a community sample of adolescents. *American Journal of Psychiatry, 144,* 931–934.

Kashani, J. H., Holcomb, W. R., & Orvaschel, H. (1986). Depression and depressive symptoms in preschool children from the general population. *American Journal of Psychiatry, 143,* 1138–1143.

Kashani, J. H., Ray, J. S., & Carlson, G. A. (1984). Depression and depressive-like states in preschool-age children in a child development unit. *American Journal of Psychiatry, 141,* 1397–1402.

Kowatch, R., & Fristad, M. A. (2006). Pediatric bipolar disorders. In R. T. Ammerman (Ed.) & M. Hersen & J. C. Thomas (Editors-in-Chief), *Comprehensive handbook of personality and psychopathology: Vol. III. Child psychopathology* (pp. 217–232). New York: Wiley.

Kowatch, R. A., Fristad, M. A., Birmaher, B., Wagner, K. D., Findling, R. L., & Hellander, M. (2005). Treatment guidelines for children and adolescents with bipolar disorder. *Journal of the American Academy of Child and Adolescent Psychiatry, 44*(3), 213–235.

Lewinsohn, P. M., Clarke, G. N., Seeley, J. R., & Rohde, P. (1994). Major depression in community adolescents: Age at onset, episode duration, and time to recurrence. *Journal of the American Academy of Child and Adolescent Psychiatry, 33,* 809–818.

Lewinsohn, P. M., Hops, H., Roberts, R. E., Seeley, J. R., & Andrews, J. A. (1993). Adolescent psychopathology: I. Prevalence and incidence of depression and other DSM-III-R disorders in high school students. *Journal of Abnormal Psychology, 102,* 133–144.

Lewinsohn, P. M., Klein, D. N., & Seeley, J. R. (1995). Bipolar disorders in a community sample of older adolescents: Prevalence, phenomenology, comorbidity, and course. *Journal of the American Academy of Child and Adolescent Psychiatry, 34*(4), 454–463.

Miklowitz, D. J. (2005). Psychological treatment and medication for the mood and anxiety disorders: Moderators, mediators, and domains of outcome. *Clinical Psychology: Science and Practice, 12*(1), 97–99.

Miklowitz, D. J., Goldstein, M. J., Nuechterlein, K. H., Snyder, K. S., & Mintz, J. (1998). Family factors and the course of bipolar affective disorder. *Archives of General Psychiatry, 45*(3), 225–231.

Peris, T. S., & Baker, B. L. (2000). Applications of the expressed emotion construct to young children with externalizing behavior: Stability and prediction over time. *Journal of Child Psychology and Psychiatry, and Allied Disciplines, 41*(4), 457–462.

Petersen, A. C., Compas, B. E., Brooks-Gunn, J., Stemmler, M., Ey, S., & Grant, K. E. (1993). Depression in adolescence. *American Psychologist, 48*(2), 155–168.

Poznanski, E. O., Grossman, J. A., Buchsbaum, Y., Banegas, M., Freeman, L., & Gibbons, R. (1984). Preliminary studies of the reliability and validity of the Children's Depression Rating Scale. *Journal of the American Academy of Child and Adolescent Psychiatry, 23,* 191–197.

Poznanski, E. O., & Mokros, H. B. (1994). Phenomenology and epidemiology of mood disorders in children and adolescents. In W. M. Reynolds & H. F. Johnston (Eds.), *Handbook of depression in children and adolescents* (pp. 19–39). New York: Plenum Press.

Tarullo, L. B., Richardson, D. T., Radke-Yarrow, M., & Martinez, P. E. (1995). Multiple sources in child diagnosis: Parent–child concordance in affectively ill and well families [Special issue]. *Journal of Clinical Child Psychology, 24*(2), 173–183.

Teare, M., Fristad, M. A., Weller, R. A., Weller, E. B., & Salmon, P. (1998). Part I: Development and psychometric properties of the Children's Interview for Psychiatric Syndromes (ChIPS). *Journal of Child and Adolescent Psychopharmacology, 8*(4), 203–209.

Tillman, R., Geller, B., Craney, J. L., Bolhofner, K., Williams, M., Zimerman, B., et al. (2003). Temperament and character factors in a prepubertal and early adolescent bipolar disorder phenotype compared to attention deficit hyperactive and normal controls. *Journal of Child and Adolescent Psychopharmacology, 13*(4), 531–543.

Tillman, R., Geller, B., Craney, J. L., Bolhofner, K., Williams, M., & Zimerman, B. (2004). Relationship of parent and child informants to prevalence of mania symptoms in children with a prepubertal and early adolescent bipolar disorder phenotype. *American Journal of Psychiatry, 161*, 1278–1284.

Weller, E. B., Weller, R. A., & Fristad, M. A. (1995). Bipolar disorder in children: Misdiagnosis, underdiagnosis, and future directions. *Journal of the American Academy of Child and Adolescent Psychiatry, 34*(6), 709–714.

Weller, E. B., Weller, R. A., Fristad, M. A., Rooney, M. T., & Schecter, J. (2000). Children's Interview for Psychiatric Syndromes (ChIPS). *Journal of the American Academy of Child and Adolescent Psychiatry, 39*(1), 76–84.

Weller, E. B., Weller, R. A., Rooney, M. T., & Fristad, M. A. (1999). *Children's Interview for Psychiatric Syndromes—Parent Version (P-ChIPS)*. Washington, DC: American Psychiatric Press, Inc.

Wozniak, J., Biederman, J., Mundy, E., Mennin, D., & Faraone, S. V. (1995). A pilot family study of childhood onset mania. *Journal of the American Academy of Child and Adolescent Psychiatry, 34*(12), 1577–1583.

Yeh, M., & Weisz, J. R. (2001). Why are we here at the clinic?: Parent–child (dis)agreement on referral problems at outpatient treatment entry. *Journal of Consulting and Clinical Psychology, 69*(6), 1018–1025.

Young, R. C., Biggs, J. T., Ziegler, V. E., & Meyer, D. A. (1978). A rating scale for mania: Reliability, validity and sensitivity. *British Journal of Psychiatry, 133*, 429–435.

Youngstrom, E. A., Findling, R. L., Calabrese, J. R., Gracious, B. L., Demeter, C., Bedoya, D. D., et al. (2004). Comparing the diagnostic accuracy of six potential screening instruments for bipolar disorder in youths aged 5 to 17 years. *Journal of the American Academy of Child and Adolescent Psychiatry, 43*(7), 847–858.

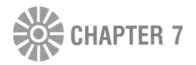

CHAPTER 7

Eating Problems

*Megan Roehrig, Steffanie Sperry, James Lock,
and J. Kevin Thompson*

Eating-related symptoms, such as under- or overeating, weight fluctuations, compensatory behaviors, or body image disturbance, are remarkably prevalent in children and adolescents. As these symptoms interact and become more pronounced, children and adolescents become increasingly vulnerable to developing eating disorders. Although lifetime prevalence estimates for eating disorders are rare, anorexia nervosa (AN) is associated with the highest mortality rate of any psychiatric disorder. Still, limited evidence is available on the psychological treatments for AN. The treatment of choice for adolescents with AN is family therapy based on the Maudsley approach. Treatment response has been promising, especially when the gap between the onset of AN symptoms and the beginning of treatment is brief. This chapter carefully describes the family-based treatment (FBT) manual developed by Lock and his colleagues for treating adolescent AN. Unlike many other treatments that emphasize etiology, intrinsic developmental deficits, and/or parental blame, FBT focuses on weight restoration and family reintegration. Using the case of "Susan" and her family, the authors describe the developmental progression of AN from cutting out sweets to "losing a little weight," and finally, to being hospitalized out of medical necessity. The authors demonstrate the treatment process through the steps of refeeding, facilitating appropriate weight gain, and the final goals of restoring family functioning and adolescent personal autonomy. The clinical guidelines are remarkably comprehensive, especially the therapeutic transcripts. Both new and experienced therapists will find the FBT approach invaluable and likely have a greater appreciation for the challenges inherent in helping youth with eating disorders.—A. R. E.

INTRODUCTION

Eating problems in youth can occur at any point across the developmental spectrum. They are relatively common in infants and young children, and are often developmentally appropriate "phases" that, although challenging, pass with time, without significant physical or developmental consequences (Bryant-Waugh, 2000). Picky or highly selective eating, food refusals, slow eating, and tantrums during eating are common manifestations in early childhood (Lewinsohn et al., 2005), and clinical intervention is not warranted in the majority of these cases. In a subgroup of infants and young children, however, the eating difficulties are significant and cause medical complications (Winters, 2003). These problems are categorized within the feeding disorder spectrum according to the *Diagnostic and Statistical Manual of Mental Disorders*, fourth edition, text revision (DSM-IV-TR; APA, 2000). According to DSM-IV-TR, feeding disorders occur in children under the age of 6 and are characterized by a persistent failure to eat adequately over at least a 1-month period, resulting in a significant weight loss or failure to gain appropriate weight. A feeding disorder is not diagnosed if an underlying medical condition is responsible for the weight problem, or if food is unavailable.

However, eating problems that are seen in older children and adolescents differ substantially from those seen in young children. Although there may be some similarities in symptom presentation (i.e., food refusal, highly selective eating), by middle childhood and beyond, the presence of significant eating problems is no longer developmentally appropriate (Bryant-Waugh, 2000). Additionally, cognitive development becomes more sophisticated as the child matures, and eating problems are more likely to have psychological underpinnings and be more characteristic of eating disorders rather than feeding disorders (Bryant-Waugh, 2000).

This chapter focuses on the description, assessment, and treatment of problems that fall on the disordered eating spectrum in older children and adolescents. Although treatment of feeding disorders is often warranted, it is beyond the scope of this chapter (for reviews, see Chatoor & Ganiban, 2003; Linscheid, 1998, 2006).

Nature of Symptom Dimensions

Upon referral, description of the presenting problem(s) may be very vague, and little information may be known about current and past eating behavior. Symptoms may broadly fall within the domains of problems related to eating, weight, compensatory behaviors, and/or body image. Interrelatedness among these symptom domains is typical, although symptoms may present in isolation in some cases. Many researchers have advocated a dimensional approach to eating problems, and a body of research has supported the continuity hypothesis of eating pathology (Chamay-Weber, Narring, & Michaud, 2005;

Fitzgibbon, Sanchez-Johnsen, & Martinovich, 2003; Franko & Omori, 1999; Stice, Killen, Hayward, & Taylor, 1998). The following section briefly reviews these four symptom dimensions and addresses the typical problems faced by clinicians.

Eating

Within the domain of eating, parents may indicate concerns with the quantity of food consumed and/or the food choices made by the child. With respect to the quantity of food consumed, parents may report concerns that the child is either undereating or overeating. Food refusal, avoidance of certain foods, and dieting are common manifestations of undereating complaints in older children and adolescents. Overeating occurs at the other end of the spectrum. Parental concerns may include binge eating, consumption of large portions, hiding food, and frequent snacking.

Problems related to the food choices made by the child or adolescent may also be reported. There may be a very limited range of foods selected by the child, and there may be almost no variety in the diet. These food choice restrictions may be based on fat and/or caloric content, food category (i.e., carbohydrates), food or brand preferences, or texture. Food choices may be dichotomized into "good" and "bad" foods, with a strict avoidance of "bad" foods. Alternatively, high-fat and high-calorie foods may dominate the client's food choices, with little to no consumption of nutrient-dense foods.

Weight

Concerns about the child or adolescent's weight status may also be brought to the attention of the clinician. Recent weight loss or failure to gain appropriate weight may be quite significant in children and adolescents and result in medical complications such as dehydration, orthostasis, bradycardia, osteopenia, impaired linear growth, and electrolyte imbalance (Katzman, 2005; Nicholls, de Bruyn, & Gordon, 2000). Underweight status may also be a concern, particularly if this is a change for the child or if there are concomitant changes in mood, eating, and exercise behaviors. Parents may also present their concerns regarding the child's recent weight gain or overweight/obesity to the child's clinician. Standardized growth charts are often useful to determine the body mass index (BMI) for age, which can screen children and adolescents for both underweight and overweight (Faith & Thompson, 2003).

Compensatory Behaviors

Any inappropriate strategy used to prevent weight gain following a binge-eating episode is considered a compensatory behavior (APA, 2000). Self-induced vomiting and misuse of laxatives, diuretics, enemas, or other medications are *purging* methods of compensatory behaviors. Excessive exercise and fasting are common *nonpurging* strategies. Self-induced vomiting and excessive exercise tend to be the more common methods of compensatory behavior in children, probably because of limited access to other methods, whereas laxative and diuretic abuse is more frequently seen in adolescents (Bryant-Waugh, 2000).

Body Image

Body image refers to the internal representation of one's physical appearance, and much attention has been given to the significant role of body dissatisfaction in eating pathology (Thompson, Heinberg, Altabe, & Tantleff-Dunn, 1999). "Body dissatisfaction" is a broad term that refers to at least some degree of dissatisfaction with one's appearance. The dissatisfaction may occur with respect to one or more body sites (i.e., thighs, stomach, chest) or relate to dissatisfaction with one's overall appearance (Cash, 2002). Extreme dissatisfaction with weight and/or shape is a core symptom of eating pathology (Thompson et al., 1999), and body dissatisfaction is becoming increasingly common in children and adolescents (Gardner, 2002).

Relationship to Specific Disorders

Four categories of eating disorders are currently listed in DSM-IV-TR (APA, 2000): anorexia nervosa, bulimia nervosa, eating disorder not otherwise specified, and binge-eating disorder. Binge-eating disorder is actually included in an appendix, "Criteria sets and Axes Provided for Further Study"; however, it is reviewed in this chapter for two reasons: It will likely be included as a bona fide eating disorder category in the next revision of DSM, and the disorder has been the subject of intense empirical study in recent years.

Anorexia Nervosa

The central feature of anorexia nervosa (AN) is a refusal to maintain body weight at or above 85% of that expected for one's age and height. In children and adolescents, this feature may manifest in either weight loss or failure to make expected weight or growth gains (Netemeyer & Williamson, 2001). Additional DSM-IV-TR diagnostic criteria include (1) an intense fear of fatness or of gaining weight, despite being underweight; (2) extreme body image disturbance, undue influence of body weight or shape on self-evaluation, or denial of the seriousness of the current low body weight; and (3) "amenorrhea," which is defined as the absence of at least three consecutive menstrual cycles (APA, 2000). Amenorrhea is the most controversial of the diagnostic criteria (Mitchell, Cook-Myers, & Wonderlich, 2005): It is not applicable to males or prepubertal females (Netemeyer & Williamson, 2001); menstrual functioning may be irregular in healthy adolescent females (citation); some very low weight patients continue to menstruate normally

(Mitchell et al., 2005); and birth control pills may be used to regulate menses in underweight patients (Bulik, Reba, Siega-Riz, & Reichborn-Kjennerud, 2005).

According to DSM-IV-TR, there are two subtypes of AN: restricting type and binge-eating/purging type (APA, 2000). In the restricting type, extreme reductions in energy balance are achieved through fasting, dieting, and excessive exercise, and binge eating and purging are absent during the current episode. In the binge-eating/purging type, binge eating, purging, or both are regularly utilized during the current episode. Purging behaviors may occur in the absence of an objective binge, and may instead occur after consumption of a small quantity of food in individuals with AN.

The epidemiology of AN in children and adolescents is largely unknown (Doyle & Bryant-Waugh, 2000). According to DSM-IV-TR, the lifetime prevalence rate for anorexia nervosa is approximately 0.5%. The peak age of onset appears to be between the ages of 15 and 19, but cases have been identified in children as young as 8 years old (Bulik et al., 2005; Lask & Bryant-Waugh, 2000). Gender differences are prominent in anorexia nervosa with women outnumbering men; however, these differences do no appear to be as significant in childhood (Doyle & Bryant-Waugh, 2000). Although the popular press has suggested that AN may be on the rise in youth, a recent review indicates that AN rates do not appear to be increasing in adolescents (Bryant-Waugh, 2006).

The course of AN is variable. It has the highest mortality rate of any psychiatric disorder with estimates around 5–6%; about half the deaths are attributable to suicide, and the rest are related to physical complications of the disorder (Agras, 2001; Herzog et al., 2000; Sullivan, 1995). On the positive side, however, Steinhausen (1995) reviewed the treatment outcome literature from the 1950s to the 1980s and found that about 33% of cases of AN improved, 20% had a chronic course, and 40% recovered. Comorbidity with major depression, obsessive–compulsive disorder, social phobia, and personality disorders is common (Thompson, Roehrig, & Kinder, 2007).

Bulimia Nervosa

The central features of bulimia nervosa (BN) include recurrent episodes of binge eating, followed by inappropriate compensatory methods to prevent weight gain (APA, 2000). A *binge-eating episode* is defined by DSM-IV-TR as having two components: (1) eating an amount of food within a discrete time period (i.e., 2 hours) that is considerably larger than most people would consume during a similar period of time under similar circumstances, and (2) a feeling of loss of control over eating during the episode. Binge-eating/purging episodes must occur on average twice a week for 3 months to meet diagnostic criteria for BN. Body image disturbance is also present in individuals with BN, and self-evaluation is "unduly influenced by body shape and weight" (APA, p. 594). These symptoms cannot occur exclusively during an episode of AN.

There are two subtypes of BN: purging type and nonpurging type (APA, 2000). In the purging type, individuals regularly attempt to prevent weight gain following a binge by "getting rid" of the food consumed by self-induced vomiting or the misuse of laxatives, diuretics, or enemas. Individuals with nonpurging type BN regularly use excessive exercise and/or fasting rather than purgative methods to compensate for binge-eating episodes.

Lifetime prevalence rates for BN are between 1 and 3%, and gender differences are found, with women outnumbering men (APA, 2000). Point prevalence rates for adolescents have been found to be 0.5% for girls and 0.3% for boys (Kjelsas, Bjornstrom, & Gotestam, 2004). Risk for BN may now be highest in 10- to 19-year-olds (Bryant-Waugh, 2006). The course is variable, and often there is comorbidity among BN and depressive, anxiety, personality, and substance use disorders (Thompson et al., 2007).

Eating Disorder Not Otherwise Specified (ED NOS)

The ED NOS category is used typically for cases in which one or more of the required diagnostic criteria are not met, yet there is evidence that the individual's level of eating disturbance meets a degree of severity that warrants clinical attention. Examples include a patient who meets all diagnostic criteria for AN except the amenorrhea criterion, or an individual who is binge eating and purging with less frequency than twice a week on average over a 3-month period. Atypical presentations also fall in the ED NOS category, such as an individual who chews and spits out, but does not swallow, large amounts of food. Most patients presenting for treatment do not meet full diagnostic criteria for AN or BN and are diagnosed with ED NOS (Mitchell et al., 2005). This is particularly true for children and adolescents with eating problems, who often do not fit neatly into DSM diagnostic criteria (Nicholls, Chater, & Lask, 2000). An estimated 0.8–14% of the general adolescent population meet criteria for ED NOS (Chamay-Weber et al., 2005).

Binge-Eating Disorder

Binge-eating disorder (BED) currently is listed in Appendix B of DSM-IV-TR as a disorder for further study and is diagnostically subsumed under ED NOS. A great deal of research has been conducted on BED over the last decade, and it will likely become a bona fide diagnosis in DSM-V (Pull, 2004). The central feature of BED is recurrent episodes of binge eating that occur in the absence of any inappropriate compensatory behaviors following the binge (APA, 2000). The binge-eating episode must also be associated with at least three of the following: (1) eating much more rapidly than normal, (2) eating until one feels uncomfortably full, (3) eating large amounts of food when one is not feeling physically hungry, (4) eating alone because one is embarrassed by food consumption, and (5) feeling disgusted with oneself, depressed, or very guilty after overeating. Symptoms must occur on average twice a week for 6 months to meet full diagnostic criteria for BED. Interestingly, there is no body image disturbance component for a diagnosis of BED.

Marcus and Kalarchian (2003) proposed modified diagnostic criteria for BED that are developmentally appropriate for children and adolescents with binge eating and based on the literature to date. According to their proposed criteria, a diagnosis of BED should be rendered if recurrent binge eating, which includes both food seeking when not hungry and loss of control over eating, occurs over at least a 3-month period and is characterized by food seeking in response to negative affect, food seeking as a reward, or sneaking or hiding food. Additionally, regular use of compensatory behaviors is absent, and the symptoms do not occur exclusively within the context of an episode of AN or BN (Marcus & Kalarchian, 2003).

Little is known about the prevalence and course of BED in children and adolescents. Binge eating appears to be more common in overweight or obese children and adolescents than in their normal-weight peers (Tanofsky-Kraff et al., 2004). In one cross-sectional study, only 1% overweight or obese children and adolescents seeking weight loss treatment met full diagnostic criteria for BED, whereas 9% admitted to overeating with a loss of control but did not meet other diagnostic criteria for BED (Decaluwe & Braet, 2003). In a sample of non-treatment-seeking normal-weight and overweight 6- to 13-year-olds, 6.2% reported objective binge eating, 3.1% endorsed subjective binge-eating episodes, 20.4% admitted to objective overeating episodes, and 70.4% had no episodes over the past 28 days (Tanofsky-Kraff et al., 2004). Loss of control over eating rather than mere overeating or dieting has been found to have a greater association with increased adiposity, disturbed eating cognitions, and depressive and anxiety symptoms in children and adolescents (Marcus & Kalarchian, 2003; Tanofsky-Kraff, Faden, Yanovski, Wilfley, & Yanovski, 2005).

Retrospective studies of adults with BED suggest that binge-eating symptoms begin between the ages of 11 and 13 in those that reported binge-eating symptoms preceding dieting behavior, whereas binge-eating symptoms develop in late adolescence for those who report dieting preceding binge-eating behavior (Marcus & Kalarchia, 2003). Much more research is needed on ethnically diverse community and clinical samples to understand the epidemiology and course of binge eating in children and adolescents.

Non-DSM Classification

DSM criteria for eating disorders have been criticized for often not sufficiently capturing the breadth of eating problems seen in children and adolescents (Nicholls, Chater, et al., 2000). The Great Ormand Street criteria (GOS) have been proposed as an alternative classification system of eating pathology that takes childhood and adolescent developmental issues and variety of symptom presentation into account (Bryant-Waugh & Lask, 1995). In addition to classic AN and BN, the GOS system identifies additional diagnoses, including food avoidance emotional disorder, selective eating, and restrictive eating (Chamay-Weber et al., 2005; Lask & Bryant-Waugh, 2000; Nicholls, Chater, et al., 2000). Food avoidance emotional disorder involves intense avoidance of food and subsequent weight loss; however, there are no disturbances or preoccupations related to weight and/or shape. Children or adolescents with selective eating present with a very narrow range of preferred foods, but their weight is within normal limits, and there are no aberrant cognitions related to weight or shape. Restrictive eating involves very little interest in food or eating in children without a mood disturbance; the weight of such children is usually in the lower end of normal range of weight, and they exhibit no body image concerns or active avoidance of food.

Differential Diagnosis and Risk Factors

Differentiating among the childhood eating disorders is a task that should be initially guided by reliance on the diagnostic criteria provided by DSM-IV-TR. As noted in our introductory material to this chapter, some of the key symptoms that indicate a specific diagnosis include the following: very low weight (AN); average weight plus binge eating, with some type of accompanying compensatory activity, such as vomiting (BN); and binge eating in the absence of compensatory activity (BED). Often a child or adolescent exhibits some of the symptoms of an eating disorder but does not meet the full criteria, in which case a diagnosis of EDNOS is appropriate.

Differential diagnosis with other DSM disorders is also a key component of any assessment. The somatoform disorder, body dysmorphic disorder (BDD), may easily be confused with an eating disorder. The primary BDD characteristic, an extreme disparagement of some aspect of appearance (weight- or non-weight-related), may be delusional (i.e., there is no evidence of a specific "defect" noted by an impartial observer). If the body site responsible for the BDD is weight-related, such as fatness disparagement associated with one's waist, hips, thighs, or other body part, then the BDD diagnosis is not appropriate when the other criteria for a specific eating disorder are met.

Another key differential is with a social phobia. One characteristic of some individuals with an eating disorder is a fear or anxiety that their physical appearance is being scrutinized and/or they feel that they are being observed by others while eating. If either of these issues is relevant, a diagnosis of an eating disorder might be entertained, depending on whether other criteria are met. The key differential here is whether the social fear is specific to issues surrounding appearance and/or food, or whether it is more general in nature, involving multiple types of social situations (wherein avoidant personality may be operating) or other specific social fears unrelated to food or appearance (e.g., speaking, dancing, etc.). It is also important to distinguish between obsessive–compulsive disorder (OCD) or obsessive–compulsive personality disorder (OCPD) and eating disorders. If the obsessions and/or compulsions are entirely food related (e.g., food hoarding, compulsive weighing or body checking, etc.), then the diagnosis is likely an eating disorder.

Because eating disorders are quite rare in childhood and adolescence, particularly AN, few studies have actually evaluated diagnosed groups to determine whether particular genetic, family, developmental, or psychological factors might aid in the task of differential diagnosis. Rather, a wealth of work has examined potential risk factors for the onset and maintenance of eating disturbances in young samples. Much of this work defines "eating disturbance" quite broadly as a constellation of dieting, binge eating, purging, and body dissatisfaction. This research can assist the clinician in targeting specific factors that may have treatment implications. In the next section, we focus on the area of risk factors, after first reviewing recent work in the area of genetics and family functioning (wherein there is a small database of direct comparisons of families with and without a child with an eating disorder).

Genetics

The area of genetics is a rapidly emerging research field that has informed our knowledge of eating disorders risk. In a review of twin studies, Klump, Kaye, and Strober (2001) concluded that 58–76% of the variance in AN was due to genetic factors; for BN the range was 54–83%. They also found that eating disturbance symptoms had a high hereditary component: 32–72% of factors such as body dissatisfaction, eating and weight concerns, and weight preoccupation were heritable, and 46–72% of dietary restraint, binge eating, and vomiting was likely heritable. Reichborn-Kjennerud et al. (2004) examined the heritability of "undue influence of weight on self-evaluation" (which is the DSM-IV-TR body image disturbance criterion for AN and BN) in a sample of over 8,000 Norwegian twins. Shared environmental factors accounted for 31% of the variance in body image disturbance, and 69% of the variance was attributed to nonshared or common environmental factors. Keski-Rahkonen et al. (2005) found significant gender differences in the heritability of drive for thinness and body dissatisfaction in a study of over 4,500 Finnish twins, with moderate to high levels of heritability in women but no heritability in males. Interestingly, Klump, McGue, and Iacono (2003) demonstrated that symptom-level eating disorder genes appear to activate during puberty.

Family Environment

A few studies have addressed family functioning for children with an eating disorder. Humphrey (1994) found greater rigidity and dependency in families with a restricting child with AN compared to families that had either a child with BN or a child of anorexic weight, who also had bulimic characteristics. Horesh et al. (1996), in a of sample adolescent girls with binge-eating disorder, found significant relations between disturbed eating patterns and parental overprotection and pressures. In a direct comparison of individuals with BN and obese binge eaters, Friedman, Wilfley, Welch, and Kunce (1997) found that troubled family functioning was higher for the BN group. Shisslak, Crago, and Estes (1995) found lower family cohesion levels for adolescents who engaged in binge eating. For more information on the issue of family environment, see the excellent review by Steinberg and Phares (2001).

Risk Factor Studies

In the last 10 years, work designed to pinpoint specific social and interpersonal risk factors for the onset of eating and body image disturbances has exploded onto the eating disorders scene (for reviews, see Field, 2004; Wertheim, Paxton, & Blaney, 2004), and the solid information these studies have yielded has been incorporated into treatment and prevention programs (Stice & Hoffman, 2004; Thompson, 2004). Thompson and colleagues (1999) have developed the tripartite influence model as one organizing theoretical framework that incorporates multiple social and interpersonal influences. In this model, three formative influences (peers, parents, and media) facilitate body image and eating disturbances directly and indirectly (by instigating social comparisons related to appearance, and by encouraging an internalization of societal standards regarding appearance) (Keery, van den Berg, & Thompson, 2004; Shroff & Thompson, 2006a, 2006b; Thompson et al., 1999).

The parental factor comprises a variety of subdimensions, including parental modeling of appearance concerns and disordered eating, along with direct communication by the parents to their children (via comments or instructions) that facilitates weight concern or disordered eating. Peer influences are similar in nature and often comprise dimensions such as appearance-focused comments and conversations or direct modeling of eating disturbances. Media influences are quite broad and may comprise information regarding disturbed eating patterns transmitted via magazines, TV, or the internet (proanorexic websites). Additionally, measures have been developed for the assessment of more abstract media influences, such as an internalization of media influence, which is an incorporation of the media's messages and images into one's belief system (namely, the importance of attractiveness; Thompson, van den Berg, Roehrig, Guarda, & Heinberg, 2004).

Prospective studies offer some of the most compelling evidence for the role of multiple factors in the onset of eating disturbances. In general, a consistent finding is that body image dissatisfaction is associated with the onset of eating disturbances (Thompson et al., 1999; Wertheim et al., 2006). Other factors that have been found to be associated in individual studies include being teased about one's weight, maternal body dissatisfaction, maternal and paternal BMI, and thin-ideal internalization (Wertheim et al., 2004). Importantly, early intervention and prevention programs have begun to incorporate the findings from risk factor work into strategies designed to prevent or reduce eating disturbances in children and adolescents (see Levine & Smolak, 2001; Levine & Harrison, 2004; Stice & Hoffman, 2004). Next, we present the case of Susan and her family.

CASE FORMULATION:
CONCEPTUAL MODEL OF ASSESSMENT AND TREATMENT

Case Presentation

Susan is a 14-year-old girl whose pediatrician referred her for treatment for weight loss and probable AN. Her mother Lola is a part-time health care professional, and her father Simon is an educator. Her younger brother Tommy is 11 years old. Susan met all usual developmental milestones and had always been healthy. She had no history of behavior problems and was well-liked by her peers throughout elementary school. Susan could best be described as timid, quietly competitive, and perfectionistic regarding her academic work. Neither Susan nor her parents reported any history of abuse, and her family environment appeared intact until she developed AN. Her paternal family history, however, was remarkable for anxiety and depression. There was no history of substance abuse on either side of the family.

Changes in Susan

Susan had been in her usual state of good health until about 8 months prior to the referral, when she began dieting and exercising. During the spring of eighth grade, Susan reported that she had decided to "lose a little" weight. She began by cutting out sweets and desserts. Her parents admired her "healthier" eating habits despite the fact that Susan did not need to lose weight. At the same time, she began regularly running with her father every other morning. Susan's weight dropped from 110 pounds (at a height of 5'3") to 100 pounds. Susan then decided to cut back on the amount of animal protein she was consuming. She felt that eating animals was immoral and began a vegetarian diet. Over the next 2 months, Susan increased her exercise regimen, for instance, by running on the days her father skipped. Her weight then dropped to 90 pounds. Susan's parents expressed concern and asked their daughter to eat more and exercise less. Susan responded by eating alone and exercising more regularly.

By the time Susan's parents took her to the pediatrician, Susan weighed 85 pounds. The pediatrician told her she needed to eat more. Although Susan told the pediatrician she continued to have her menstrual periods, her mother reported that there had been no evidence that this was so for the previous month. Susan increased her already considerable efforts in academics. Susan had always been an excellent student was but now spending excessive hours studying and restudying for tests. Although she continued to receive excellent grades, it was clear that she no longer cared about her schoolwork. Studying simply served as a good distraction from thinking about eating. She was constantly reading food labels and memorizing caloric amounts and fat grams.

In addition to losing weight and becoming overly preoccupied with food-related thoughts, Susan was spending hours in front of the mirror. She pulled at her skin and examined her stomach and thighs, disgusted at what she perceived to be fat. Susan no longer called her friends at school, because she was too preoccupied with food and weight to be concerned about them. As she continued to lose weight, Susan became increasingly isolated from both friends and family. Mealtimes, in particular, became especially tense. Susan frequently became tearful, agitated, or completely withdrew.

Changes in the Family

Over the 6-month course of Susan's illness, her family began restructuring their routines around her eating. For example, they made special shopping trips for Susan's dietary requirements. They bought low or nonfat foods, because Susan refused to eat anything else. To help her eat, the entire family began eating more vegetarian meals. Furthermore, they found themselves eating dinner at an earlier time, because Susan was afraid that if she ate later in the evening, then she would get fat.

Although Susan's family members knew that she had a problem with eating, they were uncertain how to proceed. Susan had always been a strong-willed and determined person, and it was not surprising to her parents that she would take up dieting and exercise behaviors in the same spirit. They also did not know when normal dieting as a part of adolescence became something more concerning. Many hours of family time were devoted to discussing Susan's health-related issues. Yet, out of fear of causing Susan further distress and/or creating new problems, family members delayed making a decision about intervention.

Because of the family's heightened focus on Susan, her younger brother Tommy was beginning to feel neglected. Although worried about his sister and sometimes receiving the brunt of her angry outbursts, Tommy was mostly disappointed that his parents stopped attending his athletic events. In addition, he resented mealtimes because of the intense conflict over Susan's unhealthy eating habits. Both Lola and Simon found themselves struggling to sleep and to focus on their work. The family found itself distributing its resources in an imbalanced way to accommodate the advent of Susan's AN.

When spring vacation came, the usual family ski trip was cancelled. Susan's parents felt that they could not risk taking Susan to the mountains because of the cold and the likelihood that she would exercise more rigorously. The extended family Easter dinner was also cancelled because of Susan's refusal to eat with any other family members. Susan's family had changed from a relatively high-functioning unit to one whose entire identity had been distorted. AN had become the central organizing principle.

Initial Presentation

Although Susan could not describe clearly her motivations for wanting to lose weight, she strongly believed she was healthy despite contradictory reports from her physicians. Susan acknowledged that she was lonely and had become increasingly irritable. In addition, she also reported feeling angry with her parents for bringing her in for treatment despite her objections; however, Susan freely reported her food intake.

For example, Susan reported eating half a bagel for breakfast and drinking a glass of water. In addition, she also consumed several soda crackers as a morning snack. For lunch, Susan ate half a nonfat cheese sandwich with mustard and a half-pint of nonfat milk. Her snack in the afternoon was one Jell-O cup. Susan reported that her typical dinner meal comprised a small portion of whatever her mother prepared, with the exception of meat.

During the intake, Susan reported running 2–3 miles daily until about 3 weeks earlier, when she began to feel too weak to run. At that time, her modified exercise regimen comprised 30 minutes of jumping jacks and 100 sit-ups, three times per day. She denied binge eating, intentional vomiting, and laxative or diuretic use. Susan reported minimal anxiety, but she did admit to some generalized worries regarding her academic performance and social life. She denied any history of panic attacks or depression. Finally, Susan reported that her obsessive thinking and behaviors were circumscribed around food, dieting, weight, and schoolwork, and at times resulted in sleep difficulties.

On mental status examinations, Susan appeared thin and looked younger than her age. She wore an overly large brown sweatshirt and leggings. Her short black hair was pulled back in a small ponytail. Susan's face was thin, and there were dark circles under her eyes. She made good eye contact and sat still in her chair. There were no abnormal tics or mannerisms noted. Susan spoke in a soft voice and a somewhat flat tone. Her mood was euthymic and her affect was constricted. Her thought process was linear and goal directed. Susan denied auditory or visual hallucinations. She denied suicidal or homicidal thoughts or behaviors. There was no evidence of grandiosity, frank delusions, or paranoia. On cognitive examination, Susan was alert and oriented. Her attention, concentration, memory, and abstractions were all within normal limits. As could be expected, however, Susan's insight and judgment regarding her eating disorder were poor.

Susan met with the team physician. Her ideal body weight (IBW) was calculated to be 78%. Her heart rate was 42 beats per minute; blood pressure, 85/50; and temperature, 36.1° F. Susan's lab results indicated a low complete blood count (CBC) but were otherwise within expected levels. Based on the medical presentation and the criteria for medical instability advised by pediatrics best practice, Susan was hospitalized for 8 days on a medical unit to stabilize her vital signs. During the hospitalization, Susan was cooperative. She was discharged with stable vital signs and at an IBW of 82%. Upon discharge, when outpatient care was considered medically safe, Susan's parents sought family treatment (to be discussed).

Assessment

The assessment of a child or adolescent presenting with eating-related problems is optimally achieved with the use of multiple informants and assessment techniques. The child or adolescent should be evaluated to determine his or her current health and nutritional status, as well as behaviors and cognitions surrounding food, eating, and weight. Various assessment tools and techniques for children and adolescents with eating problems are available, and some of the most commonly used assessment components and instruments are presented here.

Child Interviews

CHILD EATING DISORDER EXAMINATION

The Eating Disorder Examination (EDE; Cooper & Fairburn, 1987; Cooper, Cooper, & Fairburn, 1989; Fairburn & Cooper, 1993), a semistructured interview that is used to assess the core features of eating disorders, may be used as a diagnostic tool. The creators of the EDE advise that the interview schedule should only be used by interviewers who are knowledgeable about the defining characteristics of eating disorders, because a considerable amount of follow-up questioning is often necessary. The most recent version of the EDE (Fairburn & Cooper, 1993) not only allows for the extrapolation of individual item scores, has four subscale scores (Restraint, Eating Concern, Shape Concern, and Weight Concern) and a global score but also allows for the production of specific eating disorder diagnoses. Fairburn and Cooper (1993) provide female adult norms for the EDE subscales.

The EDE was adapted by Bryant-Waugh, Cooper, Taylor, and Lask (1996) for use with younger populations. Two primary modifications were made to the EDE in the formulation of the Child Adaptation of the EDE (ChEDE). First, two items of the EDE that assessed overvalued ideas about weight and shape were replaced by a sort task, in which the child is asked to make a list of "things that are important to you in how you see yourself or think about yourself," as well as "things that are important to you when you think about how good you are as a person" (Bryant-Waugh et al., 1996). The child is then asked to rank the items in order of importance. Second, some of the items were modified to assess intent as opposed to actual behavior to account for the fact that children and adolescents with eating disorders are still under the care of adults, which thereby makes it more difficult for them to engage in maladaptive eating behaviors (e.g., missing meals) in spite of their intent or desire to do so. In addition to these two primary modifications, minor wording changes were made throughout to make the interview more comprehensible to younger individuals.

General Psychopathology Interviews

The parent interviews that are most commonly used in the assessment of children and adolescents presenting with eating disorder symptomatology are general psychopathology interviews, such as the Diagnostic Interview Schedule for Children–2.1 (DISC-2.1: Jensen et al., 1995), the Diagnostic Interview for Children and Adolescents (DICA; Reich, Herjanic, Welner, & Gandhy, 1982), or a version of the Schedule for Affective Disorders and Schizophrenia for School-Age Children (e.g., K-SADS; Kaufman et al., 1997; Chambers et al., 1985; Ambrosini & Dixon, 1996). The K-SADS—Present and Lifetime version (K-SADS-PL; Kaufman et al., 1997) in particular allows the clinician to interview both parent and child, and combine this information before calculating total scores and making diagnoses. Using this interview schedule, the clinician is also able to obtain information about the child's present and past behavior. In addition, the K-SADS-PL provides a screener that assesses symptomatology for 20 different diagnostic areas (including eating disorders), thereby significantly reducing administration time.

In addition to a comprehensive evaluation of eating-related cognitions and behaviors, it is also important to assess for frequent comorbid conditions, such as depression, anxiety, substance abuse/dependence, dissociative disorders, OCD, and personality disorders. This is why general psychopathology interviews such as those mentioned earlier are frequently incorporated into the assessment of a child or adolescent presenting with a possible eating disorder. Nye and Johnson (1999) provide an overview of additional assessment instruments commonly used to evaluate potential comorbidity in individuals with eating disorders.

Child Self-Report Measures

CHILDREN'S EATING ATTITUDES TEST

The Children's Eating Attitudes Test (ChEAT; Maloney, McGuire, & Daniels, 1988) was adapted from the Eating Attitudes Test (EAT; Garner, Olmstead, Bohr, & Garfinkel, 1982) for use with children and adolescents. The ChEAT assesses perceived body image, obsession and preoccupation with food, and dieting behaviors. Because the ChEAT assesses only eating attitudes and dieting behavior, it is useful only as a screening instrument, not as a diagnostic tool (Christie, Watkins, & Lask, 2000), in identifying youth who are at risk for developing eating disorders, and the descriptive information provided is valuable in clinical settings as part of the establishment of individual treatment plans. The original wording of the EAT was changed to be understandable for children as young as 8 years old. Instructions are read orally, and the Likert items are completed individually by older children and are read aloud to younger children. The questionnaire takes approximately 30 minutes to complete. Normative data for the ChEAT are based on a sample of 318 children between the ages of 8 and 13 years. Relatively high internal consistency–reliability has been found, with coefficient alphas ranging from .76–.87 (Maloney et al., 1988; Smolak & Levine, 1994). The ChEAT has also demonstrated high test–retest reliability (coefficient alpha = .81; Maloney et al., 1988), and concurrent validity estimates have shown the ChEAT to be correlated with both body dissatisfaction ($r = .39$, $p < .001$) and weight management behaviors ($r = .36$, $p < .001$; Smolak & Levine, 1994).

KIDS' EATING DISORDERS SURVEY

The Kids' Eating Disorders Survey (KEDS; Childress, Brewerton, Hodges, & Jarrell, 1993) was developed for epidemiological purposes and may be used as a screening tool to identify children and adolescents who are at risk for developing eating disorders. The Eating Symptoms Inventory (ESI; Whitaker et al., 1989), an assessment of eating disorder symptomatology, has been validated in a high school sample. Childress, Jarrell, and Brewerton (1992) modified the ESI for use with younger children by shortening and simplifying the original survey. Questions are presented in a *Yes, No,* and *Don't know* format, and the survey includes a set of child figure drawings that assesses weight and body satisfaction (Childress et al., 1993). The test–retest reliability and internal consistency of the KEDS has been found to be high ($r = .83, p < .005$, coefficient alpha = .73; Childress, Jarrell, & Brewerton, 1992).

EATING DISORDER INVENTORY—CHILD VERSION

The Eating Disorder Inventory—Child Version (EDI-C; Garner, 1991a) is a frequently used self-report measure of symptoms related to AN and BN. The original EDI comprised 64 items and provided standard scores on eight subscales (Garner, Olmstead, & Polivy, 1983), including Body Dissatisfaction, Bulimia, Drive for Thinness, Ineffectiveness, Perfectionism, Interpersonal Distrust, Interoceptive Awareness, and Maturity Fears. In 1991, the EDI-2 (Garner, 1991b) was created, with an additional 27 new items that comprised three additional subscales. These provisional dimensions included Asceticism, Impulse Regulation, and Social Insecurity.

The EDI-C was created in 1991 by changing the wording of one-third of the items to make it comprehensible for children and adolescents. Unlike the EDI and EDI-2, no psychometric data have been provided for the EDI-C (Eklund, Paavonen, & Almqvist, 2005). Interestingly, the factor structure of the EDI-C is quite different from that of the EDI and EDI-2. Eklund et al. extracted a reliable, five-factor solution for the EDI-C, as opposed to the 8, and 11 dimensions suggested by the EDI and EDI-2, respectively. The factors include Drive for Thinness, Emotional Disturbance and Affective Instability, Self-Esteem, Overeating, and Maturity Fears. Overall, it appears that the EDI-C is a valid assessment of five dimensions related to eating pathology in children; however, many of the original EDI-2 items are not relevant for use with a younger population (Eklund et al., 2005).

SETTING CONDITIONS FOR ANOREXIA NERVOSA SCALE

The Setting Conditions for Anorexia Nervosa Scale (SCANS; Slade & Dewey, 1986) was created as a screening tool to help identify individuals at risk of developing an eating disorder. This 40-item measure has five component subscales (General Dissatisfaction and Loss of Control, Social and Personal Anxiety, Perfectionism, Adolescent Problems, and Need for Weight Control) that can discriminate between eating-disordered and non-eating-disordered individuals, and can identify subthreshold individuals at greatest risk for developing an eating disorder. The SCANS has been effectively used within an adolescent population (ages 11–18 years; Slade & Dewey, 1986; Felker & Stivers, 1994) to identify at-risk youth. The internal consistency–reliability of each subscale is sufficiently high, with values ranging from .66 (Perfectionism) to .90 (Need for Weight Control) across two samples.

Parent Self-Report Measures

QUESTIONNAIRE ON EATING AND WEIGHT PATTERNS— PARENT VERSION

The Questionnaire on Eating and Weight Patterns—Parent Version (QEWP-P; Johnson, Grieve, Adams, & Sandy, 1999) an extension of the Questionnaire on Eating and Weight Patterns (QEWP; Spitzer et al., 1992, 1993) and the Questionnaire on Eating and Weight Patterns—Adolescent Version (QEWP-A; Johnson et al., 1999) was designed as a parental report of binge-eating behaviors in children and adolescents. The QEWP measures provide information that can lead to a BED or BN diagnosis. Information obtained with the QEWP-P, however, does not correlate highly with that of the QEWP-A (Johnson et al., 1999) or the ChEDE interview, with the exception of eating-related distress (Tanofsky-Kraff, Yanovski, & Yanovski, 2005). This suggests that further research is needed to determine the accuracy of child-reported eating behaviors, as well as the degree to which parents are aware of their children's eating patterns.

MEDICAL EVALUATION/HISTORY

Assessment of current and past eating patterns and physical exercise habits is imperative (Ebeling et al., 2003). The occurrence of vomiting or other compensatory behaviors (e.g., use of laxatives or excessive exercising) should be noted (Greenfeld, Mickley, Quinlan, & Roloff, 1993), as well as the age of onset of restricting and/or bulimic behaviors. Careful attention should be given to age of menarche, cessation of menstruation, or failure to reach menarche. In particular, age of menarche and weight during the last regular menstrual cycle are helpful guidelines for determining the expected weight of the adolescent (Frisch & McArthur, 1974; Frisch, 1990).

In a pediatric population, it is not enough merely to monitor the weight of patients. Growth in children and adolescents should be viewed comprehensively, including assessment of deceleration or cessation of growth, degree of starvation, as noted by visual inspection (tendency to wear baggy clothing to hide thinness; lanugo hair, splitting nails, and tooth enamel defects) and pubertal irregularities (Ebeling et al., 2003; Marcus, Blanz, Lehmkuhl, Rothenberger, & Eisert, 1989). Additionally, irregularities in blood pressure and pulse rate, and signs of vasoconstriction should be noted (Marcus et al., 1989).

Both DSM-IV and the International Classification of Diseases (ICD-10) diagnostic criteria for AN require that weight be at least 15% below the expected weight for one's age (APA, 2000; World Health Organization, 1992, 1993). However, use of the BMI is limited in children and adolescents (Garn, Leonard, & Hawthorne, 1986; Hebebrand, Himmelmann, Heseker, Schafer, & Remschmidt, 1996). Even in typically developing children, BMI varies with age. Therefore, clinical attention should focus on growth trends and rate of weight loss, as opposed to absolute BMI (Nicholls, de Bruyn, et al., 2000). Take, for instance, a child who has a BMI within the normal range but has lost a substantial amount of weight over the course of the past year. Knowledge of a child's growth and weight history is highly useful in assessing the rate of weight loss. Additionally, a relative weight estimate should be used to assess the nutritional and weight status of younger patients (Parry-Jones, 1991). The relative weight of a child refers to the percentage deviation from the average weight for the child's height. This can be extrapolated directly from existing growth charts and is more useful than BMI, because it acknowledges the continuous growth that is characteristic of the developmental phases of childhood and adolescence.

ADDITIONAL ASSESSMENT CONSIDERATIONS

When working with children and adolescents who present with eating difficulties, it is generally beneficial to assess the child's readiness for change. Whereas is often useful to assess readiness for change in adults via a technique such as motivational interviewing (e.g., Kotler, Boudreau, & Devlin, 2003; Treasure & Ward, 1997), it is even more important to attend carefully to a child or adolescent's level of treatment motivation. A young child is often in treatment against his or her wishes and is being forced to seek help by parents. Additionally, the fear and denial often associated with AN in particular can hamper treatment motivation. If a child or adolescent lacks a desire to change, then treatment effectiveness is substantially hindered. Conducting a motivational assessment during the assessment phase is often valuable in determining the child's current stage of change and designing a treatment plan that addresses the apprehensions of the child or adolescent, in addition to strengthening his or her alliance with the therapist.

Link between Assessment and Treatment

A primary goal of assessment is the formulation of a treatment plan. Several areas may be considered that provide useful data for the establishment of a well-functioning, child-specific treatment plan, including determination of whether inpatient versus outpatient treatment is warranted, acknowledgment of developmental differences, establishment of the role of the family in the treatment process, and recognition of the physical and medical needs of the child or adolescent.

INPATIENT VERSUS OUTPATIENT TREATMENT

The majority of children and adolescents with eating disorders may be treated on an outpatient basis, with only a minority of patients requiring inpatient management. Patients requiring inpatient care are generally those diagnosed with AN who are experiencing physiological or psychological complications, or who have comorbid conditions (Nicholls & Bryant-Waugh, 2003). Severity of symptom presentation and medical status dictate whether the patient is appropriate for outpatient treatment or should be referred to more intensive partial hospitalization or inpatient settings. From a medical standpoint, if the patient is unstable and presenting with syncopal episodes, cardiac arrhythmias, severe fluid and electrolyte imbalances, severe dehydration, extreme fatigue, or continued weight loss, hospitalization must be the first course of action (Hill & Pomeroy, 2001). Medical complications are of particular concern in children and adolescents with eating disorders, because development and growth are not yet complete and damage may be irreparable (Katzman, 2005; Sokol et al., 2005). These complications are most commonly seen in a subgroup of patients with AN, and most patients with BN and AN may be treated effectively on an outpatient basis (Gowers & Bryant-Waugh, 2004). NICE (National Institute for Clinical Excellence, 2004) guidelines purport that the majority of both patients with AN and BN should be treated on an outpatient basis, with adequate psychological and physical management provided. The guidelines go on to suggest that if the condition of the client deteriorates, then either inpatient treatment or a more intensive form of outpatient therapy should be considered.

Meads, Gold, and Burls (2001) conducted a systematic review of the relative effectiveness of inpatient and outpatient care in the management of AN. Their main conclusions were that outpatient treatment for AN at a center specializing in eating disorders was as effective as inpatient treatment in individuals who did not require emergency intervention, and that outpatient care is generally cheaper than inpatient care. Additional care should, however, be taken to monitor adequately the physical and psychological condition of children and adolescents managed on an outpatient basis.

DEVELOPMENTAL CONSIDERATIONS

Significant differences have been found between adolescents and adults who present with eating difficulties. Fisher, Schneider, Burns, Symons, and Mandel (2001) found that adolescents, as opposed to adults, achieve a lower severity score, experience greater denial and less desire for help, and report a shorter period of more rapid weight loss. In addition, adults were more likely to report a history of bingeing and laxative use, a diagnosis of BN, and prior use of psychiatric medication and therapy. It is important for clinicians to recognize that children and adolescents with eating problems are quite distinct from the largely adult samples studied in relation to eating disorder assessment, diagnosis, and treatment to date.

For instance, developmental considerations should be made when assessing and applying formal diagnostic criteria to children or adolescents presenting with eating difficulties. Criteria for AN and BN set forth in DSM-IV-TR (APA, 2000), for example, are not always developmentally appropriate for the diagnosis of such disorders in children and in many adolescents. The large variability in the rate, timing, and degree of growth during normal puberty makes application of the weight criterion for AN very difficult (Robin, Gilroy, & Dennis, 1998). The menstruation criterion is also problematic, in that it does not apply to prepubescent girls, and prediction of when menarche would normally have occurred in an adolescent whose problematic eating behaviors began prior to the onset of puberty is often inaccurate.

In addition, the presence of an intense fear of gaining weight and body image disturbance is dependent on the cognitive functioning and abstract reasoning abilities of the child or adolescent (Robin, Gilroy, & Dennis, 1998). Higher-level processes such as abstract reasoning develop primarily during adolescence, thereby making the assessment of criteria dependent on such abilities challenging. Taking into account the cognitive level of the client is essential for not only diagnostic purposes but also treatment planning. For instance, prior to initiating cognitive-behavioral therapy (CBT) with a young patient, it is important to have some baseline assessment of his or her cognitive abilities.

In studies examining diagnostic differences between adolescent and adult individuals with eating problems, significantly more adolescents than adults fail to meet formal criteria for AN or BN in spite of having a comparable degree of psychological distress as those meeting strict criteria (Bunnell, Shenker, Nussbaum, Jacobson, & Cooper, 1990; Fisher et al., 2001). In addition, research suggests that treatment outcomes are most favorable when eating disorder symptoms are treated soon after their onset (Lask & Bryant-Waugh, 1993). Therefore, in spite of the limitations of existing diagnostic systems, it is essential that clinicians recognize the challenges associated with the assessment and diagnosis of children and adolescents with eating problems and appropriately treat even subthreshold eating disorders.

FAMILY

The family is always going to play a substantive role in the treatment of eating problems in children and adolescents, regardless of the etiology of the symptoms and treatment orientation utilized (Gowers & Bryant-Waugh, 2004; Lock, Le Grange, Agras, & Dare, 2001). Parents or caregivers generally purchase the food, are in charge of meal planning and preparation, and are often responsible for transportation to and from clinic appointments. Family issues assessed during the evaluation phase may also be essential for treatment planning and indicate whether family or individual therapy is warranted.

According to the NICE (2004) guidelines, family members, including siblings, should be included in treatment programs involving children and adolescents, including such strategies as sharing of information, behavioral management, and communication training. To maximize the inclusion of a family in treatment, a proper assessment of family functioning should first be conducted.

An essential component of a comprehensive assessment of a child who presents with eating difficulties is the family intake interview. The goal of conducting a thorough family assessment is not only the acknowledgment of familial contributing factors but also, more importantly, the recognition that family variables may be maintaining the child's difficulties (Christie et al., 2000). Present and past familial eating habits and attitudes should be assessed, as well as each family member's feelings surrounding the child's eating difficulties.

Christie et al. (2000) describe several areas of family functioning that should be considered: (1) the quality of the parental and marital relationships, (2) boundaries between family members, (3) the family atmosphere (e.g., hostile, warm, or tense), (4) the affective status and responsiveness of each individual, (5) communication processes, and (6) the presence and insight of siblings. Additionally, Le Grange (2005) provides a nice overview of family functioning measures most commonly used with the families of children with eating difficulties. Involving the family in the assessment process provides a more comprehensive view of the child, the family, and factors that may be sustaining the child's eating problems. The integration of family into the treatment process is covered more thoroughly in the treatment portion of this chapter.

PHYSICAL/MEDICAL MANAGEMENT

Patients with AN tend to have more physical complications than individuals with BN; however, these physical symptoms are generally secondary to their disturbed eating habits and malnutrition. In most cases, normalization of eating habits and restoration of weight are enough to correct the associated physical complications. Therefore, it is usually recommended that clinical attention focus on the management of the eating disorder, while closely monitoring the physical condition of the client (Fairburn & Harrison, 2003). Fairburn and Harrison, as well as Gowers and Bryant-Waugh (2004), provide a succinct overview of both the associated medical complications and the recommended physical management of eating disorders.

Treatment

Preview

The following sections detail the two most promising approaches for treating eating disorders in children and adolescents: (1) the Maudsley approach, a family-based intervention for treating AN in children and adolescents, and (2) a cognitive-behavioral approach to treating BN in adolescents. The NICE guidelines (2004) have recommended these therapeutic approaches as the first line of treatment for AN and BN, respectively. Although these two approaches are distinct and each has specific considerations that are discussed at length in later sections, their primary goals are to restore health and wellness, and to reduce eating disorder symptoms.

Several considerations are necessary for the successful treatment of eating disorders in children and adolescents. Given the complicated and pervasive nature of these disorders, treatment is generally most effective within a multidisciplinary team, including physicians, psychologists, dieticians, nurses, and/or social workers. If this is not possible, it might be helpful for the clinician to establish an ongoing relationship with a pediatrician, to consult regularly with colleagues, and/or to work with a cotherapist (if family therapy is the treatment of choice; Lock et al., 2001).

Characteristics of patients and their families must also be considered in the choice of an appropriate treatment. Lock et al. (2001) indicate that patients with AN who are under 18 years of age and live with an intact, compliant family are best suited to the Maudsley program; however, it has also been successfully adapted for nonintact families, families that are only moderately noncompliant, and weight-recovered patients and hospitalized patients. There is limited evidence that the Maudsley approach may be effective for adolescents with BN, and treatment studies are ongoing (Lock, 2004, 2006). Therefore, an adapted version of CBT that considers the patient's age, circumstances, and level of development may be a more appropriate intervention for adolescents with BN (NICE, 2004). Traditional CBT relies heavily on abstract reasoning, perspective taking, and goal setting, which can be a challenge for adolescents who are both developing higher-order cognitive abilities and struggling with issues related to autonomy. These developmental considerations must be taken into account before proceeding with CBT; however, motivation issues, struggles with autonomy, and limited abstract reasoning and goal setting abilities are a predictable part of working with adolescents, and careful understanding of the developmental changes that adolescents undergo may yield CBT treatments that match adolescents developmentally and effectively treat the eating disorder (Lock, 2005). CBT techniques, which have even been adapted for use with children with eating disorders, primarily try to help children establish a connection between their thoughts and feelings (Christie, 2000).

Context of Treatment

It should be expected at the start of treatment that the patient and perhaps even the family will deny the seriousness of the problem. Therefore, the clinician must express concern for the patient and convey the potential gravity of the situation in a serious and genuine manner (Lock et al., 2001). Regardless of the therapeutic orientation used to treat the patient, it is very important to enlist the family, including siblings, in the entire treatment process by sharing information, facilitating communication, and helping with the behavioral management plan (NICE, 2004). It is essential to establish a strong therapeutic alliance with both the parents and the patient. Initially, parents may feel overwhelmed, guilty, or frustrated by the eating disorder, and that they are to blame for it. The clinician should convey to the family that there is no single cause of the eating disorder, and that no one is to blame for it. The family's important role in the patient's recovery should be stressed, and parents may be enlisted to help their child take charge of the eating disorder (Lask, 2000).

Establishing a strong therapeutic alliance with the patient is also vital to treatment success (Constantino, Arnow, Blasey, & Agras, 2005; Pereira, Lock, & Oggins, 2006). It should be expected that many patients will minimize their eating disorder symptoms or deny there is a problem altogether. The patient's level of interest in therapy will vary, and it is common for the patient to be guarded with the therapist. To establish rapport, the initial interview with the patient should begin with open-ended, general questions about family, school, interests, and friends, posed in a warm and genuine manner that is not too familiar (Lock et al., 2001). After an initial alliance is established, questions should then proceed to problems related to eating and weight. Throughout the course of therapy, the therapist should continue to work toward maintaining a strong alliance with the patient. Oftentimes, adolescent patients want to discuss other issues in their lives (i.e., school, friends, dating) that are not related to the eating disorder. As a strategy for maintaining a strong therapeutic alliance, therapists may want to set aside a prescribed period of time (e.g., 10 minutes per session) to let patients discuss these concerns (Lock, 2005).

For patients with BN in individual therapy, Lock (2005) recommends spending extra time on alliance building by expressing interest in the adolescent's perspective and experiences, tolerating an occasional lack of attention or focus, and perhaps engaging in more frequent contact with the adolescent via phone calls between sessions. More attention to psychoeducation about the nature of the disorder, as well as the therapeutic process, may also helpful to engage adolescents in treatment; the therapist should present information in clear, concrete language and may also wish to present visual representations and to frequently check in with the patient to ensure comprehension (Lock, 2005).

Resistance to treatment and poor motivation are also common obstacles to therapy with patient with eating disorders. AN is perhaps the most notorious disorder in terms of clients' lack of motivation to change or oftentimes strong resistance to treatment. Patients with BN typically have less resistance than patients with AN, but they still tend to present with varying degrees of motivation and ambivalence toward treatment (Wilson & Schlam, 2004). Motivational interviewing prior to implementing treatment may be one strategy for increasing motivation in adolescents with eating disorders, and it may even be sufficient to induce behavioral change in a subset of patients (Gowers & Smyth, 2004; Wilson & Schlam, 2004).

Compliance with completing homework assignments may also be an obstacle in the treatment of adolescents with eating disorders. Self-monitoring records of eating behaviors, mood, and weight are a large component of CBT for BN, and patients may not comply with this homework for a variety of reasons, including difficulty understanding how to complete the task, embarrassment because of their eating patterns, fear that others will see the log, lack of time, or difficulty in labeling their experiences. Adolescents may be less skilled at self-monitoring than adults, and Lock (2005) recommends that the therapist spend extra time in early sessions completing the food record together (if it is not completed outside of session) and stressing the importance of self-monitoring. Parents are also an important resource to help with compliance issues, and their role may vary from being actively involved in the therapeutic process to being an adjunct to therapy. They should be informed of the treatment plan and may be especially helpful with food shopping, meal planning, meal monitoring, and helping the patient follow the prescribed eating routine. Parents may also become involved in implementing and completing behavior modification tasks and providing support for the patient during difficult times (Lock, 2005).

Poor academic performance or issues at school may occur during treatment of youth with eating disorders. On a practical level, the therapist may need to become involved with the school to make special arrangements for appropriate timing of meals at school and missed class time because of therapy appointments (Lock, 2005). Teachers may also be useful liaisons, helping the clinician to understand better the patient's behavior at school, as well as supporting and advocating for the student during the treatment and recovery process (Tate, 2000).

Comorbid psychiatric disorders may also represent a challenge to treatment of youth with eating disorders. Pharmacological treatment may be indicated to manage comorbid depression or anxiety or perhaps even symptoms of the eating disorder (Gowers & Bryant-Waugh, 2004). Additionally, acute crises, such as physical or sexual abuse of the patient or a suicide attempt, may occur during the course of treatment. In such cases, treatment of the eating disorder becomes secondary, and stabilization of the patient is of the utmost concern (Lock, 2005). It is important to note, however, that the clinician should not let frequent, less dire "crises of the week" interfere with the progression of treatment, because this strategy may be used by the patient to avoid working on the eating disorder.

Description of Treatment Components

COGNITIVE-BEHAVIORAL THERAPY

Cognitive-behavioral therapy (CBT) is the "gold standard" approach for adults with BN (NICE, 2004). Several randomized controlled trials (RCTs) of CBT for BN have supported the efficacy of the treatment in adults (Wilson & Fairburn, 1998). Although no study to date has conducted an RCT on an adolescent-only population, Gowers and Bryant-Waugh (2004) discuss several reasons why it may be appropriate to extrapolate the findings from the adult literature on CBT for BN to adolescents. First, many of the RCTs of CBT for BN have actually included both adolescents and adults within their sample. Second, CBT has been successfully adapted for use with adolescents in the depression and anxiety literature. Third, the core symptoms of AN and BN do not differ across the age spectrum. Last, adolescence as a developmental period is not necessarily defined by age alone, and many young adults with eating disorders may still experiences the challenges typical of adolescence.

Lock (2005; Schapman-Williams, Lock, & Couturier, 2006) adapted Fairburn's CBT manual (Fairburn, Marcus, & Wilson, 1993) to be more developmentally appropriate for use with adolescents, and preliminary data from a case series study suggest a response rate similar to that of adults. Mirroring the adult version, CBT for adolescent BN comprises approximately 20 sessions over a 6-month period and is broken down into three stages.

Stage 1. In the first stage, the primary focus is on the normalization of eating patterns, with a goal of establishing a healthy eating pattern of three meals and two snacks per day. In addition to normalizing eating patterns, the first stage of CBT for adolescent BN focuses heavily on motivation for change, development of a strong and collaborative therapeutic alliance, and psychoeducation on the nature of BN, as well as the therapeutic process. Self-monitoring of eating, compensatory behaviors, and weight is assigned for homework each week. Alternative behaviors to binge–purge episodes also may be discussed during the first stage, and the therapist can help the patient to experiment with a wide range of alternative behaviors. Approximately 10 sessions are allocated to the first stage of treatment.

Stage 2. The second stage of treatment involves continued focus on maintaining a regular eating schedule, as well as the introduction of cognitive restructuring and problem solving of issues related to body image, binge-eating–purging cycles, eating, weight, and feared foods. Self-monitoring is still a large component of treatment; however, the patient's thoughts, feelings, and beliefs become the primary focus of self-monitoring. Reintroduction of feared foods into the patient's diet is also gradually addressed. Behavioral experiments, such as going out to eat at a restaurant with friends, may also be assigned to help the adolescent become more comfortable with food, eating, and urges to binge and purge. Stage 2 of CBT for adolescent BN lasts about 7 or 8 sessions.

Stage 3. The primary focus of the third stage of treatment is relapse prevention. This is a particularly important phase for adolescents who may not have experience with chronic BN, and who may minimize the likelihood of relapse. The therapist reviews progress on BN symptoms, as well as more general developmental tasks of adolescents. Feedback and realistic expectations are provided to the patient and his or her parents, and strategies to prevent relapse are developed. Termination issues are also discussed, and the therapist should be prepared for varying responses from the adolescent relative to termination, ranging from distress to indifference.

FAMILY THERAPY

Despite the high rates of mortality and morbidity associated with AN, very few systematic research studies have been conducted on psychological treatment of AN (Le Grange & Lock, 2005). Studies that have been conducted are fraught with methodological limitations and are underpowered (Agras et al., 2004). Treatment studies of adult AN have produced discouraging results, and prognosis is poor for those with a chronic course; however, treatment response in adolescent AN has been promising (Fairburn, 2005), perhaps in part because prognosis is better when the duration between onset of AN symptoms and treatment is brief (Agras et al., 2004).

The Maudsley approach to family therapy is the most promising treatment for adolescent AN to date (Lock & Le Grange, 2005; Lock, Couturier, & Agras, 2006). Five, small RCTs of variations of the Maudsley approach have been published supporting the efficacy of this approach (Dare, Eisler, Russell, Treasure, & Dodge, 2001; Eisler et al., 2000; Le Grange, Eisler, Dare, & Russell, 1992; Robin, Siegel, Koepke, Moye, & Tice, 1994; Robin et al., 1999; Lock et al., 2006). NICE (2004) guidelines for treatment of children and adolescent AN reflect these findings and recommend family therapy as the preferred treatment to date. Research on the Maudsley approach, however, has many of the same methodological limitations as other treatment studies on AN, including small sample sizes, high attrition rates, and lack of manualization (Le Grange & Lock, 2005; Lock, Agras, Bryson, & Kraemer, 2005). A manual for the Maudsley approach, recently published by Lock and his colleagues (2001), will be important in standardizing research protocols across trials and also in helping clinicians implement outpatient family therapy with adolescents with AN. The following section provides a brief overview of the Maudsley approach, as well as the three phases of treatment (please refer to Lock et al. [2001] for an extensive guide).

THE PROCESS OF TREATMENT: STEP-BY-STEP GUIDELINES

Family-Based Treatment

Family-based treatment (FBT) sees parents as a resource in the treatment of adolescent patients with AN. Initially mobilizing parents to take action to disrupt dieting and overexercise is the first goal. The *first* phase of treatment attempts to reinvigorate the parental role in the family system, particularly as it is related to the patient's eating behaviors. In this phase, treatment is almost entirely focused on the eating disorder and its symptoms, and includes a family meal. Other goals of this phase are to develop a strong parental alliance and to align the patient with a peer or sibling subsystem. Parents are asked to work out for themselves the best way to refeed their child. The *second* phase begins after there is evidence of steady weight gain, and less difficulty eating and curtailing exercise. Treatment now focuses on transitioning responsibility for eating and exercise back to the adolescent in an age-appropriate manner. In the *third* phase, treatment is aimed at general adolescent developmental issues insofar as they have been effected by the disruptive effects of AN.

FBT differs from many other treatments for eating disorders in some of its starting points. First, the adolescent is seen as having a disorder rather than intrinsic developmental deficits. Second, the approach uses parental control to arrest the behaviors maintaining the disorder. Many parents have been told that they are to blame for the eating disorder, but FBT takes an agnostic position in this regard. Instead of focusing on etiology, FBT advocates that the therapist and family should primarily focus their attention on the task of weight restoration.

Synopsis

According to Lock et al. (2001), the Maudsley approach assumes that the adolescent is imbedded in the family, and that it is essential to involve the parents in treatment by having them take charge of the eating disorder, which has control of the adolescent with AN. The eating disorder has halted typical adolescent development, and the adolescent with AN is viewed as having regressed. Weight restoration is the primary goal of therapy, and family members are instructed to put other conflicts and issues on hold until the eating disorder is resolved. Once this has been achieved, control should be returned to the adolescent, and the remainder of therapy may then focus on typical developmental issues of adolescence within the family. The Maudsley treatment of AN typically lasts about 1 year.

Phase 1

Refeeding the patient is the sole focus of Phase 1 treatment. A family meal is conducted early on in treatment to provide direct observation of the family dynamics surrounding food and meals. The parents are encouraged to refeed their daughter in a unified manner, and the therapist is nondirective on how this goal should be achieved. Parents are encouraged to generate their own solutions for refeeding their child, and the therapist aims to provide support and encouragement to the parents, stating that they know how to help their child best. Enhancing the bond between the parental and sibling subsystems is also a large component of the first phase of therapy, and the therapist strives to reduce any guilt or blame that the family feels over the eating disorder. Phase 1 typically lasts approximately 3–5 weeks and is conducted on a weekly basis during a usual 50- to 60-minute session.

Phase 2

The second phase of the Maudsley approach begins after the patient has begun regaining weight, and the family is less in crisis over the eating disorder. The goal of Phase 2 is to restore the patient's physical health and begin to return control of eating and weight back to the adolescent. Eating disorder symptoms remain a central component of therapy; however, other family issues related to the eating disorder and adolescent development may now be reviewed and discussed. Phase 2 sessions are conducted every 2–3 weeks and may be concluded when (1) the adolescent's weight is stable, and between 90 and 100% of IBW; (2) he or she is eating regular meals without supervision; (3) the family can discuss non-eating-disordered adolescent development issues; and (4) the patient has increased peer relationships.

Phase 3

The goal of the third phase is to address more general family and adolescent issues, and to develop healthy parent–adolescent relationships in which eating disorder patterns are not the basis of interaction. Each family is unique, and issues discussed will vary from family to family. Typical topics include increased autonomy for the adolescent, establishing appropriate intergenerational family boundaries, sexuality, and future challenges associated with leaving home for college or work. This phase is brief, and only a few major themes can be addressed. Monthly sessions are generally advised.

Session 1

The first face-to-face meeting is a key session. It sets the tone for the entire therapy and the general interventions: Empowering parents, not blaming parents, externalization of illness, and focus on the eating disorder are used in various ways throughout the treatment. In preparing for the meeting, prior phone calls help to communicate the importance of everyone's attendance. The three main goals for the first session include the following:

- Engage the family.
- Obtain a focused history on the development of AN.
- Observe how the family functions (i.e., coalitions, authority structure, conflicts).

To accomplish these goals, the therapist undertakes the following therapeutic interventions:

1. Weigh the patient.
2. Set a sincere but serious tone for the session.
3. Engage each family member in discussing the development of AN.

4. Separate the illness from the patient.
5. Orchestrate an intense scene around the seriousness of the illness and difficulty in recovery.
6. Charge the parents with the task of refeeding.
7. Prepare for the next session's family meal and conclusion of session.

Weigh the Patient

Susan and her family (Lola, Simon, and Tommy) arrived for the first session. The therapist greeted them briefly in the waiting room and asked Susan to join her. She then took Susan to the scale and asked her to remove her coat and shoes before stepping on the scale. The therapist recorded Susan's weight and explained that the beginning of every session would be devoted to weighing and assessing weekly progress and/or family-related concerns. Susan was not thrilled that her weight chart would be shared with her family, and said softly, "I don't want my parents to know my weight." The therapist explained, however, that Susan's parents needed to know her weight to be able to help her. Weighing serves to provide important information that will help to set the tone for the upcoming session, as well as to facilitate rapport between the therapist and patient.

Greet the Patient and Her Family

The therapist returned to the waiting room and invited Susan's parents and brother to join her in the office, where the chairs had been arranged in a small circle. The therapist began by saying, "I am very pleased that all of you are here to help Susan in her struggle with anorexia nervosa. She will need all the help she can get in fighting this illness. Each of you will be important in helping her." The therapist then asked family members to briefly introduce themselves.

In beginning to engage patients with eating disorders and their families in treatment, the therapist is warm but serious. She ultimately wants not only to convey her concern and interest in the family but also to emphasize the dire circumstances that have brought them together. The therapist endeavors to engage all members of the family, and values and treats each with respect.

Take a History That Engages Each Family Member

The therapist asked the family members to remember how anorexia began and took its course. Lola said she remembered that Susan began running every other day with her father in the spring of the eighth grade. Simon agreed but thought things began to spiral out of hand when Susan became a vegetarian. Susan interrupted: "It began during the summer, because I wanted to be thinner when I started ninth grade." With the therapist's guidance, the family began to weave a coherent story about the development of AN in their family. This story unites the family in a single narrative about the illness and serves as a common ground for them. It is usually the first time all the family members' perspectives have been shared. During this process, it is important to make sure that no single family member monopolizes the session.

Separate the Illness from the Patient

The therapist then used the familial story to help "separate" the child or adolescent from AN. For example, the therapist said,

> "It is clear to me, as all of you describe it, that Susan today is very different than she was 8 months ago. In the past she was happy, vivacious, and interested in things besides food and weight. Now she is moody, irritable, and only interested in dieting and being thin. It is like she has been covered over by a fog. I call that 'anorexic fog' because it makes it difficult to see anything besides the issues of food and weight. When you are in a fog, you can't see what's ahead of you, and Susan has not been able to see well ahead of her. She did not anticipate having to be hospitalized. She did not anticipate that she would disappoint her parents. The fog of anorexia made it impossible. So, it is not Susan we are struggling with here, but the fog of anorexia that surrounds her that we must contend with."

In separating Susan from her anorexic behaviors and beliefs, the therapist emphasizes that Susan has minimal control over her illness. This externalization provides an opening for family members to see that they will be fighting the disorder, not their daughter/sister. The family members are desperately trying to recover their daughter/sister. Susan's parents may now take action, whereas ordinarily they might have hesitated, if they felt they were fighting Susan. In addition, the burden of some responsibility and guilt for AN is lifted off of Susan's shoulders, facilitating a stronger alignment with her therapist. Conversely, failure to achieve this alignment can increase the patient's resistance to treatment.

Orchestrate an Intense Scene Regarding the Patient's Illness

The therapist next explained the seriousness of AN in order to incite the parents' to take specific action to address Susan's starvation.

> "Anorexia nervosa has the highest mortality rate of any psychiatric illness. It has an overall mortality rate of 6–8%. Half of those deaths are because the heart stops, and the other half are due to suicide. Anorexia is hard to live with. It also causes osteoporosis, destroys skin and hair, and leads to infertility. Emotionally, those who have anorexia become depressed and anx-

ious, and seldom live up to their potential in terms of careers. Many individuals cannot go to college because they are too sick, and some may never marry. What you have told me about Susan's struggle shows me that she is headed down this track unless something is done to help her. Simon and Lola, you have tried to let Susan do this herself and her doctor has encouraged her as well. At the hospital they helped her gain weight, but she lost most of it when she came home. We must find another way."

By highlighting the severe medical and psychological sequelae of AN, the therapist aims to encourage parental anxiety. She wishes the parents to see AN as they would any other medical illness that threatens their child, so much so, that they will take decisive action without hesitation. Often this helps parents get a better handle on their anxiety and become more focused in their efforts to disrupt a child or adolescent's unhealthy dieting and excessive exercise. In this sense, anxiety is a useful motivator. As the therapist orchestrates this intervention, she must take special care to minimize guilt and blame, because these feelings discourage rather than inspire action. The specific focus is on the need to restore the adolescent's health. It is important for parents to understand that doctors, nurses, nutritionists, and even the therapist are merely facilitators of change. The parents themselves, ultimately, must be the catalysts for their adolescent's recovery.

Charge the Parents with the Task of Refeeding

The therapist next emphasized the parental role in turning the tide of the potential life-threatening direction of AN:

> "Lola and Simon, you are wonderful parents. You have brought up your children with attention and care. You love your children and you want to help them. Now, Susan needs your help to fight anorexia. You can see that she is lost in the fog and that she needs you. As her parents you are the most important resource she has to help her. The two of you, working together, need to find a way to help Susan eat again and stop exercising so she can regain her health. I will be here to help you as will Susan's pediatrician. However, you are the real experts on your family and on Susan herself."

In delivering this charge, the therapist may trigger a range of responses, from horror to anger and resentment, to relief. The therapist must strive to help family members understand that they can learn from their past efforts, and that they are the best resource to help their child or adolescent.

Prepare for the Family Picnic and End the Session

At the end of the first session, Lola and Simon were asked to bring in a meal for their daughter that would begin the process of helping her to gain weight:

"I know that it may be difficult to visualize the formidable challenge we have before us. I can only imagine how worried, tired, and frustrated you may be. But I have seen today that your family cares strongly for each other and that you have the resources to fight Susan's anorexia. On Friday, I want you, Simon and Lola, to bring a picnic lunch of sufficient nourishment, so that we can begin to reverse the starvation that has beset Susan."

Susan's parents were somewhat in shock at the end of the session, and asked the therapist what they were to do until Friday. The therapist was reassuring: "Try your best to help Susan to eat more. During the picnic, you will learn more specific steps."

In this session, the therapist uses the occasion of a family meal to learn about the current strategies the family uses to try to help their daughter, regardless of their success. This includes a thorough review of when meals are taken, who is present at them, what is generally prepared, as well as what seems to be working or not working in this regard. Within the context of the family meal, the therapist also aims to help the parents to have their daughter eat one bite more than she is prepared to eat, while making sure she feels supported by her sibling through this ordeal.

Session 2

The major goals for the second session are the following:

- Assess the family structure and its impact on parental refeeding.
- Help the parents to begin to refeed their child.
- Assess the family processes around eating.

To accomplish these goals, the therapist undertakes the following interventions during this session:

1. Weigh the patient.
2. Take a history and observe the family patterns around food preparation, food serving, and discussions about eating, especially as they relates to the patient.
3. Help the parents convince their daughter to eat at least one mouthful more than she is prepared to eat, *or* help the parents learn how best to go about refeeding their daughter.
4. Align the patient with her siblings for support.
5. End-of-session review.

Weigh the Patient

As in Session 1 and all subsequent sessions, the therapist first took Susan to a room for weighing, noting how she responded to her change in weight (whether up or down).

Take a History and Observe the Family Patterns

The therapist began the session by asking the family to begin serving and eating the meal they brought. She noted that the meal consisted of several homemade sandwiches, several packages of chips, drinks, and cookies. She also noted that Lola served the sandwiches, while Simon served the drinks. The therapist observed that Susan pushed the chips away from her place at the table and was drinking bottled water. The therapist explained: "I know it is somewhat unusual for someone to be sitting with you and not eating with you, but if I were to eat now I might get distracted from my main task at hand. Please go ahead and eat, and I will ask a few questions while you are doing that."

The therapist inquired about family routines, particularly noting when the family eats each meal, who is involved in food preparation, and which family members typically are around while the meal is being consumed. Lola said, "I make breakfast for Susan and Tommy. Susan eats cottage cheese on a half-bagel and orange juice. She doesn't like me to be there when she eats, so I leave it for her on the table. I used to make her lunch for her, but she makes her own now. I think she usually takes an apple and half a turkey sandwich."

Assist Parents in Their Efforts to Refeed the Patient

Once the therapist noted the overall pattern of mealtimes and the availability of parents, she noticed that Susan had stopped eating her sandwich. As a result, the following dialogue with the family ensued:

THERAPIST: Susan, are you finished eating now?

SUSAN: Yes. I had a big snack and I will eat more later, but I don't like this sandwich.

THERAPIST: Lola and Simon, did the two of you decide what to bring for lunch?

SIMON: Yes. We brought a turkey sandwich with mustard, water, and chips. We didn't think Susan would eat the chips or the cookies, but we brought them.

THERAPIST: Well, it looks like a healthy lunch. Why only mustard on the sandwich and water?

LOLA: That's what we thought Susan would be most likely to eat, but she didn't even finish the sandwich.

THERAPIST: Your intuitions were correct about what she needed. Now the two of you just need to help Susan eat it.

LOLA: Susan, would you please eat your sandwich?

SUSAN: (*Looks down.*)

SIMON: (*Sighs, pushing his chair back from the table.*)

THERAPIST: I wonder if it would help if you sat closer to Susan?

LOLA: (*Moves her chair closer to Susan.*)

THERAPIST: It may take a bit more than just asking. Perhaps you need to tell her to eat it.

LOLA: (*Takes a deep breath.*) Susan, eat the rest of that sandwich now.

SUSAN: (*Remains silent and looks down.*)

THERAPIST: Simon, Lola and Susan need your help. Can you sit on the other side of Susan and add your voice of encouragement to that of your wife?

SIMON: (*Moves chair to the other side of Susan.*)

LOLA AND SIMON: Susan, please eat more of your sandwich.

SUSAN: (*Begins to cry softly.*) I don't want to. Please. I don't want to. I will eat later. I promise.

SIMON: (*Pulls chair back.*)

THERAPIST: Simon, remember that anorexia is tricky and makes you feel sorry for Susan, but she is losing her life to this illness. She needs you to make sure she eats.

SIMON: (*Moves back to the table.*) Honey, (*picking up the sandwich and handing it to her*) I want you to eat that sandwich.

SUSAN: (*Takes sandwich and puts it down.*)

SIMON: (*Picks up sandwich and hands it back to her.*)

LOLA: Try to eat that sandwich Susan (*reassuring smile.*)

SUSAN: (*Picks up the sandwich and takes another bite; tears run down her cheeks.*)

One aim of this session is to help the parents make their daughter eat at least one mouthful more than she is prepared to eat. This symbolic act is important, because it sends a strong message that the parents can change the course of the disorder and leads to a sense of empowerment. It also sends a strong message to the adolescent that the severe and restricted dieting will be stopped. Of course, this single incident seldom leads to dramatic changes, but it sets the stage for what will likely be a persistent and steady erosion of the behaviors that maintain AN.

Align the Patient with Her Siblings for Support

Throughout the process, the therapist observed that Susan's younger brother Tommy remained silent and wide-eyed. In the following dialogue, the therapist works to help Susan accept her brother's support.

THERAPIST: Tommy, How would you like to help your sister?

SUSAN: (*Abruptly interjecting.*) He could stay out of it!

TOMMY: (*Looking down*). I'm sorry Susan. I don't know how to help.

THERAPIST: Tommy, it's not your role to help with feeding Susan. But there are other things you can do to make it easier on her.

SUSAN: He could be quiet!

THERAPIST: Susan, would it help you if Tommy were quieter at mealtime?

SUSAN: Yes. He makes a lot of noise eating and fidgets all the time.

THERAPIST: Tommy, for now, do you think you could try to work on those things? It might make it easier on Susan during mealtimes.

TOMMY: I'll try.

End-of-Session Review

The intention is to instill a sense of hope in family members that they can indeed help their child or adolescent overcome an eating disorder. The therapist congratulates family members on their efforts, regardless of their actual success in refeeding. The therapist closed the session by saying, "Susan you have done a wonderful job at fighting for your life today. Your parents clearly love you and will help you. Simon and Lola, it will take both of you working together to keep Susan eating for a while. You will need to be as persistent as you were today. Tommy, your sister is lucky to have you. I know you will do everything you can to support her."

The Remainder of the First Phase (Sessions 3–10)

The rest of Phase 1 consists of helping the family to bring the patient's food intake under parental control by expanding, reinforcing, and repeating some of the interventions (externalization, highlighting dangers of the disorder, confronting feelings of powerlessness and guilt) from the previous sessions. Each session comprises parental attempts at refeeding, as well as systematic guidance on how to curtail the influence of the eating disorder. As a result of this resolute focus, sessions are characterized by a considerable degree of repetition. This is necessary for the parents to become consistent in the management of their adolescent's eating behavior.

There are three goals for this part of treatment:

- Keep focused on the eating disorder.
- Continue to help the parents be in charge of eating.
- Help siblings to be supportive.

To accomplish these goals, the following interventions will be appropriate to consider during the remainder of treatment for Phase 1:

1. Weigh the patient at the beginning of each session.
2. Direct, redirect, and focus therapeutic discussion on food and eating

behaviors, and their management, until food, eating, and weight behaviors and concerns are relieved.

3. Discuss, support, and help the parental dyad's efforts at refeeding.
4. Discuss, support, and help family to evaluate efforts of siblings.
5. Continue to modify parental and sibling criticisms of the patient.
6. Continue to distinguish the adolescent patient and her interests from characteristics of AN.
7. Close all sessions with recounting of progress.

Weigh the Patient

The therapist continued to weigh Susan at the beginning of each session and maintained a careful record of her weight changes. During the first 6 weeks of therapy, Susan's weight fluctuated a great deal. However, from weeks 6 to 10, Susan's weight showed a steady increase.

Continue to Focus on Eating Behaviors and Their Management

After the family meal, feeding continues to be the focus of treatment, until the child or adolescent achieves appropriate weight gain under the new regimen. The therapist insists that Lola and Simon remain steadfast in helping Susan gain weight, until they are convinced that she will not return to anorexic behavior.

LOLA: I think we need to get at the cause of anorexia. There has to be a reason for Susan to be doing this. If we don't figure that out, her eating and gaining weight won't matter.

THERAPIST: It is hard to keep challenging Susan to eat enough. If we could really know the cause of anorexia, it might not help. We know that sun exposure causes skin cancer, but once the cancer is there, the cure is surgery, not blotting out the sun. The best way to help fight anorexia is to modify behaviors that maintain the disorder. You're doing a great job of that, and it is tiring, but you must endure.

LOLA: I know you are right, but it's so hard to keep going when Susan gets into one of her moods!

SIMON: I don't know if we are doing the right thing. She seems so sad and angry all the time.

THERAPIST: Susan is mostly sad and angry at mealtimes or when you stop her from exercising.

SIMON: That's true.

THERAPIST: During these critical times, Susan's thinking is most overcome with anorexic worries and the fog rolls in. Remember, it is not Susan that we are fighting, but the illness of anorexia that has disordered her thinking.

The therapist emphasized the need for regular, nutritionally balanced food intake and suggested that Susan's vegetarianism be suspended. Other symptoms, such as binge eating and purging, may also be subjected to parental control, if they become problematic. If this is the case, encourage parents to keep watch after a meal (e.g., watching a favorite movie on television), supervise bathroom visits, or, if necessary, lock the kitchen, when binge eating cannot otherwise be controlled.

Continue to Support the Parental Dyad's Efforts at Refeeding

In the following dialogue, because it has become clear that Lola and Simon are winning the fight against anorexia, the therapist supports and praises their efforts.

THERAPIST: Lola and Simon, tell me what you have done this past week to help Susan gain weight.

SIMON: This week Susan had difficulty on Tuesday. She went out running before we woke up. We made her stay home from school and eat more, since we were worried that it would be a setback.

Surprisingly, Susan went along with it without much fuss. We helped make arrangements to get her assignments, so she was less worried about that. Other than that, we are with her for all meals except lunch at school. Her counselor sits with her then. We think she is doing really well.

THERAPIST: It is clear that you are working together well to help Susan. An unexpected situation occurred and you were armed and ready. You have put into place a plan that makes it difficult for anorexic behaviors to get started. More importantly, if any behaviors begin again, you're prepared stop them before they become entrenched.

Evaluate Efforts of Siblings

In helping children and adolescents overcome anorexia, it is very important that all family members provide support and encouragement. An unforgiving and overly hostile sibling can easily sabotage ongoing progress. The therapist checks in with Susan's younger brother Tommy and is most pleased with his response, as is Susan.

THERAPIST: Tommy, how did you help your sister this week?

TOMMY: Well, I didn't complain about what we were eating, even though I would rather have less "healthy" meals all the time, like hot dogs. We don't get those now. I understand though. Also, I tried not to make noise when she was studying.

THERAPIST: That sounds very helpful. Do you agree Susan?

SUSAN: Sure. Especially the being quiet part. Tommy also played some games with me when I was bored at home the other night.

TOMMY: Oh yeah, I forgot! I get credit for that too!

THERAPIST: I'm most pleased to hear this. Tommy, you are playing a very important role in Susan's recovery.

TOMMY: (*Smiles.*)

Continue to Modify Any Parental and/or Sibling Criticisms

Parental criticism can have a negative impact on treatment. It can increase resistance and make refeeding more difficult. For this reason, it is important to address criticism immediately, even if it emerges from parental guilt or anxiety.

THERAPIST: Lola, how do you think Susan is doing?

LOLA: Susan is still very stubborn at times. I was very disappointed when she went running. It's like she doesn't care at all what this is doing to us.

THERAPIST: It's hard to remember that Susan has an illness that sometimes gets the better of her. What seems like Susan being stubborn is evidence that she's still struggling at times with the fog of anorexia. Isn't that true, Susan?

SUSAN: (*Looks down.*) Yes. It is very hard sometimes. I do try.

LOLA: I know you do honey. I'm sorry I get frustrated. I just want you to be well.

In this dialogue, the therapist emphasizes noncritical acceptance regarding Susan's exercising and at the same time externalizes the behavior and holds AN rather than Susan responsible.

Continue to Distinguish the Adolescent Patient and Her Interests from Those of AN

Continuing to help Susan separate her goals from those of AN ultimately improves her ability to imagine the advantages of life without this disorder. Sympathetic understanding of her plight promotes therapeutic alliance and trust. As can be expected, such trust often takes time, so the therapist should be both patient and prepared. Once this sense of trust is established, however, resistance is greatly diminished and the effectiveness of treatment enhanced.

THERAPIST: Susan, how is the fight against anorexia going for you?

SUSAN: I have some good days, but it's still very hard. I try to remember that I want to be able to stay out of the hospital and go to school, but I get very nervous about what I am eating.

THERAPIST: You are doing a great job, Susan. I like how you can see that what you want is to stay out of the hospital and go to school. These needs don't match up with anorexia. Now, you see yourself as different from anorexia.

SUSAN: I do (*speaks softly*) but I still struggle.

THERAPIST: I know, but you're also much stronger now, and you desire to be well.

End-of-Session Review

The therapist closed the session by saying, "You're all doing a wonderful job helping Susan. Lola and Simon, you are clear about your goals and have a plan that is working, as evidenced by Susan's steady weight gain during the last several weeks. Tommy, you are helping your sister, and she appreciates it. Susan, you are clearer about your struggles with anorexia, and desire to move forward with your life. This pattern of progress makes me optimistic that soon we can begin the second phase of treatment."

Beginning Phase 2: Helping the Adolescent Eat on Her Own (Sessions 11–16)

The therapist assesses the family's readiness for the second phase if:

- The patient's weight is at a minimum of about 90% IBW.
- The patient is able to eat without excessive cajoling by parents.
- The parents report feeling empowered in the refeeding process.

The major goals of the second phase of treatment are to:

- Maintain parental management of eating disorder symptoms until the patient shows evidence that she is able to eat well and gain weight independently.
- Return food and weight control to the adolescent.
- Explore the relationship between adolescent developmental issues and AN.

To achieve these goals, the therapist needs to undertake the following kinds of interventions:

1. Weigh the patient.
2. Continue to support and assist the parents in management of eating disorder symptoms, until the adolescent is ready to assume independence.
3. Assist the parents in negotiating the return of control of eating disorder symptoms to the adolescent.

4. Encourage the family to examine the relationships between adolescent issues and the development of AN.
5. Continue to modify parental and sibling criticism of the patient, especially in relation to the task of returning control of eating to patient.
6. Continue to assist siblings in supporting their ill sibling.
7. Continue to highlight the difference between the adolescent's own ideas and needs, and the demands of AN.
8. Close sessions with positive support.

At the outset of Phase 2, parents still remain in control of their adolescent's eating-related behaviors. Toward the end of this phase, however, the adolescent assumes control over her own eating. Weight maintenance is typically the goal rather than weight gain, because the adolescent is just learning to eat again on her own and slips are common. Given that the adolescent is out of immediate danger, the therapist's posture becomes more relaxed. In addition, for the first time, the therapist begins to address themes central to adolescence, in addition to ongoing management of eating-related issues.

Weigh the Patient

The therapist continued to weigh Susan at the beginning of every session. However, as Susan felt more secure about her weight, more time was devoted to discussing her general thoughts and feelings regarding family and social activities. This process helps promote an increased sense of interest and trust.

Support Parent Management of Eating Disorder Symptoms and Encourage Adolescent Independence

At this point, it is important to make sure that the adolescent is at her optimal weight or moving toward it. At the same time, support the adolescent in her efforts to assume greater responsibility for her eating behaviors.

THERAPIST: Lola and Simon, how is Susan doing with her eating?

LOLA: Susan did well during our visit to her grandmother's house. I'm starting to give her more independence about eating.

THERAPIST: In what ways are you letting Susan become more independent?

SIMON: Well, at dinner, she serves herself now. We still make everything, but she is doing a good job serving the right amount. Also, she makes her own lunch.

LOLA: Susan also eats her after school snack on her own.

THERAPIST: Susan, how do you feel about these changes?

SUSAN: I like them. They aren't big changes and I feel fine about them. . . . I could do more even.

THERAPIST: What else would you like to do?

SUSAN: I would like to buy my lunch at school again and have dinners at my friends' houses.

LOLA: I think we could try that. What do you think, Simon?

SIMON: Sounds like a good plan.

The therapist also has to make sure that family members, most notably the parents, do not relax their vigilance too quickly. She must also continue to empower parents to trust their own instincts and abilities, and to make appropriate decisions in the process of refeeding their adolescent.

Return Control of Eating Disorder Symptoms to the Adolescent

Over the next few sessions, the therapist noted that Susan's weight continued to be stable and was approaching the normal range. Lola and Simon continued to cede control carefully back to Susan, who appeared to be managing her weight with increasing autonomy. One week, however, Susan's weight fell about 2 pounds. Yet Susan's parents did not overreact, and they were able to generate solutions.

THERAPIST: What do you think happened this past week to cause this weight loss?

SIMON: I think it was because Susan started back on her soccer team. She was only practicing a little, but it was hard to tell how much to eat.

THERAPIST: Yes, as Susan begins to become more active, which is terrific, we all need to work together to help her know how much to eat. Usually, it takes more than you might imagine.

LOLA: I think that's right. Susan, do you think you could eat more before practice and then more at dinner? Because I think that would help.

SUSAN: Well, it is hard to eat too much before practice. I get a side ache. But I will eat more dinner and maybe more at lunch, so I have time to digest it.

The therapist encouraged Lola and Simon to consider this option and to support Susan in her efforts to assume greater independence over her eating at this point. Although the goal is for the adolescent to become independent in her eating, the process is an ongoing collaboration with her parents. Sometimes, the adolescent is too eager to become responsible for her eating, even if she is not fully ready to handle this endeavor. As such, the therapist attempts to create a realistic balance.

Examine Relationships between Adolescent Issues and the Development of AN

Several weeks later, during the process of being weighed, Susan freely revealed an issue that she had been struggling with for a long time. Without the sense of trust that developed with her therapist, she would likely have remained silent and been at greater risk for relapse.

SUSAN: I am nervous about eating at parties, so I just don't do it. I think that everyone thinks I'm fat, so if I eat, it just proves it.

THERAPIST: It sounds likes you worry a lot about your appearance and what others think of you. We should talk more about this with your family. Would that be OK with you?

SUSAN: I guess.

When the entire family convened, the dialogue continued.

THERAPIST: Susan and I were talking. We were discussing how nervous she gets at parties. Is that right, Susan?

SUSAN: Yes, and I was thinking about how that's one of the reasons this all started. I mean trying to lose weight. I wanted people to like me and I thought they would if I were thinner.

THERAPIST: It's hard to figure out what makes someone like someone else.

LOLA: I remember that you were worried about friends all the time. Do you think that caused the anorexia?

THERAPIST: Although these kinds of things might have triggered anorexia, I don't know if they are the cause. However, I do hear this kind of thing a lot. Kids are worried about being liked, and they think that being thinner will make them more popular.

As Phase 2 progresses, the therapist can begin to emphasize the need for age-appropriate socialization. Adolescent socialization, even to a limited degree, opens other avenues of exploration that have the potential to take precedence over AN. In this sense, the aim of therapy is to have "life" replace AN.

Continue to Modify Any Parental and/or Sibling Criticism

Throughout Phase 2, the therapist looked for even subtle signs of parental and/or sibling criticism. One such incident occurred with Simon. He became irritated with Susan's increasing use of the computer to send and receive "instant messages" from her friends.

SIMON: All Susan does is sit at the computer. She isn't getting the best grades anymore. She is wasting her time!

THERAPIST: It's difficult to see Susan developing a new set of friends outside the family and also developing priorities that may be different from your own. But Susan is still doing very well in school. She also seems much happier than before. And most importantly, the fog of anorexia is evaporating.

SIMON: (*Sighs.*) That's true. Susan is doing fine in school, and I'm very pleased that she is happier. It's an adjustment for all of us.

Continue to Assist Siblings in Supporting Their Ill Sibling

The therapist continues to work with Tommy to ensure that Susan benefits from his support. In the following dialogue, she assesses his attitude and level of understanding.

THERAPIST: How are you feeling about Susan and her recovery from anorexia?

TOMMY: I like Susan better now. She was so sad and got mad so easy before. She doesn't have as much time to play with me now, but that's OK.

THERAPIST: Tommy, as I said before, Susan is very lucky to have such an understanding brother.

SUSAN: Well sometimes he's OK (*grinning.*)

TOMMY: (*Smiles.*)

THERAPIST: Tommy, what kinds of things have you been doing to support your sister?

TOMMY: Well, I told her she looked nice in the new pants she got. . . . I went to her soccer game. They lost, but she did well.

SUSAN: (*Smiles.*)

Continue to Highlight Difference between the Adolescent's Own Ideas and Needs and Those of AN

In one meeting toward the end of Phase 2, the therapist and the family discussed an upcoming dance.

SUSAN: I want to go, but I want to look good in a dress, and that means being thinner. It is so hard to be this fat and look good.

THERAPIST: Susan, do you think your friends feel the same way you do?

SUSAN: I don't know, probably.

THERAPIST: Why do you want to go to the dance?

SUSAN: I guess to be with my friends.

THERAPIST: Are all your friends thin?

SUSAN: No, most of them are fatter than me.

THERAPIST: Susan, do you think that the strong feelings you are having now about wearing that dress are about you or about anorexia getting the better of you?

Susan: I know they are about anorexia, but they still get to me.

Therapist: I know and it's perfectly understandable. But it's so great that you can see and feel the difference. That means you're getting stronger.

As the adolescent continues to develop emotional strength, the therapist, with increased confidence, can push the cognitive split between the patient and anorexic thinking. In this way, the therapist encourages the adolescent to develop her own goals for recovery.

End-of-Session Review

As in previous sessions, the attitude of the therapist at the conclusion of sessions is warm and generally filled with praise, so that guilt, powerlessness, and feelings of inadequacy are minimized.

Starting Phase 3 of Treatment: Adolescent Issues (Sessions 17–20)

The third phase of treatment is relatively brief and aimed at examining more general issues of adolescence. This is necessary to help the family transition back to a more typical existence. A more general examination resembles the beginning of many adolescent therapies, even those for AN. The therapist creates the expectation that without the fog of AN, the adolescent can resume a more typical lifestyle that includes the usual age-appropriate trials and tribulations of this developmental period. For instance, treatment may address issues related to adolescent personal autonomy, intergenerational family boundaries, and/or reorganization of marital relationships.

The major goals for the third phase of treatment are:

- Establish that the adolescent–parent relationship no longer requires the symptoms as idiom of communication.
- Review adolescent issues with the family and model problem-solving strategies.
- Address termination issues.

To accomplish these goals, the therapist should undertake the following interventions:

1. Review adolescent issues with the family.
2. Involve the family in "review" of issues.
3. Delineate and explore adolescent themes.
4. Check the marital relationship.
5. Plan for future issues.
6. Termination.

Review Adolescent Issues with the Family

The third phase of treatment typically starts with a "minilecture" on adolescent development. Doing so allows the therapist to identify a range of themes for the family to examine. The therapist briefly described a typical adolescent developmental sequence:

> "Adolescence has three stages, each of which has a specific relationship to development and behaviors. The first stage takes place between 12 to 14 years and largely involves adjusting to the physical changes associated with puberty. As you know, getting this physical aspect of adolescence back on track has been the main focus of our work so far. The second stage, which typically begins around 14 years of age, addresses peer-related issues and the need for increased personal autonomy from parents. The third and final stage emerges around the age of 16, and involves occupational plans and the development of romantic relationships."

Involve the Family in "Review" of Adolescent Issues

The next step is for the therapist to facilitate a family discussion of general adolescent issues. In the following dialogue, the therapist uses parental adolescent experiences to frame the adolescent's struggles in a healthier context.

THERAPIST: Lola and Simon, could you please share with us your recollections of early adolescence.

LOLA: I remember that I was pretty uncomfortable when I began developing. My brothers teased me about having breasts. I didn't like having periods. I was a shrimp. Also, I wasn't that good at sports. I didn't have any real problems, but I wasn't too happy either.

THERAPIST: So, like Susan, you had some trouble adjusting to the changes associated with puberty. What about the second part of adolescence, what kind of social life did you have?

SIMON: I was a bit of a loner. I was a nerd, actually, and my few friends were like me. I was shy and didn't really know any girls.

LOLA: I had a fair number of friends. I was a sporty girl, I guess because of having those older brothers. I didn't worry too much about school like Susan does.

THERAPIST: Susan, it sounds like you share some similar experiences with both of your parents. Like your mom, the physical part of adolescence has been difficult, and like your dad, you have been lonely at times and a bit cautious about friends.

Involving family members in a review of general adolescent issues, as well as integrating their own experiences, gives the patient a healthier perspective from which to draw. More importantly, it facilitates the intergenerational connection between the adolescent and her parents.

Delineate and Explore Adolescent Themes

At this point in the treatment program, the therapist moves beyond the physical aspects of adolescence and emphasizes the importance of peer socialization.

THERAPIST: Our goal at this point is to help you become better integrated with your peers.

SUSAN: Yes, when I was listening to you talk about adolescence, I thought that was where I was.

THERAPIST: What were you thinking?

SUSAN: I thought, I want to have more friends and I want to be less worried and anxious when I go places. I want to feel more relaxed, especially with people that I don't know really well.

THERAPIST: Susan, those are excellent goals. It's such a pleasure that we can now focus on improving the quality of your friendships and helping you to feel more relaxed and secure when with others.

In this session, as well as future sessions, the therapist continues to address the family's view of the adolescent's friendships and, more importantly, how parents and siblings can help support and/or hamper the adolescent's development. The therapist, as always, is ready to provide support and guidance should problems emerge.

It appeared that Simon, in particular, was somewhat ambivalent in his efforts to promote Susan's friendships. With guidance from the therapist, as well as Lola's support, Simon gradually let go of his overprotective stance that was restricting his daughter's social development.

Check the Marital Relationship

As couples become ensconced in helping their adolescent overcome AN, it is not uncommon for them to neglect their own relationship. In the following dialogue, the therapist checks the status of Lola and Simon's marriage.

THERAPIST: Lola and Simon, can you tell me about the last time you did something special as a couple, like go out to dinner or socialize with friends?

LOLA: (*Sighs.*) In all honesty, I cannot remember. We've been so involved in taking care of Susan and have tried to pay more attention to Tommy, so he wouldn't feel left out.

SIMON: I understand it's been hard, but I still cannot help but feel lonely.

LOLA: Simon, you know that I love you. It's just that I've been so emotionally drained and exhausted.

THERAPIST: The two of you have worked so hard to help Susan recover from her anorexia, and I'm very proud of you. But now that Susan is doing better, you must once again nurture your own relationship and remember what brought you together as a couple in the first place.

LOLA AND SIMON: (*On the verge of tears, hold hands.*)

THERAPIST: I want you to make a point of spending some time alone together and focus on each other in the next 2 weeks. Can you promise to do that?

LOLA: (*Wipes her eyes and looks at Simon.*) We will.

SIMON: (*Weak smile, squeezes Lola's hand.*)

It is important that parents work on their own relationship despite the difficulty of having to cope with AN. Couples can lose touch with how they relate to each other given that so much of therapy involves joint parental action to fight AN. Sometimes, when the battle is over, couples find themselves with very little in common. Of course, this is not a good place for the couple to be, and it will not help the adolescent win the war over the long run. For this reason, the therapist should spend some time making sure that the couple is reengaging before the process of termination begins.

Planning for Future Issues

Although treatment is ending, it is important that the therapist discuss future plans and goals, as well as management of slips or potential relapse. In the following dialogue, the therapist addresses the family's concerns about future transitions and managing eating-related behaviors on their own.

THERAPIST: As you know, we will be ending our work together, but I feel that you are ready to take control on your own.

SUSAN: (*Takes a deep breath.*) I'm a little scared, but I feel ready.

THERAPIST: It's OK to be scared; everyone is at one time or another. But remember where you've been, how hard you've worked to overcome anorexia, and where you want to go.

LOLA: I think we could always find something to work on, though.

THERAPIST: Of course, there are always issues to address, but you now have the strength and skills to handle them. More importantly, you are a family that knows how to support each other, no matter what. In fighting anorexia, most other problems pale in comparison.

SIMON: But Susan, what about when you go away to college. What happens if you get sick?

SUSAN: I won't, Dad. I'm much stronger now.

THERAPIST: To some degree, this experience has helped immunize Susan against later eating-related problems. But if Susan does begin to struggle again, you are all prepared to recognize the signs. You know how to help her and would intervene as soon as possible.

LOLA: That's right (*gives Simon a reassuring smile*). We've all learned so much.

Termination

In FBT, termination is a process that begins from the outset. Ongoing goals include empowering family members to be their own agents of recovery, facilitating adolescent personal autonomy, increasing the interval between sessions, and promoting reintegration into usual adolescent life. In doing so, the therapist has prepared the family well for leaving her care. At the same time, the therapist has been with the family through a difficult ordeal and has been a source of support and guidance. There is usually a mutual feeling of gratitude and warmth. This kind of therapy is characterized by a nonhierarchical relationship between the therapist and the family. This often means that the human side of the therapist is more available than in some other forms of therapy. For all these reasons, termination has pleasant and sad overtones. The main issues are to review the course of treatment, discuss a proactive plan for potential slips, and create an expectation for further treatment gains based on the family's ongoing efforts. The therapist facilitates the last family session with the following passage:

"This is our last session and I want to review what has been accomplished. First, together you have helped Susan recover her physical and emotional health. She is now out of danger medically and has been menstruating regularly, so her bones and hormones are getting back to normal. Susan has also changed from being overly focused on weight loss and schoolwork to having a small network of friends and other interests. Lola, your energy and daily commitment to keeping things moving were indispensable. Simon, your dedication, persistence, and flexibility have given your family renewed strength and inspired action. Tommy, your support of your sister was wonderful. One more time, I'll say she is most lucky to have you. Of course, the hardest task was yours, Susan. You have overcome so much and conquered your fears. By learning to trust yourself, you have opened the channels of communication in your family and have helped create the kind of warm, loving, and supportive environment that anyone would be proud to be part of. I am so happy to see how far you've all come. I have enjoyed working with your family and am confident that you will continue to make great strides. I also hope that you will keep me informed of your progress, and if there is anything you need, will not hesitate to call me. I wish you the best."

CONCLUSIONS

Eating problems in youth are common and may occur at any point across the developmental spectrum. Eating disorders, however, although rare, are associated with some of the highest mortality rates of psychiatric disorders. In this chapter, we have reviewed a variety of issues related to the clinical assessment and management of eating problems and related disorders in youth. Treatment outcome research with this population is still in its early stages of development, yet there is intense work in the evaluation of putative risk factors, assessment strategies, and treatment approaches. In particular, cognitive-behavioral and family-based approaches are showing great promise for managing BN and AN, respectively. In the context of a clinical case, we described the developmental progression of AN and its successful treatment using Lock's FBT.

REFERENCES

Agras, W. S. (2001). The consequences and cost of the eating disorders. *Psychiatric Clinics of North America, 24,* 371–379.

Agras, W. S., Brandt, H. A., Bulik, C. M., Dolan-Sewell, R., Fairburn, C. G., Halmi, K. A., et al. (2004). Report of the National Institutes of Health workshop on overcoming barriers to treatment research in anorexia nervosa. *International Journal of Eating Disorders, 35,* 509–521.

Ambrosini, P., & Dixon, D. (1996). *Schedule for Affective Disorders and Schizophrenia for School-Age Children—Fourth Version Revised (K-SADS-IVR).* Unpublished manuscript, Medical College of Pennsylvania and Hahnemann University, Philadelphia.

American Academy of Pediatrics Committee on Adolescence (2006). Menstruation in girls and adolescents: Using the menstrual cycle as a vital sign. *Pediatrics, 118,* 2245–2450.

American Psychiatric Association (APA). (2000). *Diagnostic and statistical manual of mental disorders* (4th ed., text rev.). Washington, DC: Author.

Bryant-Waugh, R. (2000). Overview of the eating disorders. In B. Lask & R. Bryant-Waugh (Eds.), *Anorexia nervosa and related eating disorders in childhood and adolescence* (pp. 27–40). Hove, UK: Psychology Press.

Bryant-Waugh, R. (2006). Eating disorders in children and adolescents. In S. Wonderlich, J. E. Mitchell, M. de Zwann, & H. Steiger (Eds.), *Annual review of eating disorders.* Oxford, UK: Radcliffe.

Bryant-Waugh, R., Cooper, P., Taylor, C., & Lask, B. (1996). The use of the Eating Disorder Examination with children: A pilot study. *International Journal of Eating Disorders, 19,* 391–398.

Bryant-Waugh, R., & Lask, B. (1995). Eating disorders in children. *Journal of Child Psychology and Psychiatry, and Allied Disciplines, 36,* 191–202.

Bulik, C. M., Reba, L., Siega-Riz, A. M., & Reichborn-Kjennerud, T. (2005). Anorexia nervosa: Definition, epidemiology, and cycle of risk. *International Journal of Eating Disorders, 37*(Suppl.), S2–S9.

Bunnell, D. W., Shenker, I. R., Nussbaum, M. P., Jacobson, M. S., & Cooper, P.

(1990). Subclinical versus formal eating disorders: Differentiating psychological features. *International Journal of Eating Disorders, 9*, 357–362.

Cash, T. F. (2002). A "negative body image": Evaluating epidemiological evidence. In T. F. Cash & T. Pruzinsky (Eds.), *Body images: A handbook of theory, research, and clinical practice* (pp. 269–276). New York: Guilford Press.

Chamay-Weber, C., Narring, F., & Michaud, P. (2005). Partial eating disorders among adolescents: A review. *Journal of Adolescent Health, 37*, 417–427.

Chambers, W. J., Puig-Antich, J., Hirsch, M., Paez, P., Ambrosini, P. J., Tabrizi, M. A., et al. (1985). The assessment of affective disorders in children and adolescents by semistructured interview: Test–retest reliability of the schedule for affective disorders and schizophrenia for school-age children, present episode version. *Archives of General Psychiatry, 42*(7), 696–702.

Chatoor, I., & Ganiban, J. (2003). Food refusal by infants and young children: Diagnosis and treatment. *Cognitive and Behavioral Practice, 10*, 138–146.

Childress, A., Brewerton, T., Hodges, E., & Jarrell, M. (1993). The Kids' Eating Disorders Survey (KEDS): A study of middle school students. *Journal of the American Academy of Child and Adolescent Psychiatry, 32*, 843–850.

Childress, A., Jarrell, M., & Brewerton, T. (1992). *The Kids' Eating Disorders Survey (KEDS): Internal consistency, component analysis, and test–retest reliability.* Paper presented at the 5th International Conference on Eating Disorders, New York, NY.

Christie, D. (2000). Cognitive-behavioural therapeutic techniques for children with eating disorders. In B. Lask & R. Bryant-Waugh (Eds.), *Anorexia nervosa and related eating disorders in childhood and adolescence* (pp. 205–226). East Sussex, UK: Psychology Press.

Christie, D., Watkins, B., & Lask, B. (2000). Assessment. In B. Lask & R. Bryant-Waugh (Eds.), *Anorexia nervosa and related eating disorders in childhood and adolescence* (pp. 105–125). East Sussex, UK: Psychology Press.

Constantino, M. J., Arnow, B. A., Blasey, C., & Agras, W. S. (2005). The association between patient characteristics and the therapeutic alliance in cognitive-behavioral and interpersonal therapy for bulimia nervosa. *Journal of Consulting and Clinical Psychology, 73*, 203–211.

Cooper, Z., Cooper, P., & Fairburn, C. (1989). The validity of the Eating Disorder Examination and its subscales. *British Journal of Psychiatry, 154*, 807–812.

Cooper, Z., & Fairburn, C. (1987). The Eating Disorder Examination: A semistructured interview for the assessment of the specific psychopathology of eating disorders. *International Journal of Eating Disorders, 6*, 1–8.

Dare, C., Eisler, I., Russell, G., Treasure, J., & Dodge, E. (2001). Psychological therapies for adults with anorexia nervosa: Randomised controlled trial of outpatient treatments. *British Journal of Psychiatry, 178*, 216–221.

Decaluwe, V., & Braet, C. (2003). Prevalence of binge-eating disorder in obese children and adolescents seeking weight-loss treatment. *International Journal of Obesity, 27*, 404–409.

Doyle, J., & Bryant-Waugh, R. (2000). Epidemiology. In B. Lask & R. Bryant-Waugh (Eds.), *Anorexia nervosa and related eating disorders in childhood and adolescence* (pp. 41–61). Hove, UK: Psychology Press.

Ebeling, H., Tapanainen, P., Joutsenoja, A., Koskinen, M., Morin-Papunen, L., Jarvi, L., et al. (2003). Practice guideline for treatment of eating disorders in children and adolescents. *Annals of Medicine, 35*, 488–501.

Eisler, I., Dare, C., Hodes, M., Russell, G., Dodge, E., & Le Grange, D. (2001). Family therapy for adolescent anorexia nervosa: The results of a controlled comparison of two family interventions. *Journal of Child Psychology and Psychiatry, 41,* 727–736.

Eklund, K., Paavonen, E. J., & Almqvist, F. (2005). Factor structure of the Eating Disorder Inventory–C. *International Journal of Eating Disorders, 37,* 330–341.

Fairburn, C. G. (2005). Evidence-based treatment of anorexia nervosa. *International Journal of Eating Disorders, 37*(Suppl.), S26–S30.

Fairburn, C. G., & Cooper, Z. (1993). The Eating Disorder Examination (12th ed.). In C. G. Fairburn & G. T. Wilson (Eds.), *Binge eating: Nature, assessment and treatment* (pp. 317–360). New York: Guilford Press.

Fairburn, C. G., & Harrison, P. J. (2003). Eating disorders. *Lancet, 361,* 407–416.

Fairburn, C. G., Marcus, M. D., & Wilson, G. T. (1993). Cognitive-behavioral therapy for binge eating and bulimia nervosa: A comprehensive treatment manual. In C. G. Fairburn & G. T. Wilson (Eds.), *Binge eating: Nature, assessment and treatment* (pp. 361–404). New York: Guilford Press.

Faith, M. S., & Thompson, J. K. (2003). Obesity and body image disturbance. In L. M. Cohen, D. E. McChargue, & F. L. Collins, Jr. (Eds.), *The health psychology handbook: Practical issues for the behavioral medicine specialist* (pp. 125–145). Thousand Oaks, CA: Sage.

Felker, K., & Stivers, C. (1994). The relationship of gender and family environment to eating disorder risk in adolescents. *Adolescence, 29,* 821–834.

Fisher, M., Schneider, M., Burns, J., Symons, H., & Mandel, F. S. (2001). Differences between adolescents and young adults at presentation to an eating disorders program. *Journal of Adolescent Health, 28,* 222–227.

Fitzgibbon, M. L., Sanchez-Johnsen, L. A. P., & Martinovich, Z. (2003). A test of the continuity perspective across bulimic and binge eating pathology. *International Journal of Eating Disorders, 34,* 83–97.

Franko, D. L., & Omori, M. (1999). Subclinical eating disorders in adolescent women: A test of the continuity hypothesis and its psychological correlates. *Journal of Adolescence, 22,* 389–396.

Friedman, M. A., Wilfley, D. E., Welch, R. R., & Kunce, J. T. (1997). Self-directed hostility and family functioning in normal-weight bulimics and overweight binge eaters. *International Journal of Eating Disorders, 22,* 367–375.

Frisch, R. E. (1990). The right weight: Body fat, menarche and ovulation. *Baillieres Clinical Obstetrics and Gynaecology, 4,* 419–439.

Frisch, R. E., & McArthur, J. W. (1974). Menstrual cycles: Fatness as a determinant of minimum weight for height necessary for their maintenance or onset. *Science, 185,* 949–951.

Gardner, R. M. (2002). Body image assessment of children. In T. F. Cash & T. Pruzinsky (Eds.), *Body images: A handbook of theory, research, and clinical practice.* New York: Guilford Press.

Garn, S. M., Leonard, W. R., & Hawthorne, V. M. (1986). Three limitations of the body mass index. *American Journal of Clinical Nutrition, 44,* 996–997.

Garner, D. M. (1991a). *Eating Disorder Inventory–C manual.* Lutz, FL: Psychological Assessment Resources.

Garner, D. M. (1991b). *Eating Disorder Inventory–2 manual.* Odessa, FL: Psychological Assessment Resources.

Garner, D. M., Olmstead, M. P., Bohr, Y., & Garfinkel, P. E. (1982). The Eating Attitudes Test: Psychometric features and clinical correlates. *Psychological Medicine, 12,* 871–878.

Garner, D. M., Olmstead, M. P., & Polivy, J. (1983). Development and validation of a multi-dimensional eating disorder inventory for anorexia nervosa and bulimia. *International Journal of Eating Disorders, 2,* 15–34.

Gowers, S., & Bryant-Waugh, R. (2004). Management of child and adolescent eating disorders: The current evidence base and future directions. *Journal of Child Psychology and Psychiatry, and allied Disciplines, 45,* 63–83.

Gowers, S. G., & Smyth, B. (2004). The impact of motivational assessment interview on initial response to treatment in adolescent anorexia nervosa. *European Eating Disorders Review, 12,* 87–93.

Greenfeld, D., Mickley, D., Quinlan, D. M., & Roloff, P. (1993). Ipecac abuse in a sample of eating disordered outpatients. *International Journal of Eating Disorders, 13,* 411–414.

Hebebrand, J., Himmelmann, G. W., Heseker, H., Schafer, H., & Remschmidt, H. (1996). Use of percentiles for the body mass index in anorexia nervosa: Diagnostic, epidemiological, and therapeutic considerations. *International Journal of Eating Disorders, 19,* 359–369.

Herzog, D. B., Greenwood, D. N., Dorer, D. J., Flores, A. T., Ekeblad, E. R., Richards, A., et al. (2000). Mortality in eating disorders: A descriptive study. *International Journal of Eating Disorders, 28,* 20–26.

Hill, K., & Pomeroy, C. (2001). Assessment of physical status of children and adolescents with eating disorders and obesity. In J. K. Thompson & L. Smolak (Eds.), *Body image, eating disorders, and obesity in youth: Assessment, prevention, and treatment* (pp. 171–191). Washington, DC: American Psychological Association.

Horesh, N., Apter, A., Ishai, J., Danziger, Y., Miculincer, M., Stein, D., et al. (1996). Abnormal psychosocial situations and eating disorders in adolescence. *Journal of the American Academy of Child and Adolescent Psychiatry, 35,* 921–927.

Humphrey, L. L. (1994). Family relationships. In K. A. Halmi (Ed.), *Psychobiology and treatment of anorexia nervosa and bulimia nervosa* (pp. 263–282). Washington, DC: American Psychiatric Press.

Jensen, P., Roper, M., Fisher, P., Piacentini, J., Canino, G., Richters, J., et al. (1995). Test–retest reliability of the Diagnostic Interview Schedule for Children (DISC 2.1). Parent, child, and combined algorithms. *Archives of General Psychiatry, 52*(1), 61–71.

Johnson, W., Grieve, F., Adams, C., & Sandy, J. (1999). Measuring binge eating in adolescents: Adolescent and parent version of the questionnaire of eating and weight patterns. *International Journal of Eating Disorders, 26*(3), 301–314.

Katzman, D. K. (2005). Medical complications in adolescents with anorexia nervosa: A review of the literature. *International Journal of Eating Disorders, 37*(Suppl.), S52–S59.

Kaufman, J., Birmaher, B., Brent, D., Rao, U., Flynn, C., Moreci, P., et al. (1997). Schedule for Affective Disorders and Schizophrenia for School-Age Children— Present and Lifetime Version (K-SADS-PL): Initial reliability and validity data. *Journal of the American Academy of Child and Adolescent Psychiatry, 36*(7), 980–988.

Keery, H., van den Berg, P., & Thompson, J. K. (2004). An evaluation of the tripartite influence model of body dissatisfaction and eating disturbance with adolescent girls. *Body Image: An International Journal of Research, 1,* 237–251.

Keski-Rahkonen, A., Bulik, C. M., Neale, B. M., Rose, R. J., Rissanen, A., & Kaprio, J. (2005). Body dissatisfaction and drive for thinness in young adult twins. *International Journal of Eating Disorders, 37,* 188–199.

Kjelsas, E., Bjornstrom, C., & Gotestam, K. G. (2004). Prevalence of eating disorders in female and male adolescents (14–15 years). *Eating Behaviors, 5*, 13–25.

Klump, K. L., Kaye, W. H., & Strober, M. (2001). The evolving genetic foundations of eating disorders. *Psychiatric Clinics of North America, 24*, 215–225.

Klump, K. L., McGue, M., & Iacono, W. G. (2003). Differential heritability of eating attitudes and behaviors in prepubertal versus pubertal twins. *International Journal of Eating Disorders, 33*, 287–292.

Kotler, L. A., Boudreau, G. S., & Devlin, M. J. (2003). Emerging psychotherapies for eating disorders. *Journal of Psychiatric Practice, 9*(6), 431–441.

Lask, B. (2000). Aetiology. In B. Lask & R. Bryant-Waugh (Eds.), *Anorexia nervosa and related eating disorders in childhood and adolescence* (pp. 63–79). East Sussex, UK: Psychology Press.

Lask, B., & Bryant-Waugh, R. (Eds.). (1993). *Childhood onset anorexia nervosa and related eating disorders.* Hillsdale, NJ: Erlbaum.

Lask, B., & Bryant-Waugh, R. (2000). *Anorexia nervosa and related eating disorders in childhood and adolescence.* Hove, UK: Psychology Press.

Le Grange, D. (2005). Family assessment. In J. E. Mitchell & C. B. Peterson (Eds.), *Assessment of eating disorders* (pp. 150–174). New York: Guilford Press.

Le Grange, D., Eisler, I., Dare, C., & Russell, G. F. M. (1992). Evaluation of family treatments in adolescent anorexia nervosa: A pilot study. *International Journal of Eating Disorders, 12*, 347–357.

Le Grange, D., & Lock, J. (2005). The dearth of psychological treatment studies for anorexia nervosa. *International Journal Eating Disorders, 37*, 79–91.

Levine, M., & Smolak, L. (2001). Primary prevention of body image disturbances and disordered eating in childhood and early adolescence. In J. K. Thompson & L. Smolak (Eds.), *Body image, eating disorders, and obesity in youth: Assessment, treatment and prevention* (pp. 237–260). Washington, DC: American Psychological Association.

Levine, M. P., & Harrison, K. (2004). Media's role in the perpetuation and prevention of negative body image and disordered eating. In J. K. Thompson (Ed.), *Handbook of eating disorders and obesity* (pp. 695–717). Hoboken, NJ: Wiley.

Lewinsohn, P. M., Holm-Denoma, J. M., Gau, J. M., Joiner, T. E., Striegel-Moore, R., Bear, P., et al. (2005). Problematic eating and feeding behaviors of 36-month-old children. *International Journal of Eating Disorders, 38*, 208–219.

Linscheid, T. R. (1998). Behavioral treatment of feeding disorders in children. In T. S. Watson & F. M. Gresham (Eds.), *Handbook of child behavior therapy* (Vol. 1, pp. 357–368). New York: Plenum Press.

Linscheid, T. R. (2006). Behavioral treatments for pediatric feeding disorders. *Behavior Modification, 30*, 6–23.

Lock, J. (2004). Family approaches for anorexia nervosa and bulimia nervosa. In J. K. Thompson (Ed.), *Handbook of eating disorders and obesity* (pp. 218–231). Hoboken, NJ: Wiley.

Lock, J. (2005). Adjusting cognitive behavior therapy for adolescent bulimia nervosa: Results of a case series. *American Journal of Psychotherapy, 59*(3), 267–281.

Lock, J. (2006, Winter). Update on Maudsley type family therapy for eating disorders. *The Renfrew Perspective*, pp. 19–20.

Lock, J., Agras, W. S., Bryson, S., & Kraemer, H. C. (2005). Short versus long-term family treatment of anorexia nervosa. *Journal of the American Academy of Child and Adolescent Psychiatry, 44*, 632–639.

Lock, J., Couturier, J., & Agras, W. S. (2006). Comparison of long term outcomes in adolescents treated with family therapy. *Journal of the American Academy of Child and Adolescent Psychiatry, 45,* 666–672.

Lock, J., & Le Grange, D. (2005). Family-based treatment of eating disorders. *International Journal of Eating Disorders, 37*(Suppl.), S64–S67.

Lock, J., Le Grange, D., Agras, W. S., & Dare, C. (2001). *Treatment manual for anorexia nervosa: A family-based approach.* New York: Guilford Press.

Maloney, M., McGuire, J., & Daniels, S. (1988). Reliability testing in a children's version of the eating attitude test. *Journal of the American Academy of Child and Adolescent Psychiatry, 28,* 541–543.

Marcus, A., Blanz, B., Lehmkuhl, G., Rothenberger, A., & Eisert, H. G. (1989). Somatic findings in children and adolescents with anorexia nervosa. *Acta Paedopsychiatrica, 52,* 1–11.

Marcus, M. D., & Kalarchian, M. A. (2003). Binge eating in children and adolescents. *International Journal of Eating Disorders, 34*(Suppl.), S47–S57.

Meads, C., Gold, L., & Burls, A. (2001). How effective is outpatient care compared to inpatient care for the treatment of anorexia nervosa?: A systematic review. *European Eating Disorders Review, 9,* 229–241.

Mitchell, J. E., Cook-Myers, T., & Wonderlich, S. A. (2005). Diagnostic criteria for anorexia nervosa: Looking ahead to DSM-V. *International Journal of Eating Disorders, 37*(Suppl.), S95–S97.

National Institute for Clinical Excellence (NICE). (2004). *Eating Disorders: Core interventions in the treatment and management of anorexia nervosa, bulimia nervosa, and related disorders.* London: Royal College of Psychiatrists.

Netemeyer, S. B., & Williamson, D. A. (2001). Assessment of eating disturbance in children and adolescents with eating disorders and obesity. In J. K. Thompson & L. Smolak (Eds.), *Body image, eating disorders, and obesity in youth: Assessment, prevention, and treatment* (pp. 215–233). Washington, DC: American Psychological Association.

Nicholls, D., & Bryant-Waugh, R. (2003). Children and young adolescents. In J. Treasure, U. Schmidt, & E. Van Furth (Eds.), *Handbook of eating disorders* (2nd ed., pp. 415–434). Chichester, UK: Wiley.

Nicholls, D., Chater, R., & Lask, B. (2000). Children into DSM don't go: A comparison of classification systems for eating disorders in childhood and early adolescence. *International Journal of Eating Disorders, 28,* 317–324.

Nicholls, D., de Bruyn, R., & Gordon, I. (2000). Physical assessment and complications. In B. Lask & R. Bryant-Waugh (Eds.), *Anorexia nervosa and related eating disorders in childhood and adolescence* (pp. 27–40). Hove, UK: Psychology Press.

Nye, S. S., & Johnson, C. L. (1999). Eating disorders. In S. D. Netherton, D. Holmes, & C. Eugene Walker (Eds.), *Child and adolescent psychological disorders: A comprehensive textbook* (pp. 397–414). New York: Oxford University Press.

Parry-Jones, W. L. (1991). Target weight in children and adolescents with anorexia nervosa. *Acta Paediatrica Scandinavia Supplement, 373,* 82–90.

Pereira, T., Lock, J., & Oggins, J. (2006). Role of therapeutic alliance in family therapy for adolescent anorexia nervosa. *International Journal of Eating Disorders, 39*(8), 677–684.

Pull, C. B. (2004). Binge eating disorder. *Current Opinion in Psychiatry, 17,* 43–48.

Reich, W., Herjanic, B., Welner, Z., & Gandhy, P. R. (1982). Development of a structured psychiatric interview for children: Agreement on diagnosis comparing child and parent interviews. *Journal of Abnormal Child Psychology, 10,* 325–336.

Reichborn-Kjennerud, T., Bulik, C. M., Kendler, K., Roysamb, E., Tambs, K., Torgersen, S., et al. (2004). Undue influence of weight on self-evaluation: A population-based twin study of gender difference. *International Journal of Eating Disorders, 35*, 123–132.

Robin, A. L., Gilroy, M., & Dennis, A. B. (1998). Treatment of eating disorders in children and adolescents. *Clinical Psychology Review, 18*, 421–446.

Robin, A. L., Siegel, P. T., Koepke, T., Moye, A. W., & Tice, S. (1994). Family therapy versus individual therapy for adolescent females with anorexia nervosa. *Journal of Developmental and Behavioral Pediatrics, 15*, 111–116.

Robin, A. L., Siegel, P. T., Moye, A. W., Gilroy, M., Dennis, A. B., & Sikand, A. (1999). A controlled comparison of family versus individual therapy for adolescents with anorexia nervosa. *Journal of the American Academy of Child and Adolescent Psychiatry, 38*, 1428–1489.

Schapman-Williams, A. M., Lock, J., & Couturier, J. (2006). Cognitive-behavioral therapy for adolescents with binge eating syndromes: A case series. *International Journal of Eating Disorders, 39*(3), 252–255.

Shisslak, C. M., Crago, M., & Estes, L. S. (1995). The spectrum of eating distrubances. *International Journal of Eating Disorders, 18*, 209–219.

Shroff, H., & Thompson, J. K. (2006a). The tripartite influence model of body image and eating disturbance: A replication with adolescent girls. *Body Image: An International Journal of Research, 3*, 17–23.

Shroff, H., & Thompson, J. K. (2006b). Peer influences, body image dissatisfaction, eating, dysfunction, and self-esteem in adolescent girls. *Journal of Health Psychology, 11*, 533–551.

Slade, P. D., & Dewey, M. E. (1986). Development and preliminary validation of SCANS: A screening instrument for identifying individuals at risk of developing anorexia and bulimia nervosa. *International Journal of Eating Disorders, 5*(3), 517–538.

Smolak, L., & Levine, M. (1994). Psychometric properties of the children's eating attitudes test. *International Journal of Eating Disorders, 16*, 275–282.

Sokol, M. S., Jackson, T. K., Selser, C. T., Nice, H. A., Christiansen, N. D., & Carroll, A. K. (2005). Review of clinical research in child and adolescent eating disorders. *Primary Psychiatry, 12*, 52–58.

Spitzer, R. L., Devlin, M. J., Walsh, B. T., Hasin, D., Marcus, M., Stunkard, A., et al. (1992). Binge eating disorder: A multisite field trial of the diagnostic criteria. *International Journal of Eating Disorders, 11*(3), 191–203.

Spitzer, R. L., Yanovski, S. Z., Wadden, T., Wing, R., Marcus, M., Stunkard, A., et al. (1993). Binge eating disorder: Its further validation in a multisite study. *International Journal of Eating Disorders, 13*(2), 137–153.

Steinberg, A. B., & Phares, V. (2001). Family functioning, body image, and eating disturbances. In J. K. Thompson & L. Smolak (Eds.), *Body image, eating disorders, and obesity in youth: Assessment, prevention and treatment* (pp. 127–147). Washington, DC: American Psychological Association.

Steinhausen, H. C. (1995). *Eating disorders in adolescence.* New York: de Gruyter.

Stice, E., & Hoffman, E. (2004). Eating disorder prevention programs. In J. K. Thompson (Ed.), *Handbook of eating disorders and obesity* (pp. 33–57). Hoboken, NJ: Wiley.

Stice, E., Killen, J. D., Hayward, C., & Taylor, C. B. (1998). Age of onset for binge eating and purging during late adolescence: A 4-year survival analysis. *Journal of Abnormal Psychology, 107*, 671–675.

Sullivan, P. F. (1995). Mortality in anorexia nervosa. *American Journal of Psychiatry*, *152*, 1073–1074.

Tanofsky-Kraff, M., Faden, D., Yanovski, S. Z., Wilfley, D. E., & Yanovski, J. A. (2005). The perceived onset of dieting and loss of control eating behaviors in overweight children. *International Journal of Eating Disorders, 38*, 112–122.

Tanofsky-Kraff, M., Yanovski, S. Z., Wilfley, D. E., Marmarosh, C., Morgan, C. M., & Yanovski, J. A. (2004). Eating-disordered behaviors, body fat, and psychopathology in overweight and normal-weight children. *Journal of Consulting and Clinical Psychology, 72*, 53–61.

Tanofsky-Kraff, M., Yanovski, S. Z., & Yanovski, J. A. (2005). Comparison of child interview and parent reports of children's eating disordered behaviors. *Eating Behaviors, 6*(1), 95–99.

Tate, A. (2000). Schooling. In B. Lask & R. Bryant-Waugh (Eds.), *Anorexia nervosa and related eating disorders in childhood and adolescence* (pp. 323–347). East Sussex, UK: Psychology Press.

Thompson, J. K. (Ed.). (2004). *Handbook of eating disorders and obesity*. Hoboken, NJ: Wiley.

Thompson, J. K., Heinberg, L. J., Altabe, M., & Tantleff-Dunn, S. (1999). *Exacting beauty: Theory, assessment, and treatment of body image disturbance*. Washington, DC: American Psychological Association.

Thompson, J. K., Roehrig, M., & Kinder, B. (2007). Eating disorders. In M. Hersen & S. M. Turner (Eds.), *Adult psychopathology and diagnosis, fifth edition* (pp. 571–600). New York: Wiley.

Thompson, J. K., van den Berg, P., Roehrig, M., Guarda, A., & Heinberg, L. J. (2004). The Sociocultural Attitudes Towards Appearance Questionnaire–3 (SATAQ-3). *International Journal of Eating Disorders, 35*, 293–304.

Treasure, J., & Ward, A. (1997). A practical guide to the use of motivational interviewing in anorexia nervosa. *European Eating Disorders Review, 5*(2), 102–114.

Wertheim, E., Paxton, S., & Blaney, S. (2004). Risk factors in the development of body image disturbances. In J. K. Thompson (Ed.), *Handbook of eating disorders and obesity* (pp. 565–589). Hoboken, NJ: Wiley.

Whittaker, A., Davies, M., Shaffer, D., Johnson, J., Abrams, S., Walsh, B., et al. (1989). The struggle to be thin: A survey of anorexic and bulimic symptoms in a non-referred adolescent population. *Psychological Medicine, 19*, 143–163.

Wilson, G. T., & Fairburn, C. G. (1998). Treatment for eating disorders. In P. E. Nathan & J. M. Gorman (Eds.), *A guide to treatments that work* (pp. 501–530). New York: Oxford University Press.

Wilson, G. T., & Schlam, T. R. (2004). The transtheoretical model and motivational interviewing in the treatment of eating and weight disorders. *Clinical Psychology Review, 24*, 361–378.

Winters, N. C. (2003). Feeding problems in infancy and early childhood. *Primary Psychiatry, 10*, 30–34.

World Health Organization. (1992). *The ICD-10 classification of mental and behavioural disorders: Clinical descriptions and diagnostic guidelines*. Geneva: Author.

World Health Organization. (1993). *The ICD-10 classification of mental and behavioural disorders: Diagnostic criteria for research*. Geneva: Author.

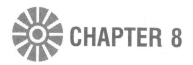 **CHAPTER 8**

Sleep Problems

Brian Rabian and Steven J. Bottjer

Sleep disturbance is one of the most common symptoms described by both children and adults. The impact of poor sleep in youth is broad and most evident in peer and family relationships, as well as in settings that require alertness, concentration, and energy to perform at optimal levels. Yet sleep problems are often misinterpreted or ignored because the resulting symptoms resemble more common behavioral problems. Sleep problems are also highly comorbid with internalizing and externalizing behavior disorders. As such, parents and educators rarely suspect that children's social–emotional, behavioral, and/or academic issues may stem from underlying sleep problems. Sleep disturbance is often viewed as a specialty best left to medical professionals. As such, many practitioners lack the necessary knowledge base to treat this population effectively. In this chapter, the authors help us understand the nature and treatment of sleep and its disorders in youth. Through the case of "Michael," they reveal how sleep problems may easily be overlooked in the midst of complex child, family, and school-related issues. Practitioners then learn how accurate identification and effective management can result in widespread behavior change.—A. R. E.

INTRODUCTION

On average, practicing clinicians tend to be less educated about sleep, including sleep architecture, developmental trends in sleep, and sleep disorders, than about pathologies such as anxiety, depression, and disruptive behavior. Professional training programs historically have neglected sleep and its disorders as a topic of study, and sleep is regarded by many in the field of mental health as a fringe interest area best left to physicians and sleep lab technicians. This

365

view fails to recognize the significant threat to healthy development posed by sleep problems, or the frequency with which sleep problems are a primary presenting concern for parents and children at community-based mental health facilities. The links between poor sleep and undesirable outcomes in academic, behavioral, emotional, and social areas of development are well established and now indisputable (for an excellent summary, see Bates, Viken, Alexander, Beyers, & Stockton, 2002) despite the fact that research on children's normal and abnormal sleep lags far behind its adult counterpart. Furthermore, there is a lack of connection between the types of sleep problems that are predominately studied in basic research settings, and those to which a clinician may be exposed. Encouraging more attention to the sleep problems experienced by young children should help to bring sleep study and practice out of the fringes and into primary settings where early identification and assessment take place.

This chapter focuses primarily on those sleep problems commonly encountered by professionals in community mental health facilities, who, along with pediatricians and physicians assistants, form the primary care "front line" that is most likely to be the first to assist parents in understanding the nature of their child's sleep problems. Perhaps more importantly, these are the professionals who show parents how these disturbances relate to other functions of the child and the family system. This is of great importance in light of data suggesting that (1) sleep disturbance is one of the most common symptoms described by children (and adults) presenting for psychiatric evaluation and treatment (e.g., Ford & Kamerow, 1989), and (2) primary care physicians do not routinely tend to screen for sleep problems, and report being more confident in treating sleep problems than in identifying and assessing them (Owens, 2001).

Our main focus is on case conceptualization utilizing assessment methods that have been established within the research domain but are applicable to the types of sleep disturbances commonly seen by mental health professionals. We cover treatment formulation that is informed by not only problem dimension but also the function of the sleep-related problem.

Nature of Symptom Dimensions

Defining what constitutes problematic sleep in children is no easy task. As mentioned earlier, far less research is available on children's sleep than on other child pathology topics, and in the research that is available, one finds significant variation in how sleep behavior is categorized. It is often difficult to compare findings across studies in the field of children's sleep because of the frequent use of laboratory-specific or study-specific definitions and measures. What qualifies as a sleep problem in Study A would not qualify as such in Study B. Sleep researchers appear to relish their role as mavericks in medicine and mental health, despite the fact that their individual tendencies have to be seen as a major contributor to the retardation of research in this area.

This lack of unanimity regarding how to define what constitutes a sleep problem reflects in part our still tenuous understanding of what constitutes "normal" sleep. The Pennsylvania State University recently hosted a small working group of distinguished researchers in the area of adult and child sleep, and those gathered acknowledged that the gaps in knowledge regarding children's, and particularly infants', sleep are enormous. We do have an understanding of the sleep stages through which all of us cycle over the course of a night's sleep and even how these stages reorganize and compensate when we are deprived of sleep for extended periods of time. What is not known, however, is how and when children are expected to settle into what constitutes more adult-like patterns of sleep. Very little is known about how myriad social and bioregulatory processes (Seifer, Dickstein, & Hayden, 1996) combine in creating a sleep experience, or how the rapidly developing physiology of the infant promotes, or is promoted by, sleep. So how should we be expected to define a nighttime arousal as problematic, when little is known about how often children at different ages typically experience arousal during the night? This state of affairs cannot be altogether surprising given that we still have no answers for even more fundamental questions: What is the function of sleep? Is it energy restoration or conservation? Memory consolidation? The extension of self-regulation? Brain growth? Emotional discharge? All of these have been argued as explanations for why we spend roughly one-third to one-half (in infants) of each day in sleep. Thankfully, we do not tackle here the question of *why* we sleep, but rather when we should consider a sleep behavior as abnormal or requiring clinical attention for a child at a given age. For a developmental context in evaluating sleep, the reader is referred to Stores's (2001) concise summary of the basic patterns of sleep and broad changes in the timing and duration of sleep throughout childhood.

Perhaps what defines a sleep experience as problematic, more so than whether or not the behavior falls within or outside epidemiological norms, is whether it is regarded by the child's parents as a problem. In other words, when a child's difficulties at night become disruptive for parents, then they become problems worthy of clinical attention. This means that the definition of a sleep problem is in large part contingent on the sensitivities and tolerances of family members who are directly or indirectly affected by it. Recognizing tremendous individual variation in sensitivities, shaped also by contextual factors such as cultural and familial expectations about children's behavior, we can begin to understand better the significant deviations, referred to earlier, across laboratories and clinical settings in how sleep behavior is labeled and measured.

Even with all of these caveats about our lack of knowledge and inconsistent approaches in how we study sleep, some commonalities may be found across conceptual frameworks put forward by those who study and treat sleep disruptions in children. A frequent distinction that is often drawn, and one that has great utility to clinicians because it reflects the common complaints brought to clinicians by parents, is that between experiences that reflect the following:

- Sleeplessness, or disruption to the quality of sleep.
- Excessive daytime sleepiness.
- Unexpected, and often unusual, physical activation during sleep.

In many cases, the third item represents sleep disruption that results from determinants that are more intrinsic or endogenous in nature (e.g., neurological or physiological arousals), and includes many of the parasomnias, such as sleep walking, teeth grinding, and night terrors. The second item, excessive daytime sleepiness, is quite often reported because it interferes with academic functioning or conflicts with parental expectations of behavior. And sleeplessness is often used to refer to disruption resulting from determinants that are more behavioral or extrinsic in nature (e.g., poor sleep hygiene or conditioning), and is most often reported because of failed parental efforts in bringing about change.

In children, sleeplessness includes bedtime or settling difficulties, such as bedtime refusal and trouble falling asleep, as well as waking during the night and waking too early in the morning, which are among the most common sleep concerns reported by parents to practitioners. These problems are particularly salient to parents, because children express their difficulties getting to sleep or staying asleep through attempts to reunify with parents (e.g., requesting to sleep in the parents' bed). Later, we talk about a model for the behavioral dimensions of sleep, developed by John Harsh and Monique LeBourgeois, that captures a number of problems best described by the label "sleeplessness." Prevalence rates for sleeplessness vary depending on the problems being considered and the manner in which they were assessed. Settling problems and night wakings, part of the group of sleep disorders known as dyssomnias (American Academy of Sleep Disorders, 2001), are most prevalent, based primarily on parental report, or are simply better known to us because they occur early in the night and typically demand engagement of the parent, therefore, presenting regularly to primary care settings.

By some estimates, prevalence rates for bedtime refusal and difficulty falling asleep are as high as 20% for children between the ages of 1 and 5 years (Hedger-Archbold, Pituch, Panabi, & Chervin, 2002; Ramchandani, Wiggs, Webb, & Stores, 2000). Rates are much lower as children develop and grow accustomed to established bedtime routines and expectations. For children in early childhood, rates for sleeplessness are reportedly around 10%, dipping closer to 5% by adolescence. Typical statements from parents reporting bedtime refusal or resistance include "It is a war just getting him into bed at night" and "She finds all kinds of reasons to put off getting ready for bed." Parents also very often report children exiting the bedroom once put to bed in order to seek reunification. Other common statements that may point to problems with initiation or maintenance of sleep and its consequences for daytime functioning include "She wakes up a lot during the night" and "None of us is getting a good night of sleep."

Excessive daytime sleepiness overlaps to some degree with nighttime problems (i.e., sleeplessness), because significant nighttime problems can leave a child well short of the sleep his or her body requires. When parents express concerns about their child's lack of energy or a tendency to "nod off" during the day, they are often relaying reports they have received from teachers about disrupted academic performance resulting from fatigue. Prevalence rates for sleepiness are around 5% for young children, and rise through adolescence. Exact figures are difficult to estimate because sleepiness is not often identified in sleep literature as a primary concern but is rather an outcome of other sleep problems. Sleepiness can result from conditions such as obstructive sleep apnea, in which a child's disrupted breathing during the night results in frequent arousals that interfere with transitions to deeper sleep. It can also result from delays or changes to the sleep–wake cycle that shift expected nighttime sleep patterns into daytime hours. Shift workers often experience reduced sleep time and quality because their bodies cannot adequately adjust to the forced changes to the sleep schedule. The perpetual sleepiness of the typical adolescent is often related to a tendency to stay up late into the night and sleep far into the day. Typical statements of parents reporting children's excessive sleepiness include "My kid is tired a lot during the day," "He is cranky all day long," and "His teacher says that he is falling asleep in class."

By "unexpected physical activation during sleep," we refer here to experiences such as night terrors, sleepwalking, and sleeptalking, which fall under the diagnostic heading of "parasomnias." The parasomnias can be broken down into subcategories according to the sleep stage in which they tend to occur, but for our purposes it is more important to note that, taken as a whole, they represent frequent and usually brief arousals from restful sleep, usually occurring within of few hours of falling asleep. These problems are less well known to us partly because their occurrence throughout the night makes them less obvious (with the exception of night terrors) to parents and other observers, and partly because some behaviors that constitute arousals, such as talking in one's sleep, are often reported by parents not as a problem but rather as an amusing novelty. Although snoring and halted breathing, which can signal the presence of sleep apnea, may also be thought of as unexpected arousals, the hallmark concern for parents of children with apnea is more likely the resulting daytime sleepiness discussed earlier. A conservative estimate of prevalence for the unexpected activations that suggest parasomnias is around 15–20% in early school-age children, with numbers dropping as children approach adolescence. Identifying true prevalence rates for problems such as the parasomnias is somewhat like attempting to hit a moving target, because most children have transient experiences in early childhood with sleep disruptions, such as sleeptalking and night terrors.

There are few clear cut boundaries between the sleep problems we discuss. For example, behavior exhibited by a child when he or she awakens at night and seeks parental attention through crying or entering the parents' bedroom can be related to the quality of parent–child negotiation of the bedtime refusal that occurred earlier in the evening. Excessive daytime sleepiness, and the changes it can bring to the sleep–wake cycle, may be related to a number of nighttime experiences, including regular apneic sleep disturbance, dyssomnia-related night wakings, or excessive delays in falling asleep. This overlap in dimensions of sleep underscores the importance of considering the function of problem behavior during assessment, as we discuss below.

Relationship to Specific Disorders

Currently, two diagnostic systems provide a framework for the classification of sleep disorders, but with different emphases. In the fourth edition, text revised, of the *Diagnostic and Statistical Manual of Mental Disorders* (DSM-IV-TR; APA, 2000), fourteen sleep disorders are broken down into four primary categories (see Table 8.1) based on etiology: (1) primary sleep disorders, which include dyssomnias and parasomnias; (2) Sleep disorders related to another mental disorder; (3) sleep disorders due to a general medical condition; and (4) other sleep disorders, which include substance-induced sleep disorder. The *International Classification of Sleep Disorders, Revised* (ICSD-R; American Academy of Sleep Disorders, 2001) groups more than 80 sleep disorders into seven primary categories (see Table 8.2). Given the unique focus of the ICSD-R and the consequent large disparity between it and DSM-IV-TR in number of sleep disorders, it should not be surprising that all of DSM-IV-TR's

TABLE 8.1. DSM Categories of Sleep

Primary sleep disorders

Primary insomnia
Primary hypersomnia
Narcolepsy
Breathing-related sleep disorder
Circadian rhythm sleep disorder
Dyssomnia not otherwise specified
Nightmare disorder
Sleep terror disorder
Sleepwalking
Parasomnias not otherwise specified

Related to another disorder

Insomnia related to another mental disorder
Hypersomnia related to another mental disorder

Due to general medical condition

Substance-induced

TABLE 8.2. ICSD Categories of Sleep

Dyssomnias

Intrinsic sleep disorders[a]	Extrinsic sleep disorders[a]	Circadian rhythm sleep disorders
Psychophysiologic insomnia	Inadequate sleep hygiene	Time zone change (jet lag) syndrome
Sleep-state misperception	Environmental sleep disorder	Shift work sleep disorder
Idiopathic insomnia	Altitude insomnia	Irregular sleep–wake pattern
Narcolepsy	Adjustment sleep disorder	Delayed sleep-phase syndrome
Recurrent hypersomnia	Insufficient sleep syndrome	Advanced sleep-phase syndrome
Idiopathic hypersomnia	Limit-setting sleep disorder	Non-24-hour sleep–wake disorder
Posttraumatic hypersomnia	Sleep-onset association disorder	Circadian rhythm sleep disorder NOS
Obstructive sleep apnea syndrome	Food allergy insomnia	

Parasomnias

Arousal disorders	Sleep–wake transition disorders	Parasomnias usually associated with REM sleep	Other parasomnias[a]
Confusional arousals	Rhythmic movement disorder	Nightmares	Sleep bruxism
Sleepwalking	Sleep starts	Sleep paralysis	Sleep enuresis
Sleep terrors	Sleep talking	Impaired sleep-related penile erections	Sleep-related abnormal swallowing syndrome
	Nocturnal leg cramps	Sleep-Related Painful Erections	Nocturnal paroxysmal dystonia
		REM sleep-related sinus arrest	Sudden unexplained Nocturnal death syndrome
		REM sleep behavior disorder	Primary snoring
			Infant sleep apnea

[a] Partial list.

sleep diagnoses are contained in ICSD-R or that they are handled with much greater specificity there. More than its counterpart, the ICSD-R appears to respect the transactional nature of childhood sleep behaviors. An example of this consideration of the parent–child exchange and the broader context may be seen in the treatment of several disorders subsumed under the broad heading of dyssomnias and subheading of extrinsic sleep disorders. Inadequate sleep hygiene and limit-setting sleep disorder both highlight specific environmental contributions to sleep problems, and, in children, recognize that sleep hygiene and limit-setting are often determined by multiple family members. As the labels imply, the emphasis is on the systemic factors that lead to sleep problems rather than on individual factors. Nevertheless, both systems focus largely on adults who experience disrupted sleep, and modifications for children are essentially left to the judgment of the clinician.

The behavioral sleep dimensions emphasized here (i.e., sleeplessness, excessive sleepiness, abnormal behaviors during sleep) are reflected across a number of formal diagnostic categories in the DSM-IV-TR. The parasomnias are defined as "disorders characterized by abnormal behavioral or physiological events occurring in association with sleep, specific sleep stages, or sleep–wake transitions" (APA, 2000, p. 630). Essentially, the parasomnias involve inappropriate activation of physiological systems during sleep, resulting in experiences such as sleep walking or "night terrors." The latter are defined as recurrent episodes of abrupt awakening from sleep, during which the child exhibits intense autonomic arousal signaling fear, but without awareness or recall of a dream. Although data regarding prevalence for parasomnias are limited DSM-IV-TR suggests that at some point during childhood, 1–6% of children experience transient sleep terrors, and between 10 and 30% of children experience an episode of sleepwalking, with 3% of children sleepwalking frequently. All parasomnias tend to peak between the toddler and pre-adolescent years, and to disappear spontaneously before adolescence. Onset tends to be without precipitants, and there is no established association between unusual nighttime behavior and other childhood disorders.

Problems with sleeplessness and excessive sleepiness are captured primarily by the dyssomnias category in the DSM-IV-TR: Dyssomnias are "disorders of initiating or maintaining sleep or of excessive sleepiness and are characterized by a disturbance in the amount, quality, or timing of sleep" (APA, 2000, p. 598). By far, the dyssomnia most relevant to our discussion of sleeplessness is primary insomnia, which is a complaint of problems initiating or maintaining restful sleep lasting at least 1 month. Over time, individuals may experience different forms of disturbance, shifting between trouble falling asleep and trouble staying asleep, and, unlike the parasomnias, problems related to insomnia tend to increase with age, particularly in adulthood. DSM-IV-TR is particularly insensitive to age in defining insomnia, offering prevalence rates only for adults. However, this insensitivity appears to be due largely to the distinction drawn between primary and secondary insomnia. According to DSM-IV-TR, primary insomnia is rare in children, typically not appearing before later adolescence, and coverage of age differences focuses almost exclusively on younger versus older adulthood. Although DSM-IV-TR recognizes the potential role of conditioning in insomnia, it fails to acknowledge explicitly the resistance behaviors at bedtime and the frequent attempts at reunification evident in so many children as part of the insomnia picture.

In topography, excessive sleepiness is reflected by the DSM-IV-TR dyssomnia called "primary hypersomnia," which is defined as excessive sleepiness lasting at least 1 month, with episodes occurring almost daily. However, sleepiness is listed within the criteria of at least three other primary sleep disorders, specifically, primary insomnia, breathing-related sleep disorder, and circadian rhythm sleep disorder. Thus, the presentation of sleepiness in a child is not diagnostically meaningful by itself, and requires a thorough assessment to determine whether sleepiness is due to a disorder or is itself the disorder (in the case of hypersomnia).

Further complicating the picture is the moderate degree of comorbidity between sleep problems and other disorders commonly presenting in children. For example, sleeplessness is common in individuals with a history of mood and anxiety disorders, and regularly presents simultaneously with symptoms of mood and anxiety in children. The latter case requires that the clinician determine whether sleeplessness is a meaningful and clinically significant behavior, independent of any other comorbid condition, or whether the use of a primary sleep diagnosis is precluded by the use of a diagnosis such as insomnia related to another mental disorder, in this case, a mood or anxiety disorder. The issues involved in making diagnostic decisions are discussed further in the next section.

Children with autism and other developmental disorders frequently have trouble settling at night and/or have inconsistent sleep–wake patterns, meeting criteria for diagnoses such as insomnia or circadian rhythm sleep disorder. Furthermore, children with severe developmental disorders may also have breathing problems that carry into the night, raising the possibility of a comorbid breathing-related sleep disorder. Learning disorders also have a significant association with sleep disorders, although the mechanism of association is not yet known. Some have speculated that a common neurological deficit may be related to both conditions, though it is also possible that learning disorders, as well as the developmental disorders mentioned earlier, interfere with the conditioning that establishes good settling practices early in childhood.

As stated earlier, within DSM-IV-TR and ICSD-R, disorders of interest are not really intended to describe the sleep of children, let alone young children, despite the fact that the first presentation of many sleep problems is quite often within the first few years of life, and certainly during the early school years. It seems important then to point out that Gaylor, Burnham, Goodlin-Jones, and Anders (2005) have attempted to fill this void, and to standardize criteria used by researchers and clinicians who address sleep problems in young children, by developing a classification scheme focused on sleep onset and night waking disturbances in infants, toddlers, and preschoolers. This scheme takes into account changing developmental expectations and distinguishes between levels of interference that characterize behavior as perturbed (i.e., one episode per week for at least 1 month), disturbed (two to four episodes per week for at least 1 month), or disordered (five to seven episodes per week for at least 1 month).

Differential Diagnosis

Parents presenting with their child at an outpatient mental health facility typically have little suspicion that the problem they are describing might lead to a diagnosis of a sleep disorder. Parents tend to view the nightly ritual of battling their child to bed or dealing with frequent reunifications as an annoying supplement to the "real" problem, such as their child's problems concentrating in school or his or her perpetual irritability. It is the job of the clinician to wade through the parents' reports and all other information with the goal of determining the independence or overlap of seemingly unrelated daytime and nighttime behaviors, and to develop an appropriate treatment program to the satisfaction of the parents and child. Ultimately, when sleep disturbance is one of the concerns expressed by a parent, the clinician is trying to determine which of the following scenarios is present:

1. A significant sleep problem exists, independent of other presenting problems, which requires intervention.
2. A sleep problem exists as a secondary symptom of another presenting problem, and direct intervention of the sleep problem may not be necessary.
3. The sleep disruption described does not rise to the level of clinical significance.

We have already acknowledged the significant overlap between sleep problems and other diagnoses commonly found in children, and that among sleep problems themselves. Where multiple disorders exist, the question is not necessarily whether only one of several potentially competing diagnostic labels is more appropriate than another, but whether the primary focus for intervention will be on one or another. Here we examine the decision-making process when considering potentially competing disorders as they relate to sleeplessness.

When considering sleeplessness, an important first distinction is between insomnia and awakenings that result from breathing-related sleep problems or circadian rhythm sleep disorder, and insomnia that results from exogenous factors, such as poor bedtime routine, overly arousing activities, or worry. A history of snoring, breathing cessation during sleep, and daily excessive daytime sleepiness, which points to breathing-related sleep problems, and circadian rhythm sleep disorder, characterized by an irregular sleep–wake schedule or delayed sleep schedule, is confused with insomnia only when an individual attempts to sleep at nonpreferred times.

When a child presents with persistent difficulty initiating sleep, the key diagnoses to consider are usually primary insomnia, one of the anxiety disorders, one of the mood disorders, or oppositional defiant disorder. The presence of significant resistance at bedtime, and the nature of that resistance, often points to anxiety related to bedtime or oppositional behavior that only happens to occur at bedtime. A child for whom difficulties settling are related to fear or worry tends to seek frequent reunification with parents and extended contact ("Can somebody lie down with me?," "Can I sleep in your bed?"), and may only exhibit crying or panic, or other symptoms of anxiety, at bedtime. Young children do not always have the ability to articulate worries, although they may express fears related to separation or to the dangers that lurk in their rooms (e.g., monsters, the dark). Because such fears are common in most children at different developmental stages, there need not be a history of long-standing and persistent anxiety at bedtime. Adolescents can better articulate their worries, though they are not always willing to share them with parents, and are more likely to keep delays in falling asleep to themselves. Thus, difficulty with sleeplessness in adolescence may appear to be a problem with daytime sleepiness, or with a sleep–wake cycle, for which the adolescent compensates by remaining in bed longer into the morning.

Oppositional behavior often presents as bedtime resistance but is less likely to result in problems awakening during the night. Children with oppositional resistance at bedtime are less likely than nonresistance children to seek contact or comfort from parents; rather, they focus on avoiding their bedroom and/or extending a desired evening activity. Although it may be difficult to distinguish between oppositional resistance and the panic resistance of the anxious child, whose fear presents as opposition in the face of an unbending parent, the nature of behaviors at times other than bedtime should offer a clue.

In the case of mood disorders, it is less likely that the child resists bedtime at all. Mood-related irritability may result in mild oppositional behavior throughout the day, but the opportunity to sleep is not a cause for strong resistance. Rather, mood problems are more likely to affect the child's ability to sleep without cognitive distraction, and delay in seeking sleep for someone with dysthymia or depression may result from excessive napping or resting during the day. Whereas anxiety related to the bedroom or to nighttime may not result in significant disruptive behavior at other times of the day, evidence of mood-related problems should be more pervasive.

The assessment process must also account for medication(s) the child is taking that potentially interfere with the ability to initiate or maintain sleep. In particular, insomnia may be brought on by medication to treat disorders such as attention-deficit/hyperactivity disorder (ADHD) especially when given late in the day, and mood disorders. Medication for the latter may also decrease the efficiency of badly needed rapid eye movement (REM) sleep.

Thus, primary insomnia and mood disorder may be diagnosed when the presenting concern is excessive daytime sleepiness, in the case of the former because difficulty falling or staying asleep has led to sleep deprivation, and in the case of the latter because of either sleep deprivation or chronic fatigue and lack of energy. However, a breathing-related sleep disorder, such as apnea, should also be considered when excessive sleepiness is present. Children who have disrupted sleep as a result of breathing problems do not typically report problems sleeping, because arousals may be subtle and falling back to sleep, instantaneous. However, daytime sleepiness is almost always present. Teachers may report problems with the child falling asleep in class, and parents are often aware of snoring or wheezing episodes during the night. Breathing-related problems do have a significant heritability, so the presence of apnea or similar conditions in one or both parents should raise a flag, and tends to be long-standing in the child's history. However, onset of breathing problems at night may be related to weight gain or allergies.

When the primary presenting complaint is about unusual behaviors that occur during night, such as yelling out or excessive restless movement, several diagnoses and problems should be considered, including nighttime panic attacks, common nightmares, parasomnias, and insomnia-related awakenings. The persistence of such behaviors is important to take into account, because parasomnias such as night terrors are experienced at least once or twice by most children and occasional nightmares are not unexpected. However, when behaviors persist, assessment should consider the child's awareness of these behaviors when awake, and when they occur during sleep. When children awaken with screaming or panic-like symptoms, ability to be soothed and recollection of dream content suggest the experience of a nightmare rather than night terror. Children experiencing night terrors typically do so in the first few hours after falling asleep and have no recollection of the episode once they are awake. Thus, night terrors do not result in subsequent anxiety related to sleeping or bedtime resistance, nor do they result in significant sleep deprivation. Nightmares, by contrast, often result in attempts to reunify with parents during the night and carryover fears. Although nighttime panic attacks are very rare in children, they are differentiated from night terrors by the child's awareness of his or her panic, and by the likely presence of panic experiences during the daytime.

CASE FORMULATION: CONCEPTUAL MODEL OF ASSESSMENT AND TREATMENT

Case Presentation

Michael A., a 6-year-old child from an African American family was referred to the Pennsylvania State University (PSU) Psychology Clinic's school-based mental health team for consultation concerning frustration tolerance issues in school and a tendency to zone out during class. Michael's first-grade teacher, Ms. R., and his school counselor were concerned that he too easily became upset in school and that this was beginning to interfere with his peer relationships and his ability to respond appropriately to his teacher's instruction. The referral was made several months into the school year, following a particularly difficult series of weeks around the Thanksgiving holiday break.

This was Michael's second year in his current school district and in the home of his biological father and stepmother, after a dramatic series of events that led Michael and his 8-year-old brother to be removed by protective services from the home of his biological mother and stepfather in a different city some distance away. Much of Michael's history prior to the move to his current home was unknown at the time of referral. What was known was that Michael and his brother ran away from home and were taken into police custody, leading to an investigation by protective services and removal from their home. Based on information available to the clinician, it appeared that Michael and brother were frequently left alone by their mother and stepfather, including evening hours, during which Michael was fed and put to bed by his brother. After running away, Michael was placed into the home of his father, a professional, and stepmother, a homemaker, with whom contact had been sporadic prior to this placement. In his current home, Michael lives with his father, stepmother, older stepbrother and younger stepsister, and his biological brother.

According to the school counselor, while Michael was in kindergarten during his first year in the school, the school worked with his parents to address a number of significant mood problems through counseling. Specifically, problems with self-esteem, loss, and crying were addressed in regular meetings with the school counselor. School personnel also worked with Michael to preteach a number of academic skills that were not in place prior to his transfer, and they attempted to address problem behaviors via a reward system. There was a significant decrease in mood symptoms over time, and Michael expressed happiness in his adjustment to his new family and city, which was considerably smaller than the previous one.

Nevertheless, at the time of referral, Michael continued to struggle with episodes of frustration, during which he would push desks or put his head down in his hands. His school instruction team expressed concern about the possibility that Michael was experiencing posttraumatic stress disorder (PTSD) and/or continuing problems with mood, and requested a consultation with recommendations for intervention, if warranted. They also emphasized that although Michael was generally pleasant in his classroom, if the resistant behavior he periodically displayed toward his teacher continued, Michael might have to face disciplinary consequences.

Assessment

Functional Behavioral Analysis

One of the primary goals of the assessment process is to weed through diagnostic material to determine whether clinically meaningful symptoms, or clusters of symptoms, are present and to differentiate between possibly competing diagnostic descriptors for the presenting problem(s); that is, the clinician's job is to determine whether a diagnosis is warranted and which diagnosis, or diagnoses, most accurately captures the problem at hand. In the case of sleep problems, this means deciding whether sleep disruption is a primary concern needing clinical attention, or whether it is likely a secondary concern that arises out of other, untreated problems. This is no small task given the myriad overlapping problems we highlighted earlier in the differential diagnosis section. Disrupted sleep is a symptom of numerous pathological conditions, and simply knowing that a child is sleepy or has trouble falling asleep does not drastically narrow down the diagnostic options facing the clinician.

The second goal of the assessment process, and one that is equally important as the first, is to identify the variables that maintain the sleep problem. Uncovering the antecedents and consequences that maintain a behavior is related to understanding the function that the behavior serves when it occurs at that moment. A single behavior, for example, trouble falling asleep, may occur, and keep occurring, for many different reasons. Does it bring attention from parents? Does it allow fearful avoidance of certain situations? Does it reflect heightened arousal related to the activities that preceded it? To answer these kinds of questions, the clinician is encouraged to conduct a functional analysis of presenting behaviors. The choices the clinician makes in picking assessment tools to evaluate a presented sleep problem should answer the question "Why this behavior now?" and highlight the importance of this process in determining what treatment, or treatments, might be most appropriate for this family, and what maintaining factors will be targeted during treatment. Unfortunately, at the present time the field offers few universally accepted measures for sleep, and instead is scattered with a variety of measures created for use within specific labs or research projects. We now turn our attention to the principal assessment tools at our disposal when children present with sleep-related problems.

The nature and timing of sleep behaviors often place significant constraints on the assessment options available to the typical clinician. Although parents and children may be instructed to monitor sleep behavior via sleep logs or diaries, and actigraphy may provide data on movement and activity during sleep, these are often crude substitutes for the physiological recordings and videotape monitoring that are a regular part of assessment in sleep labs. Moreover, although parents are often our best available reporters, they are frequently unaware of specific sleep behaviors, unless these behaviors require attention during the night. The ability to pinpoint the sleep stage(s) during which activation occurs or the frequency of undetected arousals during sleep may be important in the evaluation of particular sleep problems, such as apnea and the parasomnias. Thus, in the process of determining whether presenting sleep problems are of primary concern in the current clinical picture and the factors that help to explain their appearance, the clinician must also determine when referral to a sleep lab is warranted to allow a more refined examination of sleep processes.

Child and Parent Interviews

As stated earlier, sleep problems have historically been an afterthought to clinicians and researchers interested in childhood psychopathology, so it cannot be surprising that available structured and semistructured clinical interviews treat them as such. Several well-established broad-band interviews that exist in child and parent versions may cover diagnostic information about problems that co-occur with, or are mistaken for, sleep problems. For example, the Anxiety Disorders Interview Schedule for DSM-IV—Child Version (ADIS-IV-

C; Silverman & Albano, 1996) covers many internalizing and externalizing disorders beyond anxiety but treats sleep problems as a symptom, not as a disorder. The ADIS-IV-C includes thorough coverage of disorders, such as oppositional defiant disorder and mood and anxiety disorders, that require consideration when sleep disruption is reported. The use of an interview such as the ADIS-IV-C helps to determine differential diagnoses, but when information points to the presence of a primary sleep problem, none of the structured interviews currently available is designed to gather adequate information on sleep or on the function of sleep-related behavior. This information is typically covered in an unstructured follow-up interview by the clinician, and, in the case of a child presenting with sleeplessness, might cover the following topics:

- Does your child have a regular bedtime? Is there a typical bedtime routine? How does this routine usually start? How structured is your child's time leading up to bedtime? Describe last night's bedtime routine for me. Was that a "typical" night?
- Describe your child's activity level leading up to bedtime. Does the evening activity consist of television watching? Playing exciting games? Playing video games?
- Does your child express fears about going to bed or about his or her bedroom? What are those fears? How does your child show them to you? How do you respond when your child is scared?
- Does your child resist going to bed? How do you deal with resistance behaviors? What do you say when your child does not want to go to bed? When he or she gets out of bed? What is a typical outcome of your child's attempts to stay up?
- How new are your child's problems with sleeplessness? What kind of sleeper was he or she when younger? How did you respond to problems sleeping when he or she was younger? What did you have to do to get him or her to settle? How long has the current routine been in effect?
- What time does your child typically awaken in the morning? Is he or she difficult to awaken? Does he or she typically nap during the day? Have you heard your child snoring during sleep?
- Does your child awaken in a panic, like he or she is having a nightmare? Can he or she be calmed during these panicky times? Does your child talk in his or her sleep? Walk in his or her sleep?

These questions provide a starting point for discussion of the sleep problem areas we have emphasized here but leave a lot to the discretion of the clinician. Thus, a clinician's familiarity and comfort with sleep problems, and his or her ability to structure questions around this topic when necessary, go a long way toward determining whether sleep problems are accurately assessed. In general, however, the clinician should focus on not only the specific sleep *problems* presented but also the child's sleep history and "typical" patterns over the course of a 24-hour sleep–wake cycle. Although existing structured interviews are not geared toward evaluation of sleep, as a normal process or as a problem, the interview yield may be assisted by incorporation of better established questionnaire measures for sleep, which can also be administered in an interview format, as discussed below.

In addition to gathering information about sleep-related problems, the interview is also intended to cover behaviors, thoughts, and feelings that might be indicative of coexisting or competing diagnoses. This is important in light of the tendency to confuse primary sleep problems with depression, anxiety, and oppositional behavior. A thorough diagnostic interview is the primary means by which the clinician makes differential diagnostic decisions, but these decisions are also supplemented by the use of broad-band and focused questionnaires that provide information on the degree to which identified problem behaviors might be within normal limits for a child of a particular age.

Questionnaires

A number of broad-band measures are available for use with children and their parents, with varying degrees of coverage when it comes to sleep problems. The Child Behavior Checklist (CBCL; Achenbach, 1991) has a long-standing history, is somewhat ubiquitous in clinical settings for initial assessment, and is quite adept at discriminating between broad behavior dimensions. In addition, the parent-completed CBCL offers a number of items that assess sleep-related functioning. These items do not comprise a separate "sleep" index themselves; rather, they cut across a number of dimensions, including affective and anxiety dimensions. These sleep items include "nightmares," "overtired," sleeps less than most kids," "sleeps more than most kids during the day and/or night," and "trouble sleeping." None of these problems corresponds clearly to the sleep dimensions we discuss here (e.g., settling problems), but they do give the clinician an early indication that in addition to other behavioral and/or emotional problems in evidence, a need exists for additional follow-up regarding sleep.

The Behavior Assessment System for Children (BASC; Reynolds & Kamphaus, 2004) has gained in popularity among clinicians in recent years. Although this questionnaire makes many of the same broad-band clinical distinctions as the CBCL, the BASC also includes unique subscales not found on the CBCL, such as Self-Esteem, and Attitude Toward School/Teachers. However, because the BASC offers virtually no coverage of sleep-related functioning, it is not a useful screen for helping the clinician to identify potential sleep problems early in the assessment process.

Whereas the CBCL and the BASC demonstrate adequate sensitivity for assessing the broad "externalizing" and "internalizing" domains of functioning, the Conners Parent Rating Scale (CPRS; Conners, 1990) is adept at tapping into oppositional behaviors that may be related to bedtime refusal. With separate indices for inattention, hyperactivity, aggression, and defiance the CPRS has been shown to have better ability than other broad-band devices to discriminate between types of externalizing problems. This tool, then, might be useful when bedtime refusal and oppositional behaviors are a consideration.

When sleep problems are suspected and the assessment process must include anxiety or depression, either as contributors to sleep problems or as independent problems on their own, additional measures such as the Multidimensional Anxiety Scale for Children (MASC; March & Parker, 2004) or Children's Depression Inventory (CDI; Kovacs, 1980) should be considered. Although these measures are narrow in their coverage of anxiety and depression, respectively, the presence of a Separation Anxiety subscale and a Harm/ Avoidance subscale on the MASC adds useful information in an assessment addressing issues of bedtime resistance.

In light of the fact that sleep problems in school-age children have been associated with increased family stress (Sadeh, Raviv, & Reut, 2000), it is appropriate to include in one's assessment measures of family functioning and parenting, which might shed light on more systemic issues that may contribute to problems at bedtime and at points of contact during the night. Just as a child's internal state contributes to his or her ability to settle and comply, a parent's own level of stress and parenting practices can greatly affect a child's sleep functioning.

Tools that are useful to understand the functioning of the child's family system include the Family Environment Scale (FES; Moos & Moos, 1986), which assesses communication, conflict, and other aspects of family dynamics that may be related to behavior disturbances, and the Alabama Parenting Questionnaire (APQ; Shelton, Frick, & Wootton, 1996), which includes child and parent versions, and addresses parenting and coparenting styles, and particular practices used with an individual child. A clinician who suspects that parental psychopathology may be a contributing factor to disturbances in the child can administer a measure of adult pathology, such as the Symptom Checklist–90 (SCL-90; Derogatis, 1983), which is available in a variety of lengths.

Sleep Measures

Examples of scales that are designed for paper-and-pencil use but can be adapted to an interview format are the Sleep Disturbance Scale for Children (SCDSC; Bruni et al., 1996), the Children's Sleep Habits Questionnaire (CSHQ; Owens, Spirito, & McGuinn, 2000), the Pediatric Sleep Questionnaire (PSQ; Chervin, Hedger, Dillon, & Pituch, 2000), and the Children's Sleep–Wake Scale (CSWS; LeBourgeois, Hancock, & Harsh, 2001. The SDSC has also recently been adapted for use with preschool children, under the name Tayside Children's Sleep Questionnaire (TCSQ; McGreavey, Donnan, Pagliari, & Sullivan, 2005).

The PSQ contains more than 70 closed-ended (*Yes*, *No*, and *Don't know*) and open-ended questions to which parents respond with information about the child's medical history and current sleep behaviors. It covers a full range of sleep problems, including sleepiness, insomnia, and bedtime resistance, and appears to provide better-than-average coverage of sleep-disordered breathing, which receives less coverage on other available scales. The CSHQ, is a screening instrument that focuses on the sleep of young children, contains 45 items covering bedtime resistance, sleep onset delay, sleep duration, sleep anxiety, night wakings, parasomnias, disordered breathing, and sleepiness. The parent-reported items are scored on a 3-point scale, based on frequency of occurrence: *Rarely* (0–1 time), *Sometimes* (2–4 times), or *Regularly* (5–7 times) over a "typical," recent week. The CSWS (LeBourgeois et al., 2001; LeBourgeois & Harsh, 2001), a 43-item, paper-and-pencil measure for parents of children 2–12 years old, focuses on five functionally different behavioral dimensions of children's sleep, namely, Going to Bed, Falling Asleep, Maintaining Sleep, Reinitiating Sleep, Returning to Wake. These dimensions are based upon a developmental model of sleep (see Figure 8.1), which posits

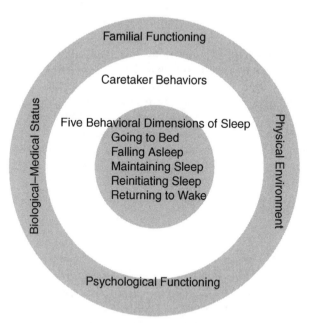

FIGURE 8.1. A behavioral model of sleep. Reprinted with permission from Monique LeBourgeois.

that sleep occurs within the context of multiple interacting factors, and emphasizes the behavioral facilitators and inhibitors of sleep during development. In addition to gauging when a child goes to bed, the CSWS has specific items about bedtime routine, how the child settles or wakes on his or her own, and the child's characteristics during these transitions, and requires parents to respond on a 6-point scale (*Never* to *Always*) about how often behaviors occurred over the past month. The CSWS has been used by B. Rabian in both research and clinical settings.

In addition to measures that touch upon the nature and frequency of disturbed sleep, it is also important that assessment include measures that gather information on the habits and practices related to evening and bedtime routines, or what is commonly referred to as "sleep hygiene." The Children's Sleep Hygiene Scale (Harsh, Easley, & LeBourgeois, 2002), developed as a companion to the CSWS, targets the frequency of behaviors comprising three domains of sleep hygiene over the past month. Parents of children 2–12 years old respond to 25 items covering their child's typical activities and routine before bedtime, disposition before bedtime, and the physical environment in which the child is going to sleep.

None of the available sleep questionnaires adequately target information about the parent–child exchanges that occur around bedtime and may be directly or indirectly related to a child's sleep. This information is largely collected during the parent, and possibly the child, interviews described earlier, and may also be targeted by other assessment tools, such as sleep logs or diaries.

Sleep Diaries

Research on children's sleep has relied much more heavily on sleep diaries than on questionnaires, and it is fair to say that most conclusions about the efficacy of treatments for children's sleep problems are based on parent-completed sleep diaries as the primary treatment outcome measure (for a summary, see Mindell, 1999). Sleep diaries may take many forms, but all share in common the goal of collecting "in-the-moment" parental reporting of settling and waking times, night awakenings, routines, daytime sleepiness, and sleep-related behaviors (see Figure 8.2. for an example). Gathering such information over 1 or 2 weeks by using a standardized, often very simple format helps to reduce the distortion and subjectivity sometimes reflected in parents' in-office recall of sleep behaviors. By including space to record evening activities and the child's response to bedtime, the sleep diary may also help to clarify the nature of antecedents to problem behaviors. In addition, if the child is old enough to complete self-report diaries for a limited number of behaviors, then it is beneficial to get such reports, because the concordance or discrepancy between parent and child reports is extremely valuable.

	Sunday	Monday	Tuesday	Wednesday	Thursday	Friday	Saturday
12:00 A.M.–1:00 A.M.	■	■					
1:00 A.M.–2:00 A.M.	■	■					
2:00 A.M.–3:00 A.M.	■	■					
3:00 A.M.–4:00 A.M.	■	■					
4:00 A.M.–5:00 A.M.	■	■					
5:00 A.M.–6:00 A.M.		■					
6:00 A.M.–7:00 A.M.							
7:00 A.M.–8:00 A.M.							
8:00 A.M.–9:00 A.M.							
9:00 A.M.–10:00 A.M.							
10:00 A.M.–11:00 A.M.							
11:00 A.M.–12:00 P.M.							
12:00 P.M.–1:00 P.M.							
1:00 P.M.–2:00 P.M.							
2:00 P.M.–3:00 P.M.							
3:00 P.M.–4:00 P.M.							
4:00 P.M.–5:00 P.M.							
5:00 P.M.–6:00 P.M.							
6:00 P.M.–7:00 P.M.							
7:00 P.M.–8:00 P.M.							
8:00 P.M.–9:00 P.M.	▒	▒					
9:00 P.M.–10:00 P.M.	▒	▒					
10:00 P.M.–11:00 P.M.	■	■					
11:00 P.M.–12:00 A.M.	■	■					

FIGURE 8.2. Sleep diary example tracking time in bed and time asleep. Blackened sections reflect time asleep. Shaded sections reflect time settling into bed.

Actigraphy and Polysomnography

Interviews, questionnaires, and diaries comprise the primary means by which the clinician outside a sleep lab collects data on a presenting sleep problem. Several other tools that assess sleep patterns and sleep problems (e.g., awakenings during the night) with the aid of modern technology are currently not utilized heavily by most clinicians in practice due to time, expense, and lack of training constraints. The simplest and least intrusive of these technology-based tools is the actigraph, a wristwatch-like device that records patterns of sleep and wakefulness during a single night and across a series of nights. The output of actigraphy corresponds well, albeit in less detail, to the output of polysomnography, but it has the advantage of portability, which allows collection of data outside of the sleep lab. Thus, the actigraph is especially useful for children, because it allows data collection while the child sleeps in his or her own bed. It is not unusual for discrepancies to exist between objective actigraphy and other measures, such as parental diaries, and the clinician must determine whether discrepant data represent complementary information that adds multiple, useful perspectives on the same behavior or inaccuracies in subjective reporting, possibly due to low motivation or low energy from sleep-deprived parents.

Polysomnography refers to the measurement (e.g., electroencephalogram [EEG], electromyogram [EMG], and electrooculogram [EOG]) of multiple physiological variables during sleep and is used to track a whole host of sleep-related processes, such as sleep onset, sleep continuity, and stages of sleep. Polysomnography is necessary in the diagnosis of only a few sleep disorders, such as sleep apnea and other breathing-related disorders, as well as the parasomnias, but it is particularly valuable in identifying the presence of subtle nighttime awakenings not captured by other assessment tools. Thus, referral to a sleep lab is sometimes necessary when the presenting problem involves excessive daytime sleepiness whose root etiology cannot be discovered through the use of an interview, questionnaire, or diary.

Videography

A recent addition to the measurement of sleep-related problems is video recording. Supplementing parent report data with actual video recording of nighttime behavior adds important objective data about the frequency of sleep behaviors, including obvious awakenings and falling back to sleep, and parental responses. Although video records historically have been underused in the evaluation of sleep because of cost and reliance on an overnight stay in a sleep lab, advances in digital recording open new possibilities for the inexpensive, continuous recording of nighttime behavior.

Case Assessment

Because Michael's referral focused on outbursts and frustrated behaviors in school, and their potential to interfere with his social and academic progress, he was originally seen through our clinic's school-based mental health consultation service, with the expectation that we would develop a behavior plan for the classroom. The assessment process originated in the school setting and included classroom observations, interviews, and questionnaires completed by Michael's teacher, Ms. R.

Ms. R. described Michael as a likable child who could be cooperative and polite, but who tended to become very frustrated easily when pushed to focus on demanding schoolwork. On several occasions, Michael's expressions of frustration, described by Ms. R. as tantrums, disrupted the classroom, prompting the school to seek consultation, with the parents consent. On the

Teacher Report Form of the CBCL, however, no significant elevations were present across the Externalizing or Internalizing subscales. When pressed, Michael's teacher acknowledged that although disruptive, his outbursts were not everyday occurrences. Ms. R. was unable to identify consistent antecedents to Michael's outbursts, other than the presentation of demanding tasks (which Ms. R. felt Michael was fully capable of handling). Several times during the interview, Michael's teacher mentioned that he routinely was brought to school late by his stepmother and often appeared to lack energy during the early part of the school day. According to Ms. R., since the very beginning of the school year, Michael had been prone to put his head on his desk and often had to be coaxed into participating in classroom activities. She felt she could sometimes anticipate that a day would be difficult for Michael when he seemed tired in the morning. During visits to Michael's classroom, we observed Michael to be a gregarious child who interacted easily, and appeared to be well-regarded by his peers. Michael could identify several friends in his classroom, and was regularly invited by his peers to play. He did not exhibit disruptive behavior during two separate observation periods, but sluggish behavior was evident, particularly in the morning.

In interviews, Michael's parents, Mr. and Mrs. A., denied the presence of outbursts or significant oppositional behaviors at home, indicating only that Michael could be mildly resistant at bedtime. Michael was quiet and could at times be short-tempered since coming to live in his current home, but these types of behaviors had improved significantly with time and individual counseling in which Michael participated through his school. Michael's parents were cooperative with efforts of school personnel to address Michael's behavior, although they viewed his disruptive behavior as likely a function of classroom management issues. Mrs. A., identified as the primary caretaker in the home, completed the CBCL. Elevations in the borderline clinical range were present for three subscales—Anxious/Depressed, Withdrawn/Depressed, and Somatic Complaints. No significant elevations were present across the Externalizing subscales. Behaviors reported to be *Very true or often true* of Michael included "feels he has to be perfect," "too fearful or anxious," "worries," "shy or timid," "withdrawn/doesn't get involved with others," "lacks energy," and "overtired." Among the DSM-oriented scales on the CBCL, a significant elevation was present for Affective Problems, primarily because Michael's mother endorsed a number of sleep-related items, such as "overtired," "sleeps more than most kids," and "trouble sleeping." She also indicated that Michael sometimes complained of stomachaches and nausea in the evening. In follow-up questioning, Mr. and Mrs. A. confirmed that they also saw the tired behavior observed in the classroom, and that they often employed a "quiet time" after school to give Michael a chance to nap or rest.

Based on the initial interviews with Michael's parents and teacher, there was little evidence to support the stated concern about PTSD. This concern was raised primarily because of Michael's largely unknown experiences while in the home of his biological mother. Furthermore, Michael's teacher provided little evidence to suggest that Michael was being deliberately oppositional in class. On the Teacher Report Form, and when pressed in a follow-up interview, she indicated that Michael's behaviors were perhaps less frequent than initially reported, and acknowledged that the intensity of Michael's upset likely influenced her perception. Ms. R. emphasized how well-liked Michael was in the school setting and indicated her willingness to help him in any way she could. She did not perceive Michael's behavior to be attention seeking (a conclusion supported by observations).

The focus of the assessment began to shift away from classroom consultation toward a broader consideration of factors that might be precipitants for Michael's poor frustration tolerance at school. Although the initial referral did not suggest a concern over sleep-related issues, this is not unusual, and the fact that this referral was initiated by the school made it less likely that sleep would be mentioned as a potential area of focus. Because his parents and teacher described Michael as often appearing tired, and because items related to his sleep were endorsed as being *Very true*, we considered the possible role that sleep-related problems might play in Michael's difficulty regulating his behavior under high task demands.

Michael's parents acknowledged that he regularly had difficulty settling at bedtime, and their interpretation was that this behavior was often willful, because none of Michael's siblings experienced similar problems. His tendency to awaken during the night to them a reflection of restlessness. The family routine prior to bedtime was reportedly "busy" and inconsistent across evenings, a situation that had worsened in recent months as Mr. A.'s workload had increased. Mr. and Mrs. A. reported that they "really slacked off" during the summer months but had fully intended to get everyone back into a great routine once the school year began. A great deal of autonomy was expected of the children during evening hours, because Mr. and Mrs. A. viewed this as their only opportunity for relaxation during the day. Despite this autonomy, Michael and his siblings were not typically overactive prior to bedtime, and watching television and stimulating games were typically kept to a minimum. Michael's resistance at bedtime typically came in the form of mild attempts to delay bedtime and a tendency to "forget" bedtime.

Michael's parents reported that they regularly kept the same early bedtime as Michael and his siblings, and that they would sometimes wake up later in the evening to find Michael still awake, with his lights on and his bedroom door open, and occasionally sitting on the stairs near the master bedroom. Although Michael appeared somewhat vigilant about keeping tabs on his parents' door, when questioned, Mr. and Mrs. A. could not identify other examples of behavior that might suggest difficulties with separation, and Michael never sought reunification with his parents after bedtime. Michael acknowledged having problems at bedtime but could not identify reasons he might be awake after bedtime. His age (6 years old) placed significant limitations on his ability to provide detailed information about his routine once he was in the bedroom. Michael denied experiencing nightmares or recurrent memories related to his previous home, and his parents could not recall his reporting nightmares to them. When discovered awake, Michael would typically report that he "can't fall asleep," but he was always compliant with his parents' directives to return to bed.

To better understand Michael's sleep behaviors and habits, his parents were asked to complete the CSWS, and the Children's Sleep Hygiene Scale. Although there was some discussion about the possibility of videotaping Michael's room at bedtime, his parents expressed reservations about doing this, and we agreed first to monitor his bedtime and sleep time via parent-completed sleep diaries before again considering videotaping. On the CSWS, Mr. and Mrs. A. indicated that Michael napped an average of four times per week for approximately an hour, and that over the last month, his bedtime had ranged from 8:00 to 10:00 P.M. Although his resistance to going to bed was viewed as a mild problem, his failure to fall asleep at "lights out" and tendency to awaken and remain awake during the night were rated as severe problems. His parents reported that although Michael did not usually fall asleep right away, he was "quiet and calm" once in bed, and only came out of the bedroom once in a while. Their ratings on the CSWS indicated that after awakening during the night, Michael was rarely visibly upset and never came out of his bedroom, called out for them, or got into someone else's bed. He was rated as being always slow-to-start in the morning, and it took him an average of 60 minutes to become alert. Because it was not their habit to go to Michael's bedroom and stay when they discovered him awake, they could report little about the quality of Michael's sleep. The Children's Sleep Hygiene Scale revealed that Michael frequency, if not always, "does things that are relaxing" in the hours before bedtime, and that, with the exception of his variable bedtime, his evening routine was typically appropriate to set the stage for going to bed at night. Mr. and Mrs. A. struggled to complete the sleep diary provided them the first week, in part because of their habit of going to bed at the same time the kids were put to bed. They acknowledged that their own fatigue made it difficult to monitor Michael's bedtime and sleep consistenly as requested, but they promised to increase their efforts for an additional week. We discussed ways to handle the diary differently during the second week, and Mr. and Mrs. A. agreed that they could trade off staying up to keep tabs on Michael. This resulted in the more complete diary they promised. Their diary (see Figure 8.3 for their report of morning and nighttime hours) confirmed not only a variable bedtime but also indicated that, contrary to what they had believed, discovering Michael awake was not indicative of his awakening after initiating sleep, but rather a delay in falling asleep for the first time. According to the diary, Michael did not tend to fall asleep for the night for several hours following bedtime, well after his parents were typically asleep. Once asleep, Michael appeared to remain asleep through the night.

	Sunday	Monday	Tuesday	Wednesday	Thursday	Friday
6:00–6:30 A.M.		■			■	■
6:30–7:00 A.M.		■			■	■
7:00–7:30 A.M.		■	▨		▨	▨
7:30–8:00 A.M.						
8:00–8:30 A.M.						
5:30–6:00 P.M.						
6:00–6:30 P.M.						
6:30–7:00 P.M.						
7:00–7:30 P.M.						
7:30–8:00 P.M.						
8:00–8:30 P.M.						
8:30–9:00 P.M.		▨			▨	
9:00–9:30 P.M.		▨		▨		
9:30–10:00 P.M.		▨		▨		
10:00–10:30 P.M.		■		▨		▨
10:30–11:00 P.M.		■		▨		■
11:00–11:30 P.M.		■		■		■
11:30–12:00 P.M.		■		■		■

FIGURE 8.3. Sleep diary completed by Michael's parents during assessment. Blackened sections reflect time asleep. Shaded sections reflect time settling into bed or waking.

Link between Assessment and Treatment

In understanding Michael's sleeplessness after bedtime and his sleepiness during the day, there were a number of factors to consider. For example, did such problems represent (1) a poor bedtime routine and/or poor limit setting by authority figures, (2) overarousal due to the evening routine, () difficulties with anxiety or mood, or (4) temperamental or idiopathic insomnia? Not enough information was available about Michael's functioning prior to coming to his current home to know whether his sleeplessness was a continuation of earlier problems or might represent a long-standing, potentially idiopathic problem. However, despite the absence of knowledge of Michael's past sleep functioning, the assessment process did uncover other factors that would begin to shape our decision-making process when considering interventions.

According to questionnaires completed by Mrs. A., Michael showed some evidence of problems with mood and anxiety. Mood was not thought to be the primary contributor to Michael's current classroom behaviors, however, because his disruptive behavior was not evident during the previous school year, when concerns over Michael's mood led to his referral to the counselor, and significant improvement in mood had been reported since the initiation of counseling. With the exception of mild resistance at bedtime and keeping his door open, Michael did not exhibit behaviors related to sleep or bedtime that were, on the surface, more obviously anxiety-based (e.g., climbing into his parents' bed, calling out to them). He denied fears (e.g., about the dark or monsters under the bed) and could not identify other ruminative thoughts that might delay sleep. In addition, if Michael did experience concerns about separation from his parents at night, as is sometimes discovered in young children who are sleepless at bedtime, these were not evident in other situations where separation was required.

To supplement the limited information available from Michael in the brief assessment process, a report from Michael's previous school counselor suggested that Michael had expressed worries related to safety and security since moving in with his parents. The counselor presumed that these worries related to experiences from his prior home, which was in an "unsafe" neighborhood. In our assessment, worries of this nature were seen as significant in light of the unstructured approach taken by Michael's parents over the past couple of months. Although Michael's parents discouraged overarousing activities in the evening, in part for their own convenience, they did not provide consistent direction to their kids. It seemed evident that one goal of intervention might be to address inconsistencies in bedtime routines and to establish a greater sense of security in the family home when the kids were being put to bed at night.

Despite the fact that the assessment process provided ample evidence of a sleep-related problem, we did not assume that sleep was the sole explanation for, or contributor to, Michael's classroom behaviors. However, we believed that the extent to which difficulties such as frustration tolerance stemmed more directly from Michael's other problems, for example mood or anxiety, might not be known until sleeplessness and related daytime fatigue were first addressed. Michael's age also played a role in recommendations, because our experience in assessment was that he was not very forthcoming about his experience of thoughts or feelings. Because we was anticipated that intervention for Michael's problems getting to sleep might be relatively brief, we recommended to his parents that we focus our attention first in this area, then assess the need for other forms of intervention as we progressed. Addressing sleep problems early would also provide Michael's parents with some immediate relief, because the assessment process had heightened their awareness of the extent of Michael's sleeplessness, and they were concerned that he was remaining awake after they had fallen asleep. Mr. and Mrs. A. had previously dismissed Michael's fatigue in school as typical of all children, but now they expressed concern that they unknowingly had contributed to Michael's school difficulties.

Michael's difficulty initiating sleep appeared to be a function of several related factors. His family acknowledged a lack of routine in the hours leading up to bedtime, and inconsistent bedtimes from night to night. For young children in particular, the establishment of a consistent sleep–wake pattern is critical in reducing risk for daytime mood and behavior problems. The fact that Mrs. A. often allowed Michael to nap or rest after school might also have made staying awake at night more likely for Michael. Below, we outline evidence for the use of parent education programs to establish or reestablish appropriate sleep patterns and describe the application of education in helping Michael and his parents. Anxiety apparently related to security or safety also appeared to play a role in Michael's remaining awake, and an approach to intervention that increased Michael's time with his parents around bedtime seemed warranted. Mr. and Mrs. A. agreed to the use of the positive routines and graduated extinction, described below, at bedtime to bring them back into greater contact with Michael, and to establish their role as guardians once Michael was in bed.

Treatment

Preview

As stated earlier, problems associated with sleep are often presented to a clinician only when they are regarded by a parent as a problem. Because of this, one obvious goal of treatment is to reduce the distress of the parent and that of the child, if present, related to sleep difficulties. The beginning of this process is often the reestablishment of more developmentally appropriate sleep patterns, or at least of conditions that should promote more normal sleep patterns (i.e., good sleep hygiene). Regardless of the form of the presenting problems, poor sleep habits very often play a key role in their maintenance. For example, difficulty falling asleep may occur for many reasons, but it can be maintained or exacerbated by allowing the child to engage in stimulating play, which includes video games, late into the evening. Similarly, excessive daytime sleepiness may result in part from inconsistent bedtimes that work against the establishment of critical sleep–wake cycles. By working with the parents and child to develop more consistent and sensible approaches to the child's nighttime routine, the clinician lays the foundation for most of the practices typically prescribed within established treatments for pediatric sleep problems.

Many of the treatment components described below center around parental education and the implementation of behavioral interventions. Both in principle and in practice, the focus of treatment for sleep problems may be very similar to treatments prescribed for parents to address common children's internalizing and externalizing behaviors. Thus, what is unique to treatment of pediatric sleep is not interventions themselves, but the venue in which they are applied and the outcomes that inform participants about efficacy.

It should also be noted that an overwhelming majority of intervention studies on childhood sleep problems have relied on parent-completed diaries or logs to evaluate outcome (Mindell, 1999). Only a handful of studies since the mid-1990s have incorporated technologies such as video recording and actigraphy to supplement parental reports. Thus, our ability to evaluate the efficacy of interventions largely implemented by caretakers is confounded in part by the fact that these same caretakers are our sole source of outcome data. Thus, parents who report changing bedtime behaviors may also be confirming that they have carried out what the intervention required, and they may be reluctant to acknowledge gaps in their application of prescribed treatment components.

Context of Treatment

Although certain sleep disorders, such as breathing-related sleep disorders, may require referral to a sleep laboratory for assessment and result in overnight stays to monitor sleep behavior and physiology, most assessment and treatment for the sleep problems discussed here are conducted on an outpatient basis. This does not mean that the context of treatment is confined to a weekly office visit, however. The established interventions for behavioral sleep problems rely heavily on homework in the form of at-home parental monitoring and implementation of intervention components, and the context of treatment is evenly divided between office and home. Unlike many interventions for which the office visit serves multiple purposes, including as a forum for experiential applications of the concepts and skills being taught, interventions for sleep problems rely on office visits largely for education and planning, with the bulk of application left to the parents at home. Stated simply, it is difficult to implement new bedtime routines in an office at 3 o'clock in the afternoon. And because of time and financial constraints, it is typically not feasible for clinicians to have a more direct presence in the home throughout the course of treatment. The use of videotape can bring the activities of the home setting to the clinician and greatly enhance his or her ability to make necessary adjustments to strategies during the course of treatment. However, the use of video can still be costly, and the perception that recording will be complicated or burdensome can contribute to noncompliant parental behavior.

When conducting treatment for pediatric sleep problems, the therapist must be particularly sensitive to the baseline fatigue presented by parents, whose own sleep has oftentimes been disrupted by their child's problems. Unfortunately, the same exhaustion that initiates the referral for treatment also contributes to significant parental noncompliance. Parents' inconsistency in carrying out homework assignments and intervention components is quite often a reflection of their own fatigue, and the therapist should be careful to avoid overinterpreting when parents "take the night off" occasionally during the course of treatment. Short-term failure in recognizing the need to provide parents with rest can lead to long-term failure of the treatment, because the parents play such a critical role in seeing that interventions are carried out in the home. Partners can negotiate nightly schedules to give each parent in turn some much needed rest, but obviously this option is not available for single parents. However, other authority figures that are a part of the parent's support network (e.g., extended family) may be asked to play a role in helping to provide respite to a weary parent. This issue is critical and must be addressed head on in light of data showing a significant association between parental compliance and treatment outcome (Mindell, 1999). The therapist should also be mindful that some sleep treatments are more difficult for parents to carry out consistently. Extinction, for example, is particularly challenging to parents when part of the prescription involves asking parents to ignore crying and pleading from their child at bedtime.

Parents often struggle with consistency, because they are asked to carry out not only intervention components but also the burden of the role of reporter for intervention data. The overwhelming majority of studies in the pediatric sleep literature have relied on diaries or logs kept by parents as the primary tool for assessing change in treatment. Because such diaries are typically recorded daily, if not multiple times per day, it is difficult for parents to sustain motivation over treatment, particularly when their child's sleep behavior is improving and their sense of urgency decreases. It is largely for this reason that a significant drop in agreement often occurs between parental reporting via diary and actigraphy recoding over the course of extended treatment. Over time, parents tend to report fewer incidents during the night, even when actigraphy suggests that arousals continue.

Although pharmacological treatment may be part of intervention for pediatric sleep problems, it is often not a consideration before better established behavioral interventions have been tried. There is evidence that the benefits provided by medication are modest at best (e.g., Richman, 1985) and that relief of sleep symptoms as a result of medication alone is usually temporary, lasting only as long as the medication is used. In terms of the problems presented here, early reliance on medication as an intervention is probably more reflective of parental distress than of patient need. Nevertheless, referral for pediatric or psychiatric consultation should be considered when sleep problems co-occur with other emotional or behavioral problems, such as anxiety or ADHD. When the timing of already-established medication is a contributing factor to presented sleep problems, for example, an evening dose of medication for ADHD interfering with a child's ability to initiate sleep, changes to pharmacological treatment may be necessary to facilitate success in treating the sleep problem.

Description of Treatment Components

There is no one-size-fits-all treatment to consider when children present with sleep-related problems. Taken as a whole, pediatric sleep problems represent well the concept of equifinality (Cicchetti & Rogosch, 1996), one of the core tenets of the developmental psychopathology field; that is, a single outcome, such as excessive daytime sleepiness, may be reached through multiple pathways, with each pathway possibly dictating a different approach to treatment. Sleepiness that is primarily the function of bouts with sleep apnea may result in treatment to ease breathing during the night, by having the child wear a CPAP (continuous positive air pressure) device. Sleepiness that is primarily the function of inadequate sleep due to excessively delayed bedtime may result in treatment to address oppositional or anxious behaviors contributing to the delay of sleep, as the case may dictate.

A number of treatment components are consistently identified in the sleep literature as worthy of consideration when planning treatment for behavioral sleep problems, but many lack adequate research support because of the extended period of professional neglect of pediatric sleep problems we mentioned earlier. Support does exist at some level for a number of therapy components, and there is also growing evidence that packaging several components together in a targeted treatment may be superior to utilizing any single component in isolation (Mindell, 1999). Mindell has identified a number of "well-established" treatments for sleep problems in children that meet the Chambless criteria (Chambless & Hollon, 1998), but, not surprisingly, these treatments, and sleep problems in general, are not yet recognized by organizations in position to disseminate information broadly to professionals and to the public. For example, Division 53 of the American Psychological Association (Society of Child and Adolescent Psychology, 2006) maintains a website for professionals and consumers that contains a section on evidence-based treatments to inform "the general public as well as practitioners regarding the most up-to-date information about mental health practice for children and adolescents." However, sleep problems are not included, along with anxiety disorders, depression, ADHD, and conduct/oppositional problems.

Mindell (1999) emphasizes that the current literature on treatment efficacy does not really take into consideration the origins of the sleep problems being treated. Emphasis has been on outcome, regardless of etiology. The treatment components described below are those we commonly employ in our work.

PARENT EDUCATION

Much of the control surrounding a child's sleep experience (e.g., bedtime, activities prior to bedtime, expected behaviors while in bed) is held by agents other than the child, namely, his or her parents. Not surprisingly, then, parent education regarding sleep, healthy sleep habits, and their role in setting the stage for good sleep has been examined as one approach to address children's sleep problems. Although parents play a role in many of the available interventions for children's sleep problems, approaches that focus on parent education are typically designed to bring about broad changes in management of the environment surrounding sleep rather than to dictate a circumscribed response (e.g., ignoring) to a specific behavior (e.g., calling out to parents from bed); that is, parent education is designed to give parents better control over the factors that can exacerbate bedtime refusal, settling problems, and prolonged night wakings. Improvement in sleep comes, then, through improvement in what it commonly referred to as "sleep hygiene," or the habits and practices that promote good sleep (see description in the treatment guidelines below).

This method typically consists of training sessions and take-home materials to educate parents about typical sleep behavior and problems that can be expected with children at various stages of development, and may include teaching parents the strategies to alleviate the problems. Although few studies have examined the efficacy of parent education (e.g., Kerr, Jowell, & Smith, 1996), parent education does meet criteria as a *well-established* prevention tool, particularly with parents of young children. A typical component of training sessions is teaching parents to chart, via the type of sleep diary or log described earlier, evening and bedtime behaviors as they occur at home to better understand the antecedents and consequences of reported sleep disturbances and related behavior problems.

EXTINCTION AND GRADUATED EXTINCTION

Extinction and graduated extinction are intervention methods employed primarily to address refusal behaviors at bedtime, including crying and tantrums, and night wakings that result in reunification attempts by the child. Collectively, they are by far the most extensively studied interventions for sleep problems in children and meet criteria for *well-established* interventions.

Extinction techniques ask the parent(s) of a referred child to adhere to a strict evening routine and bedtime, and to ignore attempts by the child to draw parental attention. Once the child is put to bed, parents are instructed to check on the child for safety reasons, then to ignore the child during subsequent wakings and/or attempts at reunification. Because parents may find ignoring their child's pleas too difficult, adherence to extinction programs is often a struggle, and some empirical studies have found that parents are unwilling to continue when assigned to an extinction group. However, early attention to parental concerns about long-term problems that may arise from letting their child cry or have a tantrum can effectively sidestep later problems with adherence.

Graduated extinction schedules are variations on the extinction model, in which a parent is instructed to respond to the child's calls at set interval points, for example, after 10 minutes have elapsed. Typically, the period of time between allowable parent "check-ins" is increased as the intervention progresses, until the child is able to settle and sleep through the night at a developmentally appropriate level. Because graduated extinction allows parents to respond in at least minimal fashion to their child's pleas, it does not generate the same problems with adherence as does extinction without contact.

In Mindell's review of intervention trials (1999), the majority of the extinction programs resulted in more changes to children's habits than to control conditions, with outcome variables including time to settle, number of night wakings, or time spent awake.

POSITIVE ROUTINES

The use of positive routines in addressing sleep problems typically is an attempt to decrease the frequency and intensity of bedtime refusal episodes. In short, the implementation of positive routines focuses on proactively changing a child's internal state at bedtime instead of altering environmental variables that may be related to sleep disturbances. The goal is to move a child into a calm state through the use of positive interactions, so that he or she can settle more easily, in contrast to experiencing an overly aroused state, immediately prior to bedtime. In published intervention trials, the protocol is typically for parents to engage the child in activities that he or she enjoys before an established, regular bedtime. Because the number of empirical trials on this technique is currently small, and the number utilizing control groups is even smaller, positive routine as an intervention falls into the category of a *promising intervention*.

SCHEDULED WAKINGS

Scheduled wakings are intervention methods designed to lessen the frequency and duration of night wakings and, more broadly, sleeplessness of a child over time. Interventions that utilize scheduled wakings require a parent to wake and comfort the child a short period of time before the child typically would awake and call for a caregiver. These scheduled wakings are faded over time to reduce the spontaneous wakings experienced by the child. With the limited number of studies available on scheduled wakings, there is no basis by which to compare its efficacy to extinction-based interventions to address night wakings, although the limited number of studies suggests that the use of scheduled wakings is *probably efficacious* in reducing night wakings in children.

It is important to note, however, that the efficacy of scheduled wakings is strongly tied to parental compliance with the intervention, which poses somewhat of a problem, because the demands of frequently waking oneself in order to wake one's child can contribute to inconsistent compliance in even the most highly-motivated parent. Although child wakings may be accomplished with alarms, it is the presence and comfort of the parent during the waking that is key to reducing reunification attempts.

RELAXATION

Intervention models that include relaxation techniques are designed to help children settle and fall asleep without difficulty by reducing arousal that can interfere with a consistent routine and with sleep. Relaxation may also be a coping strategy for children who awaken during the night, if reinitiation of sleep is difficult to achieve in a timely manner. Different methods induce relaxation to promote sleep exist, with most focused on breathing techniques or the use of mental imagery to calm oneself. Although relaxation may achieved with also be audiotapes or sound machines, the method largely relies on the individual to practice bringing about a calm self-state; thus, these techniques are employed mostly with adults or older children.

THE PROCESS OF TREATMENT: STEP-BY-STEP GUIDELINES

Preview

The assessment process of our work with Michael and his family approached the time of the local school district's holiday break, which meant incorporating a 3-week hiatus near the start of intervention. Nevertheless, Mr. and Mrs. A. felt strongly that they would like to get treatment started right away, so that Michael could begin to see the anticipated benefits of treatment as early in the spring semester as possible. Although such a lengthy break at any point during the implementation of treatment is not ideal, it may be especially problematic early a treatment designed to foster consistency, and, in the case of Mr. and Mrs. A., with parents who are very unstructured. Nevertheless, not wanting to risk a decrease in Mr. and Mrs. A.'s stated motivation to actively participate in treatment, we agreed to hold two sessions prior to the break. We anticipated that the bulk of treatment material would be covered over four or five sessions, although this may expand by several sessions depending on roadblocks encountered in treatment.

The most common roadblocks in treatments for sleep tend to be delays in applying components of treatment, and difficulty in maintaining consistency in treatment once initial gains are made. Both of these roadblocks are often direct functions of parental fatigue, and we actively promote our belief that the short-term investment of time and energy we ask to make will result in greater time and freedom in the long-term.

Session 1

Building Rapport and Establishing a Plan

Michael and his mother arrived almost 20 minutes late for the first therapy session with their therapist, John M. Mrs. A. reported that Mr. A. had mistakenly booked a meeting at work that conflicted with the session time and would not be attending the first session. John planned on meeting with Michael and his parents briefly, before spending most of his time with Mr. and Mrs. A., and he decided to maintain this structure. Later, he would address with Mrs. A. the importance of having both parents attend each session, because session time would be used to problem-solve issues relevant to both of them in treatment and a lot of material would be presented over a small number of sessions.

Although sessions would largely focus on work with Michael's parents, John initially met with Mrs. A. and Michael to describe what Michael could expect as his parents incorporated changes at home. John asked Michael what he remembered from coming to our clinic before:

MICHAEL: Answering a lot of questions.

JOHN: *(laughing) That's right. We did ask a bunch of questions, didn't we? Do you remember what some of those questions were about?*

MICHAEL: I'm not sure. School, I think.

JOHN: That's right. We asked a lot about how you like school and how things are going there. Do you remember that we also talked about how your parents said you were having trouble falling asleep at night and feeling tired in school the next day?

MICHAEL: Oh yeah.

JOHN: *(laughing)* Oh yeah. Well, we are meeting today to talk some more about sleep and about ways we might be able to help you sleep better and feel more awake at school. How does that sound?

MICHAEL: OK.

JOHN: I want us to spend a few minutes together thinking about ways that we might help you fall asleep when you want to. Do you have any ideas you can think of?

MICHAEL: *(Shrugs.)*

JOHN: Well, I thought of a way earlier. One of the things that we tell almost every kid who comes here to see us is how important it is to make sure that you are going to bed at the same time every night and waking up at the same time every morning. Does that make sense?

MICHAEL: I think so.

JOHN: We knew from what you and your parents told us that right now, and for awhile now, you really haven't had a set bedtime. I would bet that most kids in your class have a set bedtime. Do you think?

MICHAEL: I think some of my friends go to bed at 8:00 or sometime.

JOHN: What I want to do is to have you and your mom work with me today to figure out what would be a good bedtime for you. Let's put our heads together to come up with a time.

In part because Michael had quickly identified two friends who had an 8:00 P.M. bedtime, this became the first time suggested. Michael agreed that 8:00 P.M. was probably a good time, but said that he could ask even more kids in class when he went back to school. When asked whether he thought he might be able to fall asleep at 8:00 P.M., he was not sure, but he agreed to try to fall asleep at 8:00 P.M. each night.

Michael was then excused to the waiting room while John met with Mrs. A. for the bulk of the session. Because we decided that a combination of parent education and positive routines would be the primary focus of treatment, John was aware that establishing a good rapport with Mr. and Mrs. A., rather than Michael, was more important for a successful intervention. Although not a lot of time would be invested in rapport with Michael, John felt that this initial time with Michael was important to ensure that he had a good understanding of changes that would be made to his routine, and to get him on board with the goals of treatment.

John reminded Mrs. A. that they would use their time that day to establish a plan for treatment and to make sure that he addressed any concerns or questions that Mr. or Mrs. A. might have before they began the bulk of the education program in the next session. Mrs. A. had no initial questions, but she expressed her eagerness to get things started to help Michael. John reinforced her motivation to move ahead and assured her that once our team started putting pieces into place, it would not take a long time for Michael to become established in a new routine.

John used Mrs. A.'s expression of motivation to underscore the important role that she and Mr. A. would play in Michael's treatment. He emphasized that most of the work in treatments for sleep-related difficulties take place outside of session, under the supervision of the parents. John told Mrs. A. that she and Mr. A. were in the best position to make the broad environmental changes to address Michael's sleeplessness, but he stressed that this also places great responsibility on them to absorb the principles they talked about in session each week and to apply them consistently at home. He expressed confidence that they would be able to do that and referred to his role and the support he would be able to provide them in this process. Mrs. A. joked that they needed all the help they could get but indicated that they were ready to make the necessary changes.

John reinforced Mrs. A. for her motivation, then introduced discussion of sleep diaries and the role they would play in helping to monitor Michael's progress in treatment. Mrs. A. immediately laughed, recalling the difficulty she and her husband had in filling out these diaries during the assessment period. John told Mrs. A. that keeping up with the diaries was probably the hardest thing for parents to do, and that she had a lot of company. Nevertheless, he was pointed out that the diaries are critical to providing accurate information on nightly variation in routine and experiences that could if not understood and addressed, undermine success in treatment. Mrs. A. vowed to stay on top of completing the diaries, and she and John again discussed what she and her husband were to record each night. In addition to tracking when Michael went to bed and when he fell asleep, Mr. and Mrs. A. were also asked to keep a narrative each night on activities leading up to bedtime and any significant events that occurred once Michael was put to bed. Because we had Mr. and Mrs. A.'s consent to communicate with Michael's teacher about his classroom behavior, John made sure that Mrs. A. understood that he would be requesting information from Michael's teacher on the frequency and intensity of frustrated behaviors in class, and daytime sleepiness, so that the had another means of gauging the outcome of changes implemented to sleep.

John then provided a basic overview of the three-part intervention. Over the course of the second and third sessions, they would discuss sleep hygiene and cover the types activities to promote and to avoid leading up to bedtime. They would also go over any problems that had arisen in establishing new routines and talk about ways to spend more positive time with the children just prior to bedtime to help them settle down and reduce resistance behaviors. Following that, likely in Session 4, they would discuss a system for checking in on Michael after bedtime to monitor his progress in falling asleep and to establish for him that an adult in the house was still awake. For homework that week, Mrs. A. was instructed again to begin monitoring evening and bedtime routines via the sleep diary and to begin establishing 8:00 P.M. as Michael's expected bedtime. Mr. and Mrs. A. were to target 8:00 P.M. as the time for Michael to be in bed attempting to go to sleep and to make sure that at least one adult in the house remained awake for a reasonable period of time after Michael began attempting to sleep. John indicated that because they could not realistically put all pieces into place at one time, they should use their usual approach to handling sleep-related problems, until they could discuss possible new strategies together in the next session. John indicated that they would begin building more routine into Michael's new bedtime, starting the next week.

Mrs. A. promised John that she would share the information they discussed with her husband, and that both would attend the next session.

Session 2

Parent Education

Mr. and Mrs. A. both attended the second treatment session, and had been told ahead of time that it would be unnecessary to bring Michael for meetings, unless circumstances dictated otherwise. To reinforce the importance of agreed-upon homework assignments, the first thing John asked Michael's parents was how well things had gone in completing the sleep diaries. The A.'s were silent for a moment, before admitting that they had not been very consistent in keeping up with the homework. They had completed the diary, in which they were to record resistance behaviors leading up to and following bedtime, the time Michael went to bed, and the approximate time it took him to get to sleep, with only modest detail for the first two nights following the first session. However, the following evening there had been some confusion as to who was to complete the diary, and each parent had left it for the other to do. Over the course of the week, completion of the diary had caused some consternation between Mr. and Mrs. A., resulting in data being provided for only three nights. When John inquired about what the primary roadblocks to completing the diaries, Michael's parents indicated that their schedules were still very crazy and that both were simply exhausted by the time they reached the evening. Rather than cooperating and supporting each other's efforts to monitor Michael's behavior, Mr. and Mrs. A. had been viewing the diary as a sort of punishment to be avoided. John emphasized that their complaints were not unusual, and that it was understandable that given their level of fatigue, they would not want to complete the diary. Nevertheless, he reminded them that this was his primary source of information about how things were going at bedtime, and that it was simply too important to rely on faded memories in session to reconstruct events across multiple days.

John sensed that there was still something more not being discussed, and he invited the A.'s to share other thoughts that had come up during the week. Mrs. A. spoke up, reporting that they had been feeling guilty about the problems Michael was experiencing, feeling they should have recognized the problem earlier and should have done more. Their guilt was heightened when they then began to struggle to complete the sleep diary. John was supportive of their feelings, indicating that parents seen in the clinic often expressed these were feelings, but he quickly emphasized that, though currently struggling, Michael would see the benefits of their efforts sooner than they thought. He encouraged them to support each other in their ongoing efforts to implement change. John then invited them to brainstorm with him about ways to overcome the previous week's roadblocks. He suggested that a common solution to handling the question of who would fill out the sleep diaries was to negotiate who would perform the task each day right then in session. This eliminated the need for someone to "take the initiative" each day and reduced the likelihood that unspoken expectations between them would lead to further problems. Each parent got nights off during the week, which could be negotiated in advance based on both parents' schedules. John also offered to provide them with several telephone reminders during the week, if they felt that would help. Although they agreed it would, they declined and indicated that with negotiation in session, they were confident they could complete the task better in the coming week.

In the absence of diary data, Mr. and Mrs. A. were asked to estimate how well they had done in beginning to establish 8:00 P.M. as Michael's bedtime. Not surprisingly, they were somewhat inconsistent in getting Michael to bed at the same time each night. Although they got Michael into bed closer to 8:00 P.M. than they had during the assessment process, Michael nevertheless had been able to stay up until close to 9:00 P.M. on several occasions during the week. Knowing that the next session would not be held for 3 weeks and that

the break would include the holidays (a time notorious for inconsistent schedules), John asked whether they wished to begin implementation of more routine, or whether it made more sense to wait until after the holidays to start the
education portion of treatment. Mr. and Mrs. A. both felt it was important to
begin making changes and that, with the exception of 1 or 2 days around
Christmas, they would make every effort to maintain a consistent structure in
the evenings, including bedtime.

John spent the remainder of the session introducing a new concept,
emphasizing how improvement in sleep is a result of improved sleep hygiene.
They discussed the following topics:

> *Things to avoid*: lengthy naps during the day, caffeinated drinks in the
> evening, arousing activities (video games, television, rough play),
> drinking a lot of liquids, using the bed for activities other than sleep ,
> staying up past the usual bedtime, and getting out of bed at different
> times in the morning.
>
> *Things to encourage*: relaxing activities (reading), going to bed at the
> same time each night, sleeping in the same place each night, lights out,
> no loud noises, sleeping alone, and sleeping in a comfortable bed.

Although Mr. and Mrs. A. felt that many of the components of good
sleep hygiene were already in place, they also identified several things that
needed "fixing." In addition to an inconsistent bedtime, which they were
already trying to fix, they were aware that Michael sometimes drank sodas in
the evening and kept the light on when he went to bed. They were uncertain
about the frequency of several other factors; by their own admission, they
were not actively involved in providing the structure and routine in their children's evening.

As the session neared completion, John and Michael's parents agreed to
begin discussing a regular routine in which they could engage with Michael
immediately prior to bedtime. In addition to the broader changes encouraged
through the discussion of good sleep hygiene, this bedtime routine would
eliminate Michael's occasional resistance at bedtime and foster a greater sense
of security for him in the evening hours.

Session 3

Problem Solving and Expansion of Education

Both Mr. and Mrs. A. were on time for the third appointment and presented a
more complete sleep diary covering nights well through the first 2 weeks of
the break, before trailing off a bit during the most recent week. They were
clearly proud of their improvement in monitoring Michael's behavior, particularly because of the long break between sessions. John was quick to reinforce
their efforts. The diary indicated that Michael had gone to bed between 8:00

and 8:30 P.M. approximately three-fourths of the nights monitored, and had going to bed a bit later only on nights when holiday activities warranted special consideration. For example, one night Michael had requested to watch a special show on television, which ran until 9:00 P.M. on a holiday night. His parents had discussed the issue before giving Michael permission. Although it might have been preferable for Michael to maintain the 8:00 P.M. bedtime every night, this was not realistic during a long holiday break, and John preferred to praise their improved efforts and the fact that Mr. and Mrs. A. were working much more in unison to establish routines.

When queried about the floating bedtime (i.e., anywhere between 8:00 and 8:30 rather than strictly at 8:00 P.M.), Michael's parents reported that this was simply due to their own tendency to lose track of time. They laughingly reported that on several occasions, Michael had reminded them that it was past 8:00 P.M.. Although Mr. and Mrs. A. appeared to be doing better overall at establishing better sleep hygiene, they clearly lacked a routine in the period immediately prior to Michael's bedtime. As stated earlier, the implementation of positive routines focuses on proactively changing a child's internal state at bedtime instead, of altering environmental variables that may be related to sleep disturbances. The assessment process did not indicate that Michael was particularly aroused because of activities preceding bedtime, but given his tendency to worry and occasional somatic complaints at bedtime, a positive routine with direct parental involvement was seen as likely beneficial in helping him to settle into sleep. John worked with the A.'s to come up with a calm and reinforcing routine (e.g., reading books together, sharing stories from the day) that they could implement with Michael at the same time every night. Because Mr. and Mrs. A. had repeatedly commented on their own fatigue and the "busyness" in their lives, John recommended that they reserve only 15 minutes, from 7:45 to 8:00 P.M. for the positive routine. It was not necessary that both parents be present for the routine, only that at least one of them remember to do it. Mr. and Mrs. A. recognized the likelihood that, like the sleep diary, they would fail to carry out routines every day unless they first negotiated a schedule for each day of the week with John's help.

Session 4

Graduated Extinction

Mr. and Mrs. A. again reported positive results in completing the sleep diary and carrying out prescribed changes over the past week. Again, they were able to monitor Michael's bedtime and routines successfully for six nights of the week, only skipping the night immediately preceding the session, because Michael had been so consistent throughout the week. This week, Michael was in bed at 8:00 P.M. for all seven nights between sessions, and Mr. and Mrs. A. had carried out positive routines (reading for Mrs. A., and telling family stories for Mr. A.) each night.

Mr. and Mrs. A. felt that not only did Michael clearly enjoy the time he was getting to spend with them but they also enjoyed it. They raised questions, however, about how to handle the fact that their other children were now also requesting this individual time around bedtime. Although they were initially very negative about how possibly to find time in their schedules for positive individual routines with each child, John pointed out that they could carry out positive routines just as effectively as a group. They would simply have to incorporate a little extra time to negotiate an acceptable group activity, reserving the right to exercise parental authority to avoid drawn out disagreements. Mr. and Mrs. A. liked this idea, because they have been feeling bad about "neglecting" the needs of their other children. John emphasized that it was still important to have this time consistently, and to begin and end the routine in a time frame that did not throw off established bedtimes.

When queried about how Michael was doing when it came to falling asleep once in bed, Mr. and Mrs. A. reported mixed results. Although Michael was not sitting up with the lights on as he had done before, he still was not falling asleep without some trouble. They reported monitoring this behavior by listening outside Michael's door, and occasionally calling to Michael when they thought they heard noises indicating he was still awake. John introduced the concept of graduated extinction to establish further for Michael that his parents were awake and that he could allow himself to fall asleep. John instructions were that, after Mr. and Mrs. A. put Michael to bed, the parent who remained awake that evening would step into Michael's room to check on him after 10 minutes had passed. If Michael was awake, the parent would gently urge him to go to sleep, then exit the room. After 20 minutes, that parent would carry out the same routine and, if necessary, again, 20 minutes after that. These "check-ins" were intended to prevent Michael from exiting his bed to monitor activity in the house. In other children, graduated extinction might be implemented to eliminate efforts at reunification, but Michael's behavior has always stopped short of efforts to reunify with his parents. Nevertheless, graduated exposure, like positive routines, increased Michael's exposure to his parents, serving to allay his concerns about security and safety. In other words, Michael was being told to allow himself to go to sleep and let his parents take care of the parenting concerns. Mr. and Mrs. A. initially reported difficulty trading off nights to stay up longer; however, because of their improved ability to negotiate their roles on a given night and the observation that Michael's evenings were much more routine and developmentally appropriate, the trade-off far more appealing to them.

Because Michael had only recently returned to a regular routine at school after the holiday break, there was little data to be obtained from Ms. R., although she did anecdotally report to John that Michael had not been late since initiating treatment and he seemed less fatigued in school. To gauge the family's ability to maintain the routines now in place, John and the A.'s agreed that Session 5, which was anticipated to be the final session, would take place in 2 weeks, rather than 1 week, to allow Ms. R. to observe

Michael's behaviors more systematically in the classroom and to provide feedback to John.

Session 5

Graduated Extinction and Maintenance

At the start of session, Mr. and Mrs. A. were excited about how well Michael was doing with getting a consistent night's sleep. They produced diaries with data for all but two nights over the past 2 weeks, explaining that things had gotten so routine that they completely forgot to pull out the diary on two occasions. John reinforced their efforts to keep up with the diary even after forgetting once or twice and also pointed out to them that if Michael was getting a consistent night's sleep, then it was attributable to their efforts in creating consistency in the routine around bedtime and morning waking. Although this statement seems self-evident, we find often that parents are quick to attribute changes, positive and negative, to good fortune, the therapist, or forces of nature. It is important that they understand the link between the effort they have put into making changes at home and consequent changes in behavior. The current session was an opportunity for John to emphasize to the A.'s the importance of maintaining their recently acquired good sleep hygiene practices, and they were more likely to acknowledge this message if they understood the factors that had brought about change.

The diaries indicated that Michael had gone to bed at approximately 8:00 P.M. every night except two during the past week, again because Mr. and Mrs. A. wanted to give him a treat by letting him stay up to watch a desired television show one night during each weekend. This slight change to routine is fairly innocuous, but John used the opportunity to remind Mr. and Mrs. A. how easy it is to forget to keep up with the diaries, and so forth, and that, in his experience, a one-night treat might easily become two nights, and so on. They discussed further the need to be vigilant, and Mr. and Mrs. A. went so far as to suggest that they could videotape programs for Michael, so that he did not stay up later than they desired.

When asked specifically about how things had gone with "checking in" on Michael after bedtime, both Mr. and Mrs. A. thought it was helpful to Michael. For the second straight session, Michael had gone to sleep, without seeming to keep himself awake by turning the light on or opening the door. He did open the door on the one or two nights his parents had forgotten to check in as scheduled, but once either parent walked into his bedroom to urge him back to bed and sleep, Michael had remained in bed for the night. John reiterated the logic behind the graduated extinction and encouraged Mr. and Mrs. A. to be especially vigilant about not missing scheduled check-ins. John told the A.'s, "Now we want to stretch out the time between check-ins a little, so that Michael learns to tolerate more and more his quiet time in bed when attempting to fall asleep." For the coming week, the A.'s were instructed to conduct the first check-in after 15 minutes, then 25 minutes after that. In each subsequent week between that time and the next scheduled follow-up session, the A.'s were instructed to stretch out check-in times by 5 minutes per week.

John reported to Mr. and Mrs. A. that he had spoken with Michael's teacher the day before the session, and that she saw positive changes in Michael's energy in the classroom. Although she had indicated that completing a formal chart of Michael's "tired" behaviors in the class might be difficult because of demands on her time, she had agreed to note instances in which Michael was observed yawning or placing his head on his desk. She reported that only two or three times over a 2-week period did she see him engage in such behavior. Comparatively, this was a daily occurrence before treatment began. She also reported that although Michael still seemed concerned when challenged with difficult work, he had not had an outburst in class since they had returned from the holiday break. Michael still seemed periodically moody in class, but this was viewed with far less concern than by school personnel in the past. Because Michael's tantrums in class were bothersome because of their intensity, rather than their frequency, Ms. R. had been asked to rate each outburst or tantrum on a 0- to 10-point scale whenever they occurred. Because no tantrums had occurred over the past 2 weeks, no ratings were necessary.

John presented the topic of maintenance to Mr. and Mrs. A., telling them that just as changes occurring now were the result of their motivation and consistent effort in applying the principles being discussed, their own and Michael's ability to maintain these changes over time would be the result of continuing their efforts. It is very common for parents and kids to exit treatment very satisfied with how things are going, only to return to inconsistent habits. To prevent this from happening, it was important for the A.'s to remain vigilant about their evening activities and to recognize the ongoing need for routine. John related to them the analogy of someone learning to play a song on a musical instrument, then going away for several months. In one case, the person practiced the song each day during the time away and was able to play it reasonably well upon returning. In the other case, the person did not practice the song at all once away and was unable to play it at all upon returning. John indicated that they would now have an opportunity to see how well they practiced their "song" while away, and scheduled one more session 4 weeks later to see how well they maintained their current progress. His expectation was that this would be the last session of the intervention.

Mr. and Mrs. A. agreed to make changes to check-ins, as had been discussed and to continue monitoring activities using the sleep diaries between that session and the next. At John's request, Mrs. A. also took a CBCL with her to fill it out during the next few days, to reflect Michael's behavior for the past month. Although the CBCL asks respondents to think back over a 6-month period, asking Mrs. A. to summarize Michael's more recent behavior allowed John to get another index of change in Michael's functioning, without overlapping in time with Mrs. A.'s previous reports on the CBCL.

Session 6

Follow-Up

This session was intended to follow up on efforts by Mr. and Mrs. A. to maintain consistency with previously implemented strategies. With 4 weeks between sessions, the therapist should anticipate less-than-perfect effort in completion of diary and adherence to strategies. Typically, any previous movement toward improvement of nighttime functioning decreases with the decreased sense of urgency for parents to remain vigilant.

Mrs. A. had mailed back to John the CBCL she completed between meetings, so John was able to score and share with Mr. and Mrs. A. the results during this session. Although Michael was still characterized by his mother as a worrisome and shy child, none of the affective of anxiety scales approached the borderline significant range (as before), largely due to changes in the endorsement of sleep-related items.

Mr. and Mrs. A. reported doing "pretty well" in maintaining previous gains, but they did note that their monitoring via the sleep diaries had dropped off to "most nights" of the week. They expressed modest guilt about not having done better but pointed out that their poorer recording did not reflect a change in how they were approaching Michael's bedtime. Mrs. A. noted that although on a handful of nights they had allowed Michael to alter his schedule, they had otherwise kept to the 8:00 P.M. bedtime and had successfully negotiated the few points of disagreement that had arisen between them (parents). Furthermore, their contact with Michael's teacher suggested that Michael was significantly less frustrated in class and overall seemed more alert. John confirmed that he had received similar feedback from Michael's teacher. Ms. R. had provided him with some classroom ratings of the intensity of Michael's outbursts and the frequency of his "zoning out," and although ratings were recorded too inconsistently to truly chart change from week to week, the school was very pleased with the changes in Michael's engagement in the classroom and his approach to work. "Off the record," Ms. R. had shared with John her observation that Michael was not only more alert in class but he also arrived at school on time.

John reviewed the principles that had been covered in treatment, including the implementation of routine and a consistent bedtime, the use of positive routines involving parents just prior to bedtime, and the use of graduated extinction after bedtime. He reminded them about the need to maintain these new strategies and to remain vigilant about not slipping back into old practices. John also discussed a strategy with Mr. and Mrs. A. for continuing to fade out nightly check-ins, until Michael was able to fall asleep without needing them. Michael's parents pointed out that this was already occurring. Although they continued to check in after Michael had been in his room a little while, more nights than not he was already asleep, and remained so throughout the night.

John reinforced the A.'s for all of their efforts and indicated that although he was confident that they could continue the good work they had done, they could contact the clinic to schedule "booster" sessions should they later need to review the strategies they had learned.

CONCLUSIONS

We began this chapter by highlighting the general neglect of pediatric sleep problems in the fields of psychology and psychiatry. We also pointed out the need for many other areas of child psychopathology to share in this call for attention. However, as we stated earlier, the field of childhood sleep does not have the relatively long and rich background that other areas boast. Thus, it is likely to be a long time before the current state of affairs changes.

What is perhaps most striking is that the lack of funding and research in this area is not reflective of an absence of import. The limited available research consistently underscores the far-reaching implications of disturbed sleep, for the individual and for the system in which he or she operates. For children, the consequences of poor sleep are most often evident in peer and family relationships, and in settings where alertness, concentration, and energy are necessary for success (e.g., school). Too often, however, sleep-related difficulties are missed, mislabeled, or ignored because symptoms or symptom clusters fit the description of other, seemingly more common behavioral problems. The need to understand better the relationship between sleep and other behavioral concerns with which sleep shares topography is never more evident than in such cases.

The fact that sleep is still so mysterious to us is not an excuse for neglect and ultimately should not matter. We do not understand *why* some children have ADHD, any more than we understand *why* we sleep, yet this does not slow the pace of funding for ADHD research. Our understanding of the mechanics of sleep is advancing rapidly, and our attention to the related sleep topics covered in this chapter should keep pace.

Despite the lethargic pace of advancement in the area of children's sleep, we still have reason to be optimistic on some fronts. For example, efforts to identify effective interventions for pediatric sleep problems are providing scientist–practitioners more opportunities to offer hope to families whose lives have been significantly disrupted. In the case of Michael, the role of sleep easily could have been overlooked in the midst of the school's concern over classroom tantrums and the parents' initial *laissez-faire* approach. Once we identified sleeplessness as a likely contributor to several behavioral challenges presented by Michael, however, we could consider a number of intervention strategies, most of which had empirical support. The challenge for the field of child psychology (and allied fields) is to expand education in a way that recognizes the important role of sleep. This includes pushing for sleep-related research to be represented more regularly in "mainstream" professional journals, not just journals specific to sleep, and greater recognition of sleep-related processes in graduate training.

REFERENCES

Achenbach, T. M. (1991). *Manual for the Child Behavior Checklist/4–18 and 1991 profile*. Burlington: University of Vermont, Department of Psychiatry.

American Academy of Sleep Medicine. (2001). *International Classification of Sleep Disorders, Revised: Diagnostic and coding manual*. American Academy of Sleep Medicine.

American Psychiatric Association (APA). (2000). *Diagnostic and statistical manual of mental disorders* (4th ed.). Washington, DC: Author.

Bates, J. E., Viken, R. J., Alexander, D. B., Beyers, J., & Stockton, L. (2002). Sleep and adjustment in preschool children: Sleep diary reports by mothers relate to behavior report by teachers. *Child Development, 73*, 62–74.

Bruni, O., Ottaviano, S., Guidetti, V., Romoli, M., Innocenzi, M., Cortesi, et al. (1996). The Sleep Disturbance Scale for Children (SDSC): Construction and validation of an instrument to evaluate sleep disturbances in childhood and adolescence. *Journal of Sleep Research, 5*, 251–261.

Chambless, D. L., & Hollon, S. D. (1998). Defining empirically supported therapies. *Journal of Consulting and Clinical Psychology, 66*(1), 7–18.

Chervin, R. D., Hedger, K., Dillon, J. E., & Pituch, K. J. (2000). Pediatric sleep questionnaire (PSQ): Validity and reliability of scales for sleep-disordered breathing, snoring, sleepiness, and behavioral problems. *Sleep Medicine, 1*(1), 21–32.

Cicchetti, D., & Rogosch, F. A. (1996). Equifinality and multifinality in developmental psychopathology. *Development and Psychopathology, 8*(4), 597–600.

Conners, C. K. (1990). *Conners Rating Scales*. North Tonawanda, NY: Multi-Health Systems.

Derogatis, L. R. (1983). *SCL-90-R administration, scoring, and procedures manual—II*. Towson, MD: Clinical Psychometric Research.

Ford, D. E., & Kamerow, D. B. (1989). Epidemiologic study of sleep disturbances and psychiatric disorders. An opportunity for prevention? *Journal of the American Medical Association, 262*(11), 1479–1484.

Gaylor, E. E., Burnham, M. M., Goodline-Jones, B. L., & Anders, T. (2005). A longitudinal follow-up study of young children's sleep patterns using a developmental classification system. *Behavioral Sleep Medicine, 3*(1), 44–61.

Harsh, J. R., Easley, A., & LeBourgeois, M. K. (2002). An instrument to measure children's sleep hygiene [Abstract]. *Sleep, 25*, A316.

Hedger-Archbold, K., Pituch, K. J., Panahi, P., & Chervin, R. D. (2002). Symptoms of sleep disturbances among children at two general pediatric clinics. *Journal of Pediatrics, 140*(1), 97–102.

Kerr, S. M., Jowett, S. A., & Smith, L. N. (1996). Preventing sleep problems in infants: A randomized controlled trial. *Journal of Advanced Nursing, 24*, 938–942.

Kovacs, M. (1980). Rating scales to assess depression in school-aged children. *Acta Paediatrica, 46*, 305–315.

LeBourgeois, M., Hancock, M., & Harsh, J. (2001). Validation of the Children's Sleep–Wake Scale (CSWS). *Sleep, 24*, 219.

LeBourgeois, M., & Harsh, J. (2001). A new research measure for children's sleep. *Sleep, 24*, 213.

March, J. S., & Parker, D. A. (2004). The Multidimensional Anxiety Scale for Children (MASC). In M. Maruish (Ed.), *The use of psychological testing for treatment planning and outcomes assessment: Vol. 2. Instruments for children and adolescents* (3rd ed., pp. 39–62). Mahwah, NJ: Erlbaum.

McGreavey, J. A., Donnan, P. T., Pagliari, H. C., & Sullivan, F. M. (2005). The Tayside Children's Sleep Questionnaire: A simple tool to evaluate sleep problems in young children. *Child: Care, Health and Development, 31*(5), 539–544.

Mindell, J. A. (1999). Empirically supported treatments in pediatric psychology: Bedtime refusal and night wakings in young children. *Journal of Pediatric Psychology, 24*(6), 465–481.

Moos, R. H., & Moos, B. S. (1986). *Family Environment Scale manual* (2nd ed.). Palo Alto, CA: Consulting Psychologists Press.

Owens, J. A. (2001). The practice of pediatric sleep medicine: Results of a community survey. *Pediatrics, 108*, E51.

Owens, J. A., Spirito, A., & McGuinn, M. (2000). The Children's Sleep Habits Questionnaire (CSHQ): Psychometric properties of a survey instrument for school-aged children. *Sleep, 23*(8), 1043–1051.

Ramchandani, P., Wiggs, L., Webb, V. V., & Stores, G. (2000). A systematic review of treatment of settling problems and night waking in young children. *Western Journal of Medicine, 173*(1), 33–38.

Reynolds, C. R., & Kamphaus, R. W. (2004). *Behavior Assessment System for Children, Second Edition (BASC-2)*. Bloomington, MN: Pearson Assessments.

Richman, N. (1985). A double blind trial of sleep problems in young children. *Journal of Child Psychology and Psychiatry, and Allied Disciplines, 26*, 591–598.

Sadeh, A., Raviv, A., & Reut, G. (2000). Sleep patterns and sleep disruptions in school-age children. *Developmental Psychology, 36*(3), 291–301.

Seifer, R., Sameroff, A. J., Dickstein, S., & Hayden, L. C. (1996). Parental psychopathology and sleep variation in children. *Child and Adolescent Psychiatric Clinics of North America, 5*(3), 715–727.

Shelton, K. K., Frick, P. K., & Wootton, J. (1996). Assessment of parenting practices in families of elementary-age children. *Journal of Clinical Child Psychology, 25*, 317–329.

Silverman, W. K., & Albano, A. M. (1996). *Anxiety disorders Interview Schedule for DSM-IV: Child Version, Parent Interview Schedule*. San Antonio, TX: Psychological Corporation.

Society of Clinical Child and Adolescent Psychology and the Network on Youth Mental Health. (2006, August 1). *Evidence-Based treatments for children and adolescents*. Retrieved August 1, 2006, from *www.wjh.harvard.edu/7Enock/Div53/EST/index.htm*.

Stores, G. (2001). *A clinical guide to sleep disorders in children and adolescents*. Cambridge, UK: Cambridge University Press.

Index

Academic performance. *See also* School issues
   ADHD and, 170–171
Achenbach System of Empirically Based Assessment, 175–176
Actigraphy, for assessing sleep problems, 384–385
Activity scheduling, in treatment of negative affect, 241–242
Acute stress disorder, *versus* BPD, 274–275
ADIS-IV-C/P. *See* Anxiety Disorders Interview Schedule for DSM-IV, Child and Parent Versions
Affect and Arousal Scales, 229–230
Affective instability, mood disorders and, 265, 276
Agoraphobic avoidance, 4–5
Alabama Parenting Questionnaire, for assessing sleep problems, 381
Anorexia nervosa
   adolescent issues and, 349–350, 353–354
   assessment, 321–329
      child interviews in, 322–323
      child self-report measures in, 323–325
      developmental considerations in, 327–328
      link with treatment, 326–329
      parent self-report measures in, 325–326
   case presentation, 319–321
   DSM-IV-TR criteria for, 312–313
   epidemiology and course, 313
   mortality rate for, 309, 338
   separating illness from patient, 337–338, 346–347
   subtypes of, 313
   treatment, 329–356
      cognitive-behavioral therapy in, 332–334
      context of, 330–332
      family-based treatment in, 334–336
      future issues in, 355–356
      inpatient *versus* outpatient, 327
      parental relationship and, 354–355
      parents' role in, 339, 341–342, 344–346, 348–349
      preview of, 329–330
      session 1, 336–340
      session 2, 340–343
      sessions 3–10, 343–347
      sessions 11–16 (helping adolescent eat on her own), 347–352
      sessions 17–20 (adolescent issues), 352–356
      siblings' role in, 342–343, 345–346, 350–351
      termination of, 356
      weight criterion for, 326
Anorexia nervosa/bulimia, social anxiety and, 59
Antidepressants, manic symptoms and, 271

Anxiety. *See also* Negative affect
  bodily symptoms of, 78
  framing as helpful emotion, 33
  physiological hyperarousal and, 214
  social. *See* Social anxiety
  three-component model of, 34–35
Anxiety disorders
  ADHD comorbidity with, 162–163
  case formulation: assessment, 11–28
    behavioral observations in, 22–24
    child self-report measures in, 16–18
    fear and avoidance hierarchy in,
      15–16
    intake and functional behavioral
      analysis in, 13–14
    link with treatment, 25
    medical evaluation in, 21–22
    parent self-report measures in, 18–
      21
    psychosocial history in, 11–13
    self-monitoring in, 24
    self-report measures in, 14–15
  case formulation: treatment
    BDI phase, 33–38
    CDI phase, 28–33
    components, 26–28
    context, 26
    PDI phase, 38–44
    termination, 44
  comorbidities with, 1–2, 218–219
    with ADHD, 157
  differential diagnosis of, 7–11
    GAD, OCD, and SAD, 10–11
    SAD *versus* PD, 7–8
    SAD *versus* PTSD, 9
  heterogeneity of symptoms in, 2
  self-report of, 228–230
  symptom dimensions, 2–4
  worry and somatic complaints in, 1–2
Anxiety Disorders Interview Schedule
      for Children for DSM-IV-TR, 63,
      69
Anxiety Disorders Interview Schedule
      for DSM-IV, Child and Parent
      Versions, 13, 227, 233
Anxiety Disorders Interview Schedule for
      DSM-IV—Child Version, for
      assessing sleep problems, 378–379
Anxiety reduction, focus on, 1

Anxiety-provoking situations, feelings
      and behaviors in, 34–35
Apnea, sleep, 369
  daytime sleepiness and, 394
Asperger syndrome, attention problems
      in, 160–161
Assertiveness training, in treatment of
      social anxiety, 82, 91, 92f
Assumptions, learned, 103–104
Attachment theory, mental illness and,
      169–170
Attention-deficit/hyperactivity disorder,
      109, 112–113, 128. *See also*
      Inattentiveness
  assessment. *See* Inattentiveness,
      assessment
  versus bipolar disorder, 271–272
  as disorder of intention *versus*
      attention, 159
  inattentiveness in, 157
  versus learning disabilities, 160
  medications for, sleep problems and,
      375
  neurocognitive deficits in, 157
  in parents of children with BPD, 270–
      271
  as performance *versus* skills deficit,
      159
  sleep problems and, 393
Auditory processing disorder, ADHD
      comorbidity with, 161–162
Autism
  attention problems in, 160
  sleep problems and, 373
Avoidance behaviors
  phobic, 105–107
  in three-component model of anxiety,
      34–35
Avoidant personality disorder, 109

B

BATs. *See* Behavior avoidance tests
BDD. *See* Body dysmorphic disorder
BDI. *See* Bravery-Directed Interaction
Bedtime resistance, 374–375, 386–387,
      400
  daytime sleepiness and, 394

Behavior Assessment System for Children, for assessing sleep problems, 380
Behavior Assessment System for Children—2, 122, 176
Behavior avoidance tests, 148
  in assessment of negative affect, 231
  in assessment of obsessive thoughts, 124–125
Behavior rating scales, for ADHD-related symptoms, 175–177
Behavioral avoidance, negative affect and, 213
Behavioral inhibition, 55–56
Behavioral instability
  mania/depression and, 273
  mood disorders and, 265, 276
Behavioral observations
  in anxiety disorders assessment, 22–24
  in mood disorders assessment, 287
  in negative affect assessment, 230–233
  in obsessive thoughts assessment, 123–124
Beliefs, core, 103–104
Binge-eating disorder
  diagnostic criteria for, 314–315
  family environment and, 317
Binge-eating episode, defined, 313
Biological factors, in ADHD, 166–168
Bipolar disorder. See also Mood disorders
  versus acute stress disorder/PTSD, 274–275
  versus ADHD, 271–272
  in children, controversy over DSM-IV-TR criteria, 266–267
  versus conduct disorder, 273–274
  diagnostic difficulties, 264–265
  DSM-IV-TR description of, 265–267
  DSM-IV-TR types of, 265–267
  early-onset, comorbidity with ADHD, 164–165
  versus intermittent explosive disorder, 274
  versus major depressive disorder/dysthymic disorder, 272–273
  misdiagnosis of, 267

versus oppositional defiant disorder, 273
versus psychotic disorder, 275
Body dissatisfaction, 312
Body dysmorphic disorder, 102
  assessment of, 123
  comorbidities with, 109
  course of, 110
  differential diagnosis, 110–112, 111f
  versus eating disorders, 316
  genetic factors in, 110
  prevalence rate, 109
  treatment, family variables in, 131–133
Body image, eating problems and, 312
Body image dissatisfaction, eating disorders and, 318
Body image disturbance, DSM-IV-TR criteria for, 317
Brain structure, ADHD and, 167
Bravery Ladder, 15–16
  application of, with SAD, 38, 42–44
  explanation of, 36–37
Bravery-Directed Interaction, 33–38
  assessment of, 38
  coaching sessions for, 36–38
  focus of, 27
  teaching session for, 33–35
Breathing, halted, 369
Brief Rating Inventory of Executive Function, 174–175
Bug-in-the-ear, 30–31, 41, 43
Bulimia nervosa
  DSM-IV-TR criteria for, 313–314
  individual therapy for, 331
  subtypes of, 314
Bullying, dealing with, in Cool Kids program, 82

C

Case assessment, for assessing sleep problems, 385–388
Catastrophic thinking, cognitive restructuring for, 241
CDI. See Child-Directed Interaction
Central auditory processing disorder. See Auditory processing disorder

Chair warning, 40
Chemical imbalances, in ADHD, 167
Child and Adolescent Psychopathology Scale, 122
Child and Adolescent Social and Adaptive Functioning Scale, 64–65
Child Anxiety and Depression Scales, Revised, 229
Child Anxiety Impact Scale, 65
Child Anxiety Sensitivity Index, 17–18
Child Behavior Checklist, 18–19, 122
    for assessing sleep problems, 380
Child-Directed Interaction, 28–33
    assessment of, 33
    coaching sessions in, 30–33
    focus of, 27
    rules of, 29
    teaching session for, 28–30
Childhood Illness Attitude Scales, 123, 126
Children's Automatic Thoughts Scale, 65
Children's Depression Inventory, for assessing sleep problems, 381
Children's Depression Rating Scale—Revised, 281, 282t
Children's Eating Attitudes Test, 323
Children's Interview for Psychiatric Syndromes, 280–281, 287, 288t
Children's PTSD Inventory, 9
Children's Sleep Habits Questionnaire, 381
Children's Sleep Hygiene Scale, 383, 388
Children's Sleep–Wake Scale, 381–383, 387–388
Children's Yale–Brown Obsessive–Compulsive Scale, 18, 121, 126
CHT. See Cognitive hypothesis-testing model
Circadian rhythm sleep disorder, 374
Classical conditioning, fear and avoidance behaviors and, 106
Clinical interviews. See Diagnostic interviews
Cognitive abilities, Cattell–Horn–Carroll theory of, 172

Cognitive Assessment System, 173
Cognitive biases, negative affect and, 224
Cognitive changes, mood disorders and, 265, 276
Cognitive hypothesis-testing model
    for assessing ADHD, 190–191, 191t
    for assessing inattentiveness, 178–200, 178f
    in assessment and treatment of inattentiveness, 179–187, 184t
    in assessment and treatment of inattentiveness with executive function deficit, 188–200
    inattentiveness and, 156
    intellectual measure in, 183
Cognitive restructuring
    in treatment of negative affect, 241
    in treatment of social anxiety, 79–80, 84–87
Cognitive-behavioral therapy
    for bulimia nervosa, 332–334
    for obsessive thought disorders, 131, 135
    for social anxiety, 70–72. See also Cool Kids program
Cognitive–neuropsychological assessment, of ADHD-related symptoms, 172–175
Commands, parental approach to, 39–40
Communication, nonverbal/verbal, in MFPG approach, 300–302
Compensatory behaviors, eating problems and, 311–312
Compulsions, 105–106. See also Obsessive-compulsive disorder
    features of, 6
    in OCD, BDD, and HC, 105–106
    self-monitoring of, 141f
Conduct disorder, versus BPD, 273–274
Conners Continuous Performance Test—II, 175
Conners Parent and Teaching Rating Scales—Revised, 176
Conners Parent Rating Scale, 122
    for assessing sleep problems, 381

Contingency management, in treatment of social anxiety, 80–81, 87–88

Continuous positive air pressure device, for sleep apnea, 394

Control, perceptions of, negative affect and, 223–224

Cool Kids program
cognitive restructuring in, 79–80
context of, 72–74
contingency management in, 80–81
gradual exposure in, 81–82
muscle relaxation in, 78–79
obstacles, 74–76
problem solving in, 80
rationale for, 77–78
social skills in, 82

Coping strategies, replacing safety signals with, 4

Core beliefs, 103–104

Cyclothymia, description of, 266

D

Delis–Kaplan Executive Function System, 174

Delusional disorder, 109

Delusions, 275

Depression. *See also* Major depressive disorder; Negative affect
behavioral instability and, 273
in children, 218
comorbidities with, 218–219
double, 218
parental, 221
prevalence of, 56–57
self-report of, 228–230
versus social anxiety, 60–61

Depressive disorders. *See also* Major depressive disorder
comorbidity with ADHD, 157
negative affect and, 214
in youth, 213

Developmental coordination disorder, case study of, 179–187

Developmental disorders, sleep problems and, 373

Diagnostic and Statistical Manual of Mental Disorders, fourth edition, text revision. *See* DSM-IV-TR

Diagnostic Interview for Children and Adolescents, 323

Diagnostic Interview Schedule for Children—2.1, 322

Diagnostic interviews
in assessment of negative affect, 226–227
child/parent, in assessment of sleep problems, 378–380
in differential diagnosis, 63
for eating disorders, for children, 322
general psychopathology, 322–323
in obsessive thoughts assessment, 118–121
social anxiety assessment, 63–67
tools for, 13–14

Differential Abilities Scales, 173

Discipline, parental approach to, 39–40

Diuretics, misuse of, 311

Double depression, 218

Doubting, 104–105

DSM-IV-TR
anxiety disorders in, 213
negative affect and, 216
BPD in, 265–267
eating disorders in, 312
feeding problems in, 310
GAD in, 219–220
major depressive disorder in, 219–220
relevant anxiety disorders in, 4
sleep disorders in, 370–373, 370t

Du Salle, Legrand, 105

Dyadic Parent–Child Interaction Coding System, 23–24

Dyadic Parent–Child Interaction Coding System-II, 23–24

Dysomnias, 370
DSM-IV-TR definition of, 372

Dysthymia, comorbidity with ADHD, 163–164

Dysthymic disorder
versus bipolar disorder, 272–273
in children, 218
DSM-IV-TR description of, 268

E

Eating Disorder Examination, 322
Eating Disorder Inventory—Child
    Version, 324
Eating disorders
  assessment, of child's readiness to
    change, 326
  versus body dysmorphic disorder, 316
  with depression, *versus* social anxiety,
    61–62
  in differential diagnosis, 111, 111f
  differential diagnosis of, other DSM
    disorders in, 316
  DSM-IV-TR criteria for, 312–315
    developmental considerations and,
      328
  family environment and, 317–318
  non-DSM classification of, 315–316
  not otherwise specified, 314
  prevalence of, 309
  risk factor studies of, 318
  social anxiety and, 59
  with social phobia, 316–317
  treatment, with family-based therapy,
    334–336
Eating problems, 309–364. *See also*
    Anorexia nervosa; Bulimia
    nervosa; Eating disorders
  assessment, 321–329
    child interviews in, 322–323
    child self-report measures in, 323–
      325
    link with treatment, 326–329
    parent self-report measures in, 325–
      326
  case presentation, 319–321
  compensatory behaviors and, 311–312
  differential diagnosis/risk factors,
    316–318
  genetic factors in, 317
  relationship to specific disorders,
    312–316
  symptom dimensions, 310–312
  treatment, 329–356
    cognitive-behavioral therapy in,
      332–334
    comorbidity and, 332

context of, 330–332
  family-based treatment in, 334–
    336
  homework assignments in, 332
  NICE guidelines for, 328–330
  preview of, 329–330
  resistance to, 331
  session 1, 336–340
  session 2, 340–343
  sessions 3–10, 343–347
  sessions 11–16 (helping adolescent
    eat on her own), 347–352
  sessions 17–20 (adolescent issues),
    352–356
  therapeutic alliance in, 331
  weight and, 311
  in young children *versus* older
    children/adolescents, 310
Emotion
  negative affect and, 214
  tripartite model of, 214, 216, 217f,
    221–222, 253
Enemas, misuse of, 311
ERP. *See* Exposure with response
    prevention exercises
Executive function deficits, 156
  in auditory processing disorder,
    161
  in autism *versus* Asperger syndrome,
    160–161
  with inattentiveness, case study of,
    188–200
  in pervasive developmental disorders,
    160–161
Exercise, excessive, 311–312, 320–321
Exposure, in treatment of negative
    affect, 240, 247
  school-based, 247–249
Exposure with response prevention
    exercises, in treatment of
    obsessive thoughts, 126–127,
    129–130, 147, 150
Expressed emotion, definition and
    significance, 270
Externalizing disorders, comorbidity
    with ADHD, 157
Extinction schedules, for sleep problems,
    395–396, 403–406

Extraversion, Eysenck's concept of, 221–222

Eyberg Child Behavior Inventory, 19–20

F

Family
  of child with anorexia nervosa, 320
  in diagnosis of mood disorders, 269–270
  psychiatric history of, ADHD and, 165–166

Family engagement
  in treatment of eating disorders, 328–329
  in treatment of social phobia, 237–238

Family environment
  anorexia nervosa and, 341
  eating disorders and, 317–318
  negative affect and, 222–223

Family history, in assessment of mood disorders, 279–280, 280f

Family History—Research Diagnostic Criteria Interview, 279–280

Family variables, and treatment of obsessive thoughts, 131–133

Family-based therapy
  for eating disorders, 334–336
  for eating problems, 309

Fasting, 312

Fear and avoidance hierarchy, 15–16, 36
  in treatment of negative affect, 244–245, 245f

Fear of Abandonment, 16

Fear of Being Alone, 16

Fear of physical illness, 2
  decreased, 44
  disruptions due to, 2–3
  panic/separation anxiety and, 8

Fear Survey Schedule for Children—Revised, 18, 121

Feeding disorder spectrum. See also Anorexia nervosa; Bulimia nervosa; Eating disorders
  in DSM-IV-TR, 310

Feelings, in three-component model of anxiety, 34

Feelings management, in MFPG, 294–295, 301

FIND strategy, for assessing mood disorders, 276–277

Five-second rule, 40

Fix-It List, 292

Fluoxetine, for social anxiety, 77

Fluvoxamine, for social anxiety, 77

FPI. See Fear of physical illness

Frequency of Calamitous Events subscale, 16

Functional behavioral analysis, in assessment of sleep problems, 377–378

G

Generalized anxiety disorder, 228
  versus ADHD, 162
  biological factors in, 220–222
  comorbidities with, 218
  course of, 110
  with depression, versus social anxiety, 61
  differential diagnosis, 110–112, 111f, 219–220
  features of, 5
  OCD and SAD and, 10–11
  versus social anxiety, 61
  social anxiety and, 58
  treatment, family variables in, 131–133

Genetic factors
  in ADHD, 166–167
  in eating disorders, 317
  in GAD and MDD, 220–221
  in OCD, BDD, and HC, 110

Genograms, in assessment of mood disorders, 279–280, 280f

Get ready checklist, in treatment of ADHD, 198–199, 199f

Good behavior chart, 196–197, 196f

Gradual exposure, in treatment of social anxiety, 81–82, 88–91, 90f

Great Ormand Street criteria for eating disorders, 315–316
Group A beta-hemolytic streptococcal infection, 112

H

Hallucinations, 275
Handwriting intervention, response to, 186f, 187
Harsh, John, 368
Homework, in treatment of ADHD, 198–199, 198f
Hypersexuality, BPD and, 274–275
Hypersomnia, primary, 372
Hypochondria, 127
 comorbidities with, 109
 course of, 110
 differential diagnosis, 110–112, 111f
 genetic factors in, 110
 prevalence rate, 109
 treatment, family variables in, 131–133
Hypochondriasis, 102, 118
Hypomania, description of, 266

I

Ideation, overvalued, 107
 and treatment of obsessive thoughts, 130–131
Inattentiveness, 156–211. *See also* Attention-deficit/hyperactivity disorder
 anxiety disorders and, 162–163
 assessment, 171–178
  cognitive–neuropsychological, 172–175
  with personality inventories, 177–178
  social–emotional, 175–177
 auditory processing disorder and, 161–162
 in autism *versus* Asperger syndrome, 160–161
 case presentation: Lisa, 188–200,

 190t, 191t, 193t, 194t, 195f, 196f, 198f, 199f
 case presentation: Thomas, 179–187, 181f, 182t, 184t, 186f
 case study of, 179–187
 cognitive hypothesis-testing model and, 156
 conceptual model of, 178–200
 differential diagnosis of, 165–171
  biological factors in, 166–168
  historical antecedents in, 165–166
  psychological factors in, 168–169
  psychosocial factors in, 169–171
 with executive deficits, case study of, 188–200
 mood disorders and, 163–165
 pervasive developmental disorders and, 160–161
 prevalence of, 156
 specific learning disabilities and, 158–160
 symptom dimensions, 157–165
Insight, 107
Insomnia
 primary, differential diagnosis of, 375–376
 versus sleeplessness, 374
Intermittent explosive disorder, *versus* BPD, 274
International Classification of Sleep Disorders, Revised, 370–373, 371t
Interviews, child/parent, in assessment of mood disorders, 280–283, 282t, 284t

K

Kids' Eating Disorders Survey, 324

L

Laxatives, misuse of, 311
Learning
 ADHD and, 170–171
 superstitious, 40

Learning disabilities
  comorbidity with ADHD, 157, 158–160
  nonverbal (right-hemisphere), 158
  attention/executive problems in, 160–161
  prevalence of, 158
  social deficits and, 170
Lebourgeois, Monique, 368
Life events, negative affect and, 223

M

Macquarie University, Cool Kids program at, 72–74
Major depressive disorder, 281. *See also* Depression; Mood disorders
  biological factors in, 220–222
  versus bipolar disorder, 272–273
  in children, 218
  comorbidity with ADHD, 164
  diagnostic difficulties, 264–265
  differential diagnosis of, 219–220
  DSM-IV-TR description of, 267–268
  social anxiety and, 59
Mania, 281
  behavioral instability and, 273
Mania Rating Scale, 281, 283, 284t
Manic episode, DSM-IV-TR definition of, 265–266
Mathematics disorders, 159
Maudsley family therapy, 309
  for anorexia nervosa, 334
  indications for, 330
  overview of, 334–336
  step-by-step guidelines for, 336–356
Medical conditions, comorbidity with ADHD, 165
Medical evaluation, in anxiety disorders assessment, 21–22
Medical history, for eating disorders, 325–326
Medication grid, 285f
Medication history, in assessment of mood disorders, 283
Medications
  manic symptoms and, 271
  in MFPG, 292–293

for sleep problems, 393
sleep problems and, 375
for social anxiety, 77
Menstruation, cessation of, anorexia nervosa and, 328
Methylphenidate (Ritalin), for ADHD and DCD, 180, 181f
MFPG program. *See* Multifamily psychoeducation group
Millon Adolescent Personality Inventory, 177
Minnesota Multiphasic Personality Inventory—Adolescents, 177
Monitoring, in assessment of negative affect, 232–233
Mood disorders, 264–308. *See also* Bipolar disorder; Dysthymic disorder; Major depressive disorder
  assessment, 276–290
    behavioral observations in, 287
    child/parent interviews in, 280–281, 282t, 283, 284t
    differential diagnosis in, 287, 288t
    family history in, 279–280, 280f
    link with treatment, 287
    medication/treatment history in, 283, 284f, 285f
    psychoeducational–neuropsychological testing in, 283
    time line for, 277, 278f, 279
  case presentation, 276
  comorbidity with ADHD, 163–165
  conceptual model of, 275–290
  differential diagnosis of, 268–271
    bipolar disorder *versus* acute stress disorder/PTSD, 274–275
    bipolar disorder *versus* ADHD, 271–272
    bipolar disorder *versus* conduct disorder, 273–274
    bipolar disorder *versus* intermittent explosive disorder, 274
    bipolar disorder *versus* major depressive disorder/dysthymic disorder, 272–273

Mood disorders, differential diagnosis of
    (cont.)
  bipolar disorder *versus* oppositional
    defiant disorder, 273
  bipolar disorder *versus* psychotic
    disorder, 275
  and family history of mental illness,
    269–270
  not otherwise specified
    description of, 266
    DSM-IV-TR description of, 268
  sleep problems and, 375
  symptom dimensions, 265
    DSM-IV-TR diagnoses and, 265–
    268
  treatment, 288–303
    components of, 289–290
    follow-up to, 303
    preview of, 288–289
    session 1, 291–292
    session 2, 292–293
    session 3, 293–295
    session 4, 295–297
    session 5, 298–300
    session 6, 300–301
    session 7, 301–302
    session 8, 302–303
Moodiness. *See also* Mood disorders;
    specific disorders
  in bipolar disorder, 265–267
  in dysthymic disorder, 268
  in major depressive disorder, 267–
    268
MRS. *See* Mania Rating Scale
Multidimensional Anxiety Scale for
    Children, 17
  for assessing sleep problems, 381
Multifamily psychoeducation group,
    264
  as adjunctive intervention, 288
  in assessment and treatment of mood
    disorders, 275–304
  components of, 289
  framework/goals
    for children's group, 290
    for parent group, 289–290
  session 1, 291–292
  session 2, 292–293
  session 3, 293–295
  session 4, 295–297
  session 5, 298–300
  session 6, 300–301
  session 7, 301–302
  session 8, 302–303
Muscle relaxation, teaching, for social
    anxiety, 78–79
Mutism, selective, social anxiety and, 58

N

Negative affect, 212–263
  assessment, 226–234
    behavioral observations and tests
      in, 230–233
    case assessment in, 227–228
    diagnostic interviews in, 226–227
    link with treatment, 233–234
    self-report measures in, 228–230
  case presentation, 224–226
  in Clark and Watson's tripartite
    model, 214, 217f
  cognitive components of, 213
  and comorbidity among anxiety,
    depressive, and other Axis I
    DSM-IV-TR disorders, 219
  differential diagnosis of, 219–224
    biological factors in, 220–221
    psychosocial factors in, 223–224
    temperament in, 221–222
  dimensional conceptualization of,
    benefits of, 215–216
  inappropriate, 216–217
  in normal emotional experience, 216
  onset/course, 217–218
  physiological indicators of, 213
  prevalence, 215, 217
  relationship to specific disorders,
    216–219
  symptom dimensions, 213–216
  treatment, 234–244
    activity scheduling in, 241–242
    case summary, 252
    cognitive restructuring in, 241
    exposure in, 240
    family engagement in, 237–238
    maintenance and relapse prevention
      in, 251–252

preview, 234–236
problem solving in, 242
psychoeducation in, 239–240
relaxation in, 242–243
self-monitoring in, 240
session 1: building rapport, 244
session 2: constructing fear
    hierarchy, 244–245
session 3–4: psychoeducation, 246
session 5: school-based exposure,
    247–249
therapeutic breakthrough in, 251
therapeutic complications in, 250–
    251
troubleshooting in, 243–244
unanticipated events in, 238
youth engagement in, 236–237
Negative reinforcement, 107
NEPSY, 173–174
in assessment of inattentiveness,
    191t
Neurocognitive deficits, in ADHD, 157
Neuroticism, Eysenck's concept of,
    221–222
NICE guidelines, for eating problems,
    328–330
Night terrors, 369, 372, 376
Nightmares, 376
Nonverbal (right-hemisphere) learning
    disabilities, attention/executive
    problems in, 160–161
Nonverbal (right-hemisphere) learning
    disability, 158

O

Obsessions
forms and classification, 103–104
health, differential diagnosis of, 110–
    111
in OCD, BDD, and HC, 105–106
Obsessive Compulsive Cognitions
    Working Group, 104
Obsessive thoughts, 102–155
assessment, 118–127
    behavioral observations/behavioral
        avoidance tests in, 123–125
    clinical interviews in, 118–121

differential diagnosis decision tree
    in, 113f–114f
link with treatment, 125–127
case presentation, 112–118
symptom dimensions, 103–107
    compulsions and phobic avoidance
        behaviors, 105–107
    differential diagnosis of, 110–112,
        113f–114f
    doubting, 104–105
    obsessions, 103–104
    overvalued ideas/unrealistic
        thoughts, 107
    relationship to specific disorders,
        107–110
    shifting, 107
treatment, 127–151
    biopsychosocial model in, 127–
        128
    comorbidity and, 129–130
    components of, 135
    context of, 128–129
    family variables and, 131–133
    hierarchies in, 142–150, 144f
    intensive, 134
    multiple settings and, 134–135
    overvalued ideation and, 130–131
    points of resistance in, 142, 146
    relapse prevention in, 150–151
    session 1, 136–139
    session 2, 139–142
    sessions 3 and 4, 142–146
    session 5, 146–148
    sessions 6–10, 148
    session 11, 148–150
    sessions 12–15, 150–151
    therapist/therapy variables and,
        133–134
Obsessive–compulsive disorder, 118,
    120. See also Body dysmorphic
    disorder; Hypochondriasis;
    Obsessive thoughts
ADHD comorbidity with, 162–163
chronicity of, 218
comorbidities with, 109
course of, 109
developmental constraints and, 2
differential diagnosis, 110–112, 111f
versus eating disorders, 316–317

Obsessive–compulsive disorder *(cont.)*
features of, 5–6
GAD and SAD and, 10–11
genetic factors in, 110
heterogeneity of symptoms, 2
prevalence rate, 109
treatment
family variables in, 131–133
therapist/therapy variables and,
133–134
Obsessive–compulsive personality
disorder, *versus* eating disorders,
316–317
Operant conditioning, fear and
avoidance behaviors and, 106
Oppositional-defiant disorder, 281
versus BPD, 273
parent–child interaction therapy for, 1
Overvalued Ideas Scale, 130
Overvalued ideation
in OCD, BDD, and HC, 107
and treatment of obsessive thoughts,
130–131

P

PA. *See* Positive affect
PANDAS. *See* Pediatric autoimmune
neuropsychiatric disorder
associated with streptococcal
infections
Panic, developmental constraints and, 2
Panic attacks
comorbidity with SAD, 7–8
DSM-IV-TR definition of, 4
nighttime, 376
Panic disorder
versus ADHD, 163
criteria for, 4–5
physiological hyperarousal in, 214
versus SAD, 7–8
Parasomnias, 369, 370
DSM-IV-TR definition of, 372
Parent education, about sleep problems,
394–395
Parent interviews, in obsessive thoughts
assessment, 120
Parental Expectancies Scale, 65

Parent–child interaction therapy. *See
also* Bravery-Directed Interaction;
Child-Directed Interaction;
Parent-Directed Interaction
for oppositional defiant disorder, 1
for separation anxiety disorder, 25–44
BDI phase of, 33–38
CDI phase of, 28–33
context of, 26
monitoring progress of, 27–28
overview of, 26–27
PDI phase of, 38–44
termination of, 44
Parent-Directed Interaction, 38–44
coaching sessions for, 42–44
focus of, 27
teaching session for, 38–42
termination of, 44
Parenting factors, in ADHD, 168–170
Parenting Stress Index, 20–21
Parents
anxious/depressed, and negative affect
in children, 222–223
eating disorders and, 318
in Maudsley family therapy, 336–337
encouraging anxiety in, 339
focusing on eating behavior
management, 344–345, 348–349
focusing on modifying criticisms,
346, 350–351
refeeding task and, 339, 341–342
in multifamily psychoeducation group
approach, 289–303
sleep problems and, 392–393, 397–
308
in treatment of eating problems, 331
and treatment of obsessive thoughts,
131–133
in treatment of social anxiety, 71–73,
74–76
in treatment of social therapy, 238
Paroxetine, for social anxiety, 77
PCIT. *See* Parent–child interaction
therapy
PDI. *See* Parent-Directed Interaction
Pediatric autoimmune neuropsychiatric
disorder associated with
streptococcal infections, 112
Pediatric Sleep Questionnaire, 381–382

Peer relations, ADHD and, 170
Penn State Worry Questionnaire for Children, 229
Personality inventories, for ADHD-related symptoms, 177–178
Personality Inventory for Children—II, 177
Personality Inventory for Youth, 177
Pervasive developmental disorders, comorbidity with ADHD, 160–161
PH. *See* Physiological hyperarousal
Phobias
    resolution of, without treatment, 218
    social. *See* Social phobia
Phobic avoidance, 2
    eliminating, 1
Phobic avoidance behaviors, 105–107
Physiological hyperarousal, 216
    in Clark and Watson's tripartite model, 214, 217f
    in panic disorder, 214
    temperament and, 222
Polysomnography, for assessing sleep problems, 384–385
Positive affect, 216
    assessing, 229
    in Clark and Watson's tripartite model, 214, 217f
    emotions in, 213
Positive and Negative Affect Schedule for Children, 229–230
Positive behavior system, 196–199, 196f, 198f
Posttraumatic stress disorder
    versus ADHD, 163
    versus BPD, 274–275
    features of, 6
    versus SAD, 9
Problem solving
    in MFPG approach, 298–300
    for sleep problems, 402–403
    in treatment of negative affect, 242
    in treatment of social anxiety, 80
Psychoeducation. *See also* Multifamily psychoeducation group
    in treatment of negative affect, 239–240, 246
    in treatment of obsessive thoughts, 142

Psychoeducational–neuropsychological testing, in assessment of mood disorders, 283
Psychological factors
    ADHD and, 168–169
    in negative affect, 223–224
Psychosocial factors
    in ADHD, 169–171
    in negative affect, 222–223
Psychotic disorder, *versus* BPD, 275
Purging behaviors, 311

Q

Questionnaire on Eating and Weight Patterns—Parent Version, 325

R

Reading disorders, 159
Relaxation scripts, for social anxiety, 78–79
Relaxation techniques
    for sleep problems, 397, 402
    in treatment of negative affect, 242–243
Revised Behavior Problem Checklist, 122
Revised Child Anxiety and Depression Scales, 229
Revised Child Manifest Anxiety Scale, 18
Rewards, in treatment of ADHD, 196–199
Ritalin. *See* Methylphenidate (Ritalin)
Routines, positive, for sleep problems, 396
Rumination, depression and, 224

S

SAD. *See* Separation anxiety disorder
Safety signals
    excessive reliance on, 3–4
    functions of, 3–4
    identification and gradual elimination of, 3–4
    types of, 3, 3t

Safety Signals Index, 16
Schedule for Affective Disorders and
     Schizophrenia for School-Age
     Children, 323
School, exposure therapy in, for
     negative affect, 247–249
School issues
  with bipolar disorder, 270–271
  with eating problems, 332
School Refusal Assessment Scale, 18
Screen for Child Anxiety Related
     Emotional Disorders, 64, 122,
     126
Seeking safety behaviors, 1–52
  generalized anxiety disorder and, 5
  impetus for, 3
  obsessive–compulsive disorder and, 5–
     6
  panic disorder and, 4–5
  PTSD and, 6
  SAD and, 4
Selective mutism
  versus social anxiety, 60
  social anxiety and, 58
Self-destructive behavior, in PTSD
     versus SAD, 9
Self-monitoring
  in anxiety disorders evaluation, 24
  in assessment of obsessive thoughts,
     125
  of compulsions, 141f
  in treatment of negative affect, 240
Self-monitoring intervention, response
     to, 185, 186f
Self-report measures
  for anxiety disorders, 14–15
  in assessment of negative affect, 228–
     230
  broad- versus narrow-band, 228
  child, 16–18
     for eating disorders, 323–325
  fear and avoidance hierarchy, 15–16
  in obsessive thoughts assessment,
     121–122
  parent, 18–21
     for eating disorders, 325–326
Self-report of Personality, 177
Separation Anxiety Assessment Scale—
     Child Version, 16–17

Separation Anxiety Assessment Scale—
     Parent Version, 18
Separation Anxiety Assessment Scales—
     Child and Parent Versions, 16
Separation anxiety disorder, 225
  causes of, 33–34
  features of, 4
  GAD and OCD and, 10–11
  heterogeneity of symptoms, 2
  versus panic disorder, 7–8
  PCIT for, 1
  versus PTSD, 9
  resolution of, without treatment, 218
Serotonin, in OCD, 137–138
Service provider grid, 286f
Setting Conditions for Anorexia
     Nervosa Scale, 324–325
Sexuality, BPD and, 274–275
Shifting, inability for, 107
Shyness. See also Social anxiety
  prevalence of, 53
Sleep
  developmental model of, 382–383,
     382f
  "normal," 367
  physical activation during, 368–369,
     376
  research on, 366–367
Sleep apnea, 369
  daytime sleepiness and, 394
Sleep diaries, 383, 384f, 389f, 399–403,
     405
  parent-completed, 392
Sleep disorders
  breathing-related, 372
  circadian rhythm, 374
  comorbidities of, 373
  DSM-IV-TR criteria for, 370–373,
     370t
  ICSD categories of, 370–373, 371t
  with medical condition, 370
  with other mental disorder, 370
  primary, 370
  sleep-related, 392
  substance-induced, 370
Sleep Disturbance Scale for Children,
     381
Sleep hygiene, 400, 402
Sleep measures, 381–383

Sleep problems, 365–410
    assessment, 377–391
        actigraphy and polysomnography
            in, 384–385
        case assessment in, 385–388
        child/parent interviews in, 378–380
        functional behavioral analysis in,
            377–378
        link with treatment, 389–391
        questionnaires in, 380–381
        sleep diaries in, 383, 384f, 389f
        sleep measures in, 381–383
        videography in, 385
    in BPD/MDD, 272–273
    breathing-related, 375–376
    case presentation, 376–377
    comorbidities with, 393
    differential diagnosis of, 373–376
    medication-related, 375
    relationship to specific disorders,
        370–373, 370t
    research on, 408
    resistance at bedtime, 374–375
    routine bedtime and, 398–402
    symptom dimensions, 366–370
    treatment, 391–408
        components of, 393–397
        context of, 392–393
        preview of, 391–392
        session 1: building rapport, 397–
            400
        session 2: parent education, 400–
            402
        session 3: problem solving/
            expanding education, 402–403
        session 4: graduated extinction,
            403–405
        session 5: graduated extinction/
            maintenance, 405–406
        session 6: follow-up, 407–408
        step-by-step guidelines, 397–408
Sleepiness
    daytime, 368–369, 375–376
    causes of, 394
    excessive, 372
Sleeplessness, 368–369
    DSM-IV-TR definition of, 372
    versus insomnia/breathing-related
        sleep problems, 374

Sleeptalking, 369
Sleepwalking, 369, 372
Snoring, 369, 375
Social anxiety, 53–101
    assessment, 62–71
        functional behavioral analysis in,
            62–69
        link with treatment, 69–71
    case presentation, 62
    characteristics of, 54–55
    comorbidity and differential diagnosis,
        59–62
        eating disorders and depression,
            61–62
        GAD and depression, 61
        social phobia and depression, 60–
            61
        social phobia and GAD, 61
        social phobia and selective mutism,
            60
    developmental course, 55–57
    relationship to specific disorders, 57–
        59
        eating disorders, 59
        generalized anxiety disorder, 58
        major depressive disorder, 59
        selective mutism, 58
        social phobia, 57–58
    social phobia and, 57–58
    symptom dimensions, 54–55
    synonyms for, 54
    treatment, 72–92. See also Cool Kids
        program
        and awareness of bodily symptoms
            and relaxation, 78–79
        cognitive restructuring in, 79–80
        components of, 77
        context of, 72–74
        contingency management in, 80–81
        goal setting in, 83
        gradual exposure in, 81–82
        including parents in, 71–73
        medication in, 77
        obstacles to, 74–76
        problem solving in, 80
        rationale for, 77–78
        session 1, 82–84
        session 2, 84–87
        session 3, 87–88

Social anxiety, treatment *(cont.)*
   session 4, 88–90
   sessions 5–9, 90–91
   session 10, 91–92
   social skills in, 82
Social Anxiety Scale for Children—
   Revised, 64
Social deficits
  ADHD and, 170
  learning disabilities and, 170
Social phobia, 228
  comorbidities with, 218
  versus eating disorders, 316
  measures of, 64
  versus social anxiety, 60
  social anxiety and, 57–58
  treatment, 235–237
Social Phobia and Anxiety Inventory for
  Children, 64, 67
Social Skills Rating System, 177
Social skills training, in treatment of
  social anxiety, 82
Social withdrawal, negative affect and,
  213
Social–emotional assessment, of ADHD-
  related symptoms, 175–178
Sociocultural factors, in obsessive
  thoughts disorder, 128
Somatic complaints, and fear of
  consequences, 2
Spence Children's Anxiety Scale, 64, 67
State–Trait Anxiety Inventory for
  Children, 18, 121
Sticky thoughts, 119
Stimulants
  for ADHD, 192–193, 193t, 194t,
   195, 195t
  for ADHD and DCD, 180, 181f
  manic symptoms and, 271
Stop, Think, Plan, Do, Check
  framework, 298–300
Student Behavior Survey, 177
Subjective units of distress, in treatment
  of obsessive thoughts, 127
Substance abuse, 109
Suicide attempts, negative affect and,
  213
Superstitious learning, 40

Symptom Checklist-90, for assessing
  sleep problems, 381
Symptom-self exercise, 293

T

Tayside Children's Sleep Questionnaire,
  382
Teacher interviews, in obsessive
  thoughts assessment, 121
Teasing, dealing with, in Cool Kids
  program, 82, 91
Temperament
  ADHD and, 167–168
  negative affect and, 221–222
  in pediatric bipolar disorder, 270
Test of Variables of Attention, 175
Therapeutic alliance, in treatment of
  eating problems, 331
Thinking, Feeling, Doing exercise, 295–
  297
Thought, in three-component model of
  anxiety, 34
Thoughts
  discussion of, in treatment of social
   anxiety, 83–84
  unrealistic, 107
Time lines, in assessment of mood
  disorders, 277, 278f, 279
Time-out procedures, SAD and, 40–42
Time-out room, 41
Tool Kit, 295, 296, 298
"Top 10 Things Kids Worry About,"
  114–115
Tourette syndrome, 109
  in differential diagnosis, 111, 111f
Trauma, child/family member exposure
  to, 9
Tripartite model of emotion, 214, 216,
  217f, 221–222, 253
Troubleshooting, in treatment of
  negative affect, 243–244

U

Unrealistic thoughts, 107

V

Videography, for assessing sleep problems, 385
Vomiting, self-induced, 311–312

W

Wakings, scheduled, for sleep problems, 396
WCE. *See* Worry about calamitous events
Wechsler Intelligence Scale for Children–IV, 172
  in assessment of ADHD, 182–183, 182t
  in assessment of inattentiveness, 191t
    working memory, executive function, 189–190, 190t
Weekly Record of Anxiety at Separation, 24, 31, 35, 42

Woodcock–Johnson Tests of Cognitive Abilities, 172
Woodcock–Johnson–III, in assessment of inattentiveness, 191t
Worry
  anxiety and, 224
  in GAD, 10
  spheres of, 2
Worry about calamitous events, 2
  decreased, 44
  disruptions due to, 2–3
  with SAD and PD, 8
Worry bullies, 119, 138–145
Worry scale, 83, 89f
WRAS. *See* Weekly Record of Anxiety at Separation
Written expression disorders, 159–160

Y

Youth engagement, in treatment of social phobia, 236–237